HEALTH PROMOTION
Philosophy, Prejudice and Practice

HEALTH PROMOTION
Philosophy, Prejudice and Practice

Second Edition

David Seedhouse
*Auckland University of Technology, New Zealand
and Middlesex University, London, UK*

John Wiley & Sons, Ltd

Other Wiley Editorial Offices

John Wiley & Sons Inc., 111 River Street, Hoboken, NJ 07030, USA

Jossey-Bass, 989 Market Street, San Francisco, CA 94103-1741, USA

Wiley-VCH Verlag GmbH, Boschstr. 12, D-69469 Weinheim, Germany

John Wiley & Sons Australia Ltd, 33 Park Road, Milton, Queensland 4064, Australia

John Wiley & Sons (Asia) Pte Ltd, 2 Clementi Loop #02-01, Jin Xing Distripark, Singapore
129809

John Wiley & Sons Canada Ltd, 22 Worcester Road, Etobicoke, Ontario, Canada M9W 1L1

Wiley also publishes its books in a variety of electronic formats. Some content that appears
in print may not be available in electronic books.

Library of Congress Cataloging-in-Publication Data

Seedhouse, David, 1956–
    Health promotion : philosophy, prejudice, and practice / David Seedhouse. – 2nd ed.
        p. cm.
    Includes bibliographical references and index.
    ISBN 0-470-84732-8 (alk. paper) – ISBN 0-470-84733-6 (pbk. : alk. paper)
    1. Health promotion – Philosophy. 1. Title.
RA427.8.S44 2004
613'.01–dc22
                                                            2003057623

British Library Cataloguing in Publication Data

A catalogue record for this book is available from the British Library

ISBN 0 470 84732 8 ppc
ISBN 0 470 84733 6 pbk

Typeset in 10/12pt Palatino by Dobbie Typesetting Ltd, Tavistock, Devon
Printed and bound in Great Britain by TJ International, Padstow, Cornwall
This book is printed on acid-free paper responsibly manufactured from sustainable forestry
in which at least two trees are planted for each one used for paper production.

FOR DEAR HILARY, CHARLOTTE AND PENELOPE

IN MEMORY OF MY BEAUTIFUL GRANDMOTHER, JESSIE SEEDHOUSE

Contents

About the Author

PROFESSOR DAVID SEEDHOUSE, BA (HONS), PhD (Manchester)

David Seedhouse is a practical philosopher, intensely interested in health matters. He has written or edited 13 books and produced over 200 book chapters, journal papers and other articles. His most successful books are *Health: The Foundations for Achievement* and *Ethics: The Heart of Health Care*, both of which are in their second editions. His latest book is *Total Health Promotion: Mental Health, Rational Fields and the Quest for Autonomy.*

Professor Seedhouse has researched and written extensively about:

- The Philosophy of Health
- Health Care Ethics
- Medical Ethics
- Health Promotion
- Mental Health and Illness
- Ethical Decision-making
- Values-based Decision-making

David is Professor of Health and Social Ethics at Auckland University of Technology, New Zealand (where he directs the National Centre for Health and Social Ethics www.healthethics.info). David is also a popular keynote conference speaker and visiting professor in 13 different countries, and is widely noted on the internet.

Preface to the Second Edition

CATEGORICAL AND HYPOTHETICAL HEALTH PROMOTION

The first edition of *Health Promotion: Philosophy, Prejudice and Practice* is often read as arguing that conventional health promotion has so many theoretical and ethical deficiencies that it should be abandoned. But this is not the point. In fact conventional health promotion can be a good thing and there are many reasons why there ought to be more of it.

Conventional health promoters (the Magpie Profession) want to eliminate or alleviate pain, disease and certain social obstacles in order to enable people to live safer and more fulfilled lives. These admirable ambitions are shared by foundations health promotion (the unconventional form of health promotion advocated in this text). There is a crucial difference, however: conventional health promotion assumes that its particular interpretation of health is the only correct understanding, while the foundations theory openly appreciates that there are different interpretations of health and many alternative ways to live a fulfilled life.

Health Promotion: Philosophy, Prejudice and Practice is essentially a plea for tolerance. It makes tough criticisms of conventional health promotion's academic inadequacies, and exposes a massive ethical crisis most conventional health promoters continue to ignore. But these objections are not meant to overthrow established health promotion. Rather they are made so that conventional health promotion can grow and flourish as a philosophically mature discipline.

Most of conventional health promotion's conceptual and ethical errors could be remedied overnight were the movement's leaders to accept the intellectual and moral primacy of **hypothetical** over **categorical** health promotion.

Categorical health promotion (the type advocated by all official health promotion bodies) presupposes that:

1. Health is an objective state
2. It is practically and morally good to behave in ways that create health
3. Given 1 and 2, health promoters can evaluate any given practice as either categorically good or categorically bad for health
4. It is ethical to promote health because health is a universally desirable goal.

By contrast, **hypothetical health promotion** is based on the demonstrable facts that:

1. There is no objectively true understanding of health

2. All categorical statements to the effect that practice A is good for health, practice B is bad for health and so on, are nothing more than logical extensions of unprovable assumptions about the nature of health

3. Different individuals and peoples hold different beliefs about how best to live. In the light of this social reality it is an unreasonable imperialism to claim that only those behaviours which conform to a particular health promoter's idea of health are truly healthy.

Assertions about 'how people should live' cannot arise spontaneously from the evidence; rather they must be chosen (knowingly or unknowingly) according to the asserter's instincts, values, and ways of classifying the world (her prejudices, in other words). Take, for example, the apparently straightforward health promoting declaration many of us heard repeatedly as children:

> Eat your greens, young man/woman. You'll never grow big, healthy and strong unless you do.

There is evidence in favour of this assertion. Green vegetables are a good source of beta carotene and vitamin C, and there is research that indicates that eating broccoli (particularly the sprouted seeds) may help protect against some forms of cancer (see http://www.cancer.org/docroot/NWS/content/NWS_3_1x_Broccoli_and_Cauliflower _Help_Fight_Cancer.asp for example). But this does not make it categorically true that eating your greens is good for your health. All anyone can say is:

> If you want to grow up without vitamin C deficiency, and if you want slightly to increase your chances of avoiding bladder cancer as an adult, then you should eat your greens, young man/woman.

I have chosen not to tell my own my children to 'eat their greens' because I do not believe that this approach is good for their health. When I picture my children's health I see them standing on a stage that looks like roughly this:

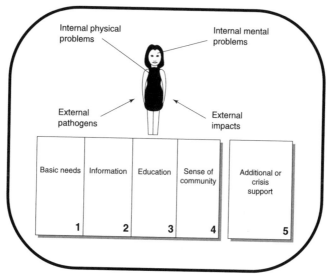

THE STATE OF HEALTH OF AN INDIVIDUAL OR A GROUP

Figure I   The foundations conception of health

As I understand it, my role as a father is to help create the highest possible degree of health for both Charlotte and Penny. In part, this means ensuring their physical robustness by providing them with a nutritious diet in order to avoid a range of possible problems (this aspect of my health promotion task is represented in Fig. 1 by the person/group standing on the platform, together with the relevant arrows). But this is not the whole story. The way I see it, promoting my children's health means that I should work to build up their mental strength, their confidence, their social skills, and their understanding of the world's splendour, confusion, joy and pain. And this means that I am constantly aiming to help them to make their own decisions – I am encouraging their independence as best as I know how. I occasionally tell them that such and such food is good for them in certain ways, too much fat may be bad for them, and so on. But I also want them to trust their instincts about what to eat, and I want them to know that their judgements matter. In fact, to insist on them eating their greens would most likely be BAD for their foundational health: they would probably not eat their greens as a matter of principle in any case; I would be undermining their ability to choose for themselves; I would be underestimating their intelligence; and I would be hiding behind commands rather than connecting with them directly.

Categorical health promotion says:

Health is X. It is good to act in ways that will make you Xey.

Hypothetical health promotion says:

IF you think health is X and IF X is what you want THEN you should do A, B, C etc.

This simple distinction is the basis of *Health Promotion: Philosophy, Prejudice and Practice*. Understand it and you understand the whole book. *Health Promotion: Philosophy, Prejudice and Practice* is NOT against health promotion, rather it applauds the idea that we should try to bring about a world where people can live more meaningful, creative lives on their own terms.

Despite my criticisms of the official health promotion crusade, I remain profoundly committed to health. Indeed I would go so far as to say that I am MORE committed to health than ANY of the Magpie Profession. How can this be? Just like anyone else committed to health, I am committed to MY idea of it. The difference is that I admit it, I own up to it. I am committed to a PREJUDICED idea of health. I am committed to the idea that healthy people possess the foundations for living a life THEY choose to live, and I am committed to the idea that certain foundations are better than others for this purpose. I cannot prove my preferences to be better than those of anyone else because such preferences lie ultimately in the realm of values and politics, not science or medicine.

But how can I claim to be MORE committed to health than members of the Magpie Profession? After all, they have official titles. They are health leaders, managers, doctors, nurses, policy-makers, health promoters with degrees in the subject. I am merely an academic interested in the philosophy of health. And yet I believe that I CAN claim to be more committed to health than the members of the Magpie Profession because I have bothered to work out what I think about health. I have reflected carefully on my prejudices, I have explored their logic, I have defined health explicitly, I have come up with a graphic and still growing theory of health (not a doctrine and not commandments, but a theory). And, like all useful theories, this theory continues to spawn further theories and practical approaches to health promotion.

In sum, this book criticises conventional health promotion in order to help it develop theoretically, morally and practically. Read with an open mind it is obvious that the book proposes a powerful synergy between the foundations and conventional (essentially medical) understandings of health. If this synergy is to flourish the Magpie Profession must accept and correct four fundamental errors.

Firstly, the fact that a way of life benefits one person or group of people does not mean it will necessarily benefit others. I like to swim regularly. I think it is good for my health. Yet the majority of people have no wish to spend their leisure time staring at the bottom of a chlorinated pool, and unless trained to swim energetically and with correct technique they stand to gain little if any physical benefit. Part of my path to health could be the road to depression, disease and failure for someone else.

Secondly, the conventional view of health promotion devalues ways of living which conflict with medical interpretations of health (a point made persuasively by several 'anti-healthism' campaigners in recent years).[7,46] For instance, conventional health promotion cannot recommend Buddhism as a 'healthy lifestyle' because dissociation from everyday reality (the ultimate aim of Buddhist practice) and preoccupation with death (part of the core of Buddhist philosophy) are regarded as symptoms of psychiatric illness by Western doctors. Nor can mainstream health promotion endorse mountain climbing, riding fast motorbikes, hang-gliding, drinking strong beer or eating cream cakes, even though each of these activities can be gorgeously fulfilling in their place.

Thirdly, establishment health promotion has no interest in ethical reflection. Ethics is a never-ending process of deliberation aimed at producing defensible ways of living in a world shared with other sentient beings. But this is not how official health promotion sees it. For conventional health experts 'being ethical' means behaving in ways most likely to maintain personal health (conventionally understood) and encouraging or possibly even coercing other people to behave the same way.

Fourthly, the entire edifice of conventional health promotion is built on a philosophical mistake. The Magpie Profession thinks health is a concrete state. And yet it takes only a moment of open-mindedness to realise there can be no such thing. 'Health' and 'healthy' are merely words human beings use to describe states and behaviours we value positively. Different human beings value different things. Consequently we do not always agree which states and behaviours to label 'healthy', and there is no way any of us can prove the others wrong. Nor should we try to do so, for to claim that one understanding of health is the only true way to think of it is akin to the claim that there is one and only one true comprehension of love or justice or the value of childhood.

HOPES FOR THE SECOND EDITION

This second edition has been lightly edited for style and sense, includes notes to exercises for teachers and lecturers previously published separately, and incorporates the innovative rational field template more fully explained in a companion publication, *Total Health Promotion: Mental Health, Rational Fields and the Quest for Autonomy* (Wiley, 2002). It offers an extensive additional dialogue in which James and Diane have entered into a partnership as rational field health promoters, and demonstrate how the rational field idea can be used to promote health in practice.

My hopes for (and reasons for writing) this second edition are twofold. Firstly, health promotion is essentially a practical task. However elegant or philosophically accomplished health promotion theories are, they will remain impotent unless they can be turned into workable plans and strategies. The rational field theory explained in this second edition finally bridges the gap between the foundations theory and practical health promotion. Armed with the rational field template, and other decision-making tools, health promoters can now readily apply the foundations theory of health to promote health.

Secondly, though the book's thesis is obviously correct, *Health Promotion: Philosophy, Prejudice and Practice* has been largely ignored by senior health promotion practitioners and decision-makers, and by the World Health Organization in particular. In my opinion establishment health promotion should urgently address the considerable social implications of its promoting a version of health in the supposed interests of millions of citizens without consulting us or obtaining our consent. If establishment health promotion will accept and act upon the simple arguments contained within this text, it will make a massive step toward the democratisation of health practice and public health.

Torbay, Auckland
New Zealand
New Year's Day 2003

Preface to the First Edition

On my first day as a health promotion officer my boss asked me what I would like to do. I asked him what the options were. 'Anything that promotes health' he replied, 'I'll tell you what we do here at the moment if you like.' He explained that he was the 'resource person'. He saw himself as a spider, whose role was to distribute information to all corners of his web. His own manager was Dr Roberts, the District Medical Officer, whom I would see only occasionally – so long as I didn't try to change anything. Helen was support person for the health visitors and district nurses, who were always dropping in for pamphlets, videos and a cup of tea. Denise, he said, had the most active job. 'She is LAY, look after yourself, and mostly runs exercise groups around the town. Karen is nutrition, Nigel is community development and Jane is our information officer. How do you feel about drugs and alcohol?' (It is most probably my imagination but I seem to recall that at this very point in our conversation Denise burst into the room in her pink leotard and black leggings – we were in the kitchen – and 'warmed down' vigorously in front of the sink, apparently oblivious to my boss and I.) Becoming more anxious by the minute about my latest career-move, I said that drugs and alcohol might suit, but could I do some research first? 'Naturally' answered Harry, and so it was that I became the 'drugs person' in our Unit.

It turned out to be an interesting job, working with kind, friendly people. Probably because the situation was so happy I had plenty of time to think about what I was doing. Not only was I able to reflect on the many scientific, legal and ethical questions raised by work to counter 'drug misuse', but I was also free to try to work out how I might have made a more *deeply* rational decision about what to do as a health promotion officer.

The truth is that I fell into the 'drug misuse' work because it was there. I decided to do it because it meant I could do some reading and research into a new subject, and because some of the existing health promotion materials seemed so unlikely that I was sure I must be able to do better. My decision was thus purely pragmatic. It was not based in the slightest on a belief that 'I should do this because it is the best contribution I can make to *health promotion as a whole*' since I had no idea what *health promotion as a whole* was. I had already written on the philosophy of health, and so knew that Harry's suggestion that I should do 'anything that promotes health' was no answer. I knew health to be a rich and deeply controversial idea, and therefore knew that the same must apply to health promotion. But that only made it harder to work out how I could make a philosophically justified decision about my role.

I discovered, through speaking with other health promoters, that everyone else in the field had chosen what to do on practical grounds too: they were good at something, the health authority desired a particular project, they could be effective, it was good experience, clients wanted it. But although many of these health promoters were deeply committed to promoting healthy lives, none could explain *why* in any way much beyond platitude: 'obviously a healthy life is better than a sick one', 'we must add years to life and life to years', 'people have a right to health', or 'the goal of health promotion is health for all', was the best most could manage.

But if 'health' is a deeply contestable notion, then so too are these slogans. Is a 'healthy' life in permanent unemployment better than a 'sick' one with a good job? What *sort* of 'life' should be 'added to years' – a happy one, a demanding one, an exciting one, a cautious one? Who says people have a right to health? Is this a legal right? A moral right? If health can mean 'not being sick' does it make sense to say that people have a *right* not to be sick? Do I really have a right not to catch a cold? What *is* Health for All? If 'health' can have different meanings, and if some of these are incompatible (as they are), then isn't Health for All a logical impossibility?

THERE ARE NO OBVIOUS CONCLUSIONS IN HEALTH PROMOTION

These questions hovered constantly in my thoughts. But, like most other inquisitive health promotion workers, I had to leave them there in order to concentrate on my practical tasks. Had I had the time and experience to think about the philosophy of anti-drugs health promotion I would probably have discovered the roots of health promotion then not now, 11 years later. At the time I quickly (too quickly) formed the opinion that there is only one intelligent approach to drugs and health promotion. I decided first that health promoters should be aware that it is a universal characteristic of human beings that if we find substances which allow us some temporary relief from life's grind, many of us will use them. I concluded secondly that health promoters should recognise that the distinction between legal and illegal drugs is an arbitrary one. And thirdly I reasoned that health promoters must appreciate that if you make something illegal not only do you automatically make it attractive to some, but you instantly create new classes of problem: in this case the 'drug abuser' and the things he will do to gain access to his chosen drug, and a new brand of criminal – the supplier of the illegal substance.

I thought then that these things were plain as day, and that anyone who held an alternative view was just wrong. However – even though I hold the same opinions about illicit drugs today – I have come to realise that the matter is in fact not simply obvious, and that those who disagree with me cannot, and most certainly should not, be cursorily dismissed. Health promotion is far more important than that. There are deeper reasons for my belief that free-thinking people should not be prevented from choosing to use drugs – and deeper reasons for the contrary beliefs too.

I now realise that these different beliefs – like every other belief about what is right and wrong in health promotion – rest in different *political outlooks*. Speaking roughly, my views about drug use emanate from my philosophical conviction that mature and competent citizens ought to be permitted by the state to behave as they wish so long as they do no harm to others, and that the role of good government is to enable all citizens to choose as freely as possible by giving them as much unbiased information as possible. Equally, the prejudices of those who are horrified by illicit drug use stand – in one way or another – on alternative views of what society should be. For instance, a person opposed to 'drug misuse' is likely – though not certain – to believe that the central pillars of any decent society are social order and the rule of law, that the use of illicit drugs is subversive and damaging to work and family ethics, and that for these reasons it is essential that the use of such mind-altering substances is minimised.

HEALTH PROMOTION IS ESSENTIALLY PREJUDICED

I recognise now that however factually compelling the evidence seems, all forms of health promotion must *first* be prejudiced. Each form will use evidence in its practices, but none will be initially *directed* by that evidence. Each type of health promotion is based on a point of view about the ways people should and should not behave, and ultimately therefore on some notion of the good society. And since the good society can be thought of in very different ways, and since health promoters inevitably hold a wide range of political philosophies, health promotion is riddled with deep theoretical tensions. Yet health promotion's practical surface rarely reflects its inner turmoil. And this not only makes life extremely difficult for the reflective health promoter, but so long as the rifts and faults remain largely ignored by mainstream health promotion the discipline is prevented from maturing. Only when the philosophical discussion of health promotion's basic purposes has become commonplace will this have happened.

This book is meant for all those health promoters who feel as I did in 1985. It is for those who want to promote health from a firm theoretical base but who find themselves caught in an uneasy 'no-man's land' – intermittently tossed between rebellion, capitulation and some sort of compromise. *Health Promotion: Philosophy, Prejudice and Practice* cuts through the rhetoric of health promotion to reveal its conceptual roots, and so provides an accessible map of health promotion to working health promoters. Armed with this map, any health promoter who sets out to achieve a particular practical goal will not only be able to select a path she can defend theoretically, but will be fully aware of the many philosophical and political assumptions she sanctions as she chooses it. And, once thoughtful health promoters have gained sufficient confidence to discard the suffocating rhetoric, so the theoretical side of health promotion will begin to flourish, and health promotion will finally come of age.

Eden Park
Auckland
New Zealand
January 1996

Acknowledgements

FIRST EDITION

But for the exhaustive support of Ian Buchanan this book would never have seen the light of day. Its words are mine alone, I take full responsibility for everything in its pages, yet Ian's insights and knowledge were so much a part of the book's creation that in many ways it belongs to him too.

I am also deeply grateful to Hannelore Best and Alan Cribb for taking the considerable trouble to read and comment on the book in manuscript form.

It was both a privilege and a pleasure to be able to write this book in a happy, tranquil environment. For this I must pay credit to Auckland University's old-fashioned respect for academic research, and thank all my friends in the Department of Psychiatry and Behavioural Science for their gentle presence, encouragement and humour. I am, however, especially grateful to those colleagues who do not see health promotion as I do, yet who continue to exhibit an extraordinary level of tolerance to my sometimes vehement criticisms. All of these things have undoubtedly promoted my health.

SECOND EDITION

I am grateful that sufficient people have read, used and purchased *Health Promotion: Philosophy, Prejudice and Practice* for it to merit a second edition. I especially thank those teachers and students of health promotion who have been sufficiently open-minded to recognise conventional health promotion's practical and ethical flaws, and brave enough to explore my criticisms and suggestions for better ways forward.

I would also like to thank Professor Max Abbott of Auckland University of Technology for his wise and patient support for my work.

Introduction

In the rush to make the world a better place many health promoters have forgotten how to think. There are exceptions, but most health promotion writers, and nearly all conventional health promotion campaigns, assume very much more than they ought to. Typically they take for granted – when they should not – that health is something everyone desires equally, that choosing targets for health raises few moral difficulties, that any method which might improve health is justifiable, and that a united health promotion movement is crusading for a healthier world.

WE KNOW WHAT WE ARE AGAINST, SO WE MUST KNOW WHAT WE ARE FOR

Many of its devotees think of health promotion as the front line in the attack on a tired 'biomedical model' obsessed with disease and illness. Only the most radical health promoters are wholeheartedly set against medicine – most accept that clinicians have a place in the fight for health – but the great majority are opposed to (what they see as) the continuing medical dominance of health creation. Many health promoters revere the supposedly seminal Lalonde Report which protests that: '...the traditional view of equating the level of health...with the availability of physicians and hospitals...' is 'inadequate'.[1] The report has such high status within health promotion that it has become an article of faith that too much attention is paid to medicine, and too little to environment, biology and lifestyle.

MEDICINE IS NEGATIVE?

Forward-thinking people find Lalonde's simple statements persuasive because for the most part medical work is obviously done to remedy *negative* states of affairs. As a general rule doctors work to relieve existing problems – to restore people to the states they were in before undesirable changes occurred. *Positive* in medicine usually means no more than 'as you were', and this sort of positive rarely satisfies the idealistically inclined.

What's more, 'as you were' is itself sometimes the cause of disease and illness. People are regularly detoxified only to recommence a life of heavy drinking on discharge. Patients

Health Promotion, Second Edition: David Seedhouse
© 2004 John Wiley & Sons, Ltd: ISBNs 0 470 84732 8 (HB); 0 470 84733 6 (PB)

receive helpful psychiatric treatment, but have no choice but to live in situations which trigger psychotic episodes. Clinicians provide therapy for respiratory problems but can only look on as patients are ferried back to houses which feed their diseases. Understandably, many health promoters see such medical interventions as inadequate and temporary cover for cracks which only structural change can properly mend.

It seems obvious to these health promoters that *positive health* means much more than back to neutral. And left like this – without worrying too much about the detail of fundamental change – health promotion can be inspiring. Unlike medicine, health promotion is still young enough to talk of rebellion and the possibility of a better world – and so has an instant appeal to those who are determined to shake things up.

HEALTH PROMOTION IS POSITIVE?

It is easy to be carried away by the excitement generated by being against something, and just as easy to imagine that by being explicitly opposed to bad practice you know automatically what you mean by good practice. But unfortunately it is almost always easier to be against things – to be against unemployment, against war, against exploitation, against illness – than to prescribe detailed and workable alternatives.

UNHAPPINESS THERAPY VS HAPPINESS PROMOTION: A PARALLEL

Health promotion's problem can be most readily seen by drawing a parallel.

Imagine a society where 95% of the national happiness budget goes into unhappiness treatment and palliation. Over the years, thanks partly to such generous funding, a large group of professional unhappiness therapists has evolved. In collaboration with a resourceful happiness industry (with which the therapists have a symbiotic relationship) a store of techniques has been developed to combat unhappiness in all its forms and contexts. The unhappiness therapists are especially good at diagnosing and classifying the many different unhappinesses, and have even reached the stage where they are able to cure some of the simpler and more commonly occurring types and syndromes.

All is well with the world of unhappiness therapy. Then, one day, a visionary – call him Mr L – decides he must voice a protest at this undue focus on unhappiness. Just look at how much money we are spending on *misery*, he says. Look at all the labels we have dreamt up to categorise it, look at all these expensive machines we have invented to treat unhappiness when we refuse to invest in tackling its wider causes. Just look at the years we spend training our young people to become *specialists in unhappiness*. Is this really what we want? Should we be concentrating so many of our resources on rescuing people from drowning? Wouldn't it be more sensible to prevent people falling into rivers in the first place? Better still, shouldn't we be improving people's lives so they never have to face the dangerous rivers at all? Surely it makes more sense to aim for happiness rather than try to cure misery. Surely it's time to change gear. From now on we should all concentrate on promoting happiness.

Mr L's rallying call strikes quite a chord: it seems revolutionary but simple, radical *and* down-to-earth, and so has a very broad appeal. A new cause is born and quickly attracts disciples committed to creating happiness any way they can. Those with training in communication skills set out to help people be more open with each other; those experienced in horticulture dedicate themselves to helping people establish low-maintenance gardens; converts to the cause with training in literature dedicate themselves to teaching people to use libraries more efficiently, and to choose books most likely to create well-being; accountants offer free budgeting services to those citizens with the lowest incomes; scribes help people compose wittier letters to their friends – there seems no end to the happiness promotion possibilities.

But, despite the very best efforts of the happiness seekers, not everyone is content. Indeed, before long happiness promoters themselves decide they deserve better social status. Many want to belong to a profession, and some even start describing themselves as happiness experts – instigators of an emerging discipline, founders of the *new happiness movement*. Equally inevitably, some unhappiness therapists feel threatened by this trend, and resolve to work out what to do about it.

They discuss strategy. One possibility would be to try to incorporate happiness promotion within their own hierarchies. Another would be to ridicule the whole idea. Or they might do whatever it takes to ensure that happiness promotion funding is always dedicated to unhappiness prevention. They might even say that happiness promotion was their idea in the first place.

But the leading unhappiness therapists are wise, and do not see the need to resort to panic measures. They realise that happiness promotion contains the seeds of its own destruction and tell their juniors not to be concerned. Not all unhappiness therapists are reassured, however, so their leaders patiently explain the strengths of unhappiness therapy, and point out happiness promotion's Achilles' heel. They tell their anxious colleagues that unhappiness therapy is enormously resilient because:

a. unhappiness is a state which deviates negatively from statistical norms and is therefore a definable and measurable condition. Any deviation *below* normal standards of mental disposition and general behaviour can be quantified
b. generally speaking, unhappiness may be treated by paying attention to a specific problem or set of problems (*remove* the problem and the unhappiness will be cured)
c. successful therapy is *demonstrable* – success is either a return to normal or the alleviation of the unhappiness symptoms (even if the root problem cannot be eliminated)
d. so long as unhappiness therapists seek mostly to help people who present with and define their own problems it is possible to minimise ethical controversy. Although there has been a recent history of academic research into the ethics of unhappiness therapy this is nothing compared to the furore that will ensue once ethicists realise just how deeply controversial and value-soaked happiness promotion is.

Senior unhappiness therapists know that happiness promotion is *not* the mirror-image of unhappiness therapy (even though it is true that the removal of problems that are making people miserable *can* increase happiness). They also realise that happiness promotion is highly unstable, because:

a. happiness can be achieved in an infinite number of ways. Therefore it is meaningless to say that happiness is a positive deviation from normal standards. Happiness is impossible to define objectively, and is therefore impossible to quantify precisely

b. it is one thing to seek to promote happiness by trying to prevent unhappiness, but quite another to attempt happiness promotion *independent* of unhappiness therapy. In the latter case happiness promotion instantly loses its moorings *and* its bearings. Without the focus on observable problems happiness promotion becomes a hopelessly open-ended task (should anyone be able to define happiness? Can anything be happiness promoting? Surely not. But then what is the core of happiness promotion practice? Why pick one set of happiness targets rather than any other?)

c. successful happiness promotion is impossible to demonstrate conclusively because the nature of happiness is contestable. You might think you are happy but it is always open to someone else to disagree with you. You might think you are unhappy but score well according to some researchers' 'happiness indicators'. Such disputes are impossible to resolve in the absence of hard evidence – and sooner or later happiness promotion must leave hard evidence behind

d. so long as happiness promotion proceeds without the explicit consent of those who might be affected by it – as by its nature it very often must – happiness promotion will be plagued with ethical problems.

Having had these points spelt out the unhappiness therapy profession breathes a collective sigh of relief. Its members can now see that unless the happiness movement works out a solid theoretical set of justifications for what it wants to achieve it will eventually sink without trace. No one with any sense will take it seriously for long and it will, after all, turn out to be a passing fad.

HEALTH PROMOTION NEEDS A THEORY OF HEALTH PROMOTION

The parallel with this world and the imaginary one should be obvious. The analogy captures the essential differences between medicine as work for health (it sets out mainly to remedy negatives) and health promotion as work for health (it sets out mainly to establish positives). The wise words of the senior unhappiness therapists illustrate the enormous intellectual hurdle health promotion must climb if it is to become a serious, theoretically based discipline. Either health promoters must think out proper theories of health promotion's purpose, or health promotion will eventually disappear under a sea of empty words and vacant phrases.

It boils down to this. The practices of science, education, engineering and law – indeed all established professional practices – are partly based on a multitude of detailed theories about *how* to perform specific techniques. There are, for example, theories about the most efficient way to extract vitamins from plants;[2] about how best to teach languages to small groups,[3] about how to calculate the optimum relationship between bridge span and support required,[4] and about ways in which it is acceptable to extend the common law.[5] Any profession which has to deal with complex practical problems will inevitably develop theoretically based procedures to address them. And this is equally true of health promotion, which employs a wide range of problem-solving methods borrowed from other disciplines. But unlike health promotion, most other professions have developed a deeper level of theory.

Mature human enterprises are shaped by theories of *purpose*. Professions worthy of the name take the trouble to think out substantial theories about *why they do what they do*. Science, education, technology and law each have carefully crafted and well-established philosophies. Of course each profession has *several* theories about its nature and purpose, and there are disagreements between advocates of the different schools. But this is all to the good since it is necessary for each competing philosophical school to develop the very best justification for its account of the profession's purpose, and for its description of best practice. A plurality of rationales is a sign of a reflective profession (or at least of a profession where serious reflection is a constant possibility). Moreover, where theoretical pluralism exists any researcher or policy-maker worth her salt should feel duty-bound to explain what basic *kind* of advance or change she is seeking. That is, she should feel obliged to indicate which theoretical tradition her practical proposal is built on.

But at the moment this is not possible in health promotion. Fundamental theoretical reflection cannot take place. Although health promotion has many theories of *process* (theories about how best to perform procedure X, theories about why method A is more effective in achieving goal C than method B, and so on) it possesses not one sustained account of its *purpose*. Theories of health promotion of equivalent substance to theories of jurisprudence or the nature of science are strikingly absent. There is much vague talk, countless gestures to a healthier world for everyone, but scant attention to the bed-rock question 'what is the *point* of promoting health?' And unless this situation changes health promotion is surely heading for a fall.

THE PURPOSE OF THIS BOOK

This book is an attempt to show the source and full nature of the difficulties facing health promotion theorists and practitioners, and to offer a theoretically sound way forward – to indicate one route by which a serious discipline might come into being. Basically, the book argues that health promotion does not just happen in some neutral way, nor is health promotion always unquestionably a good thing. Rather all health promotion is prejudiced – every aspect of health promotion is based ultimately on human values of some kind and is, therefore, essentially political – even if health promoters are unaware of it. The foundations theory of health promotion offered in Part Three of this book is no exception. However, it makes a virtue of its prejudice by openly acknowledging it and by using it to set limits on those health promotion interventions carried out under its auspices.

The foundations theory is one suggestion only. There are potentially many different theories of health promotion. If the field is to mature, other thinkers must offer theoretically justified ways forward too. Not only that, but there must be deep and continuing dialogue between the different theorists, and there must then either be unity in the profession or – as is much more likely – markedly different *types* of health promotion must emerge. And as this happens health promotion must also remain (or become) of practical use. This is clearly a tall order, yet it is not out of the question: perhaps this book will come to be seen as a marker of the beginning of the end of health promotion's adolescence.

THE DIALOGUES

Health Promotion: Philosophy, Prejudice and Practice is thought-provoking, educational and above all accessible. In this second edition, the more academic analysis of health promotion is interspersed with seven dialogues between Diane, a young journalist, and various characters she meets as she researches health promotion. At first Diane knows very little about the subject. However, she learns quickly, and becomes increasingly perturbed by her failure to see the ultimate reason for health promotion. From Diane's point of view, unless she can understand the profession's overall purpose, she is unable to make proper sense of the specific health promotion tasks she learns about.

It is hoped that at least some readers currently employed as, or studying to be, health promoters will identify with Diane as she struggles to come to terms with health promotion's multiple models, indicators, and targets. At some stage in their careers all inquisitive health promoters will have experienced something of Diane's disorientation and will have asked – or have dearly wanted to ask – the questions she poses.

The dialogues and the more conventional text are linked. As each dialogue or set of dialogues ends Diane consults a philosopher, and the formal text which follows should be read as the philosopher's direct response to Diane's inquiries. If, as is intended, the reader feels a sense of shared interest with Diane, it should seem that the philosopher is talking immediately to you.

THE EXERCISES

Health Promotion: Philosophy, Prejudice and Practice offers 11 carefully prepared exercises. These may be attempted separately, and have been designed for independent study. However they will prove most useful if they are undertaken in discussion with other health promoters or health promotion students, as the book is read through.

The Exercises are accompanied by notes for teachers and lecturers. The notes offer advice on the best ways to generate rich and stimulating student discussion. In the first edition these notes were offered in a separate booklet. They are offered as part of the main text in this edition – in edited form – since their advice has proved to be equally useful to students, practitioners and other readers.

The Magpie Profession

Health Promotion on Offer: All Models Available

SCENE ONE

A telephone rings in a well-appointed foyer.

RECEPTIONIST: Good morning. Willesville Public Health Directorate. How can I help you?

DIANE: Hi, my name is Diane Grant. I'm a reporter with the *Chronicle*. I'm hoping to do a feature on health promotion and I've been told that your Director is the man to speak to. Could you put me through to him do you think?

RECEPTIONIST: Mr Alpine is very busy. However, you may speak with his secretary. I'm putting you through . . .

SECRETARY: Good morning. Willesville Public Health Directorate. Miss Bowman speaking. How can I help you?

DIANE: (*Introduces herself as before*) I wonder if I could speak with Mr Alpine for a few moments?

SECRETARY: Mr Alpine is very busy. Perhaps I can help you. What exactly do you want to know?

DIANE: What health promotion is. Who does it in Willesville. What goes on. Who benefits. How much it costs. Who approves of it. Who doesn't. Couldn't I speak to Mr Alpine?

SECRETARY: No. Mr Alpine has meetings all day. But I think I can point you in the right direction, Ms Grant. Many people in Willesville are health promoters. Some work in hospitals. Some work for the local authority. Some work for the Community Trust. And there are some in Willesville who think of themselves as health promoters but who are not actually called health promoters.

DIANE: I would be grateful, Miss Bowman, if you could tell me where I could find the largest group of health promoters. That would make my job easier.

Health Promotion, Second Edition: David Seedhouse
© 2004 John Wiley & Sons, Ltd: ISBNs 0 470 84732 8 (HB); 0 470 84733 6 (PB)

SECRETARY: Of course. In that case I suggest you contact James Campion, our District Health Promotion Officer, on 528-7952. He's in charge of the Willesville District Health Promotion Unit. I'm sure he'll have time to see you. You may say that Mr Alpine's secretary gave you his name. Good morning.

SCENE TWO

A group of youngish adults are sitting – on plastic chairs at least a size too small even for the slightest of them – in a semi-circle in a spacious room with a polished wood floor. The room resembles a small gym bare of equipment and has only one window, a large one which looks out onto the backside of a row of small shops with flats above. Other chairs are stacked against the scuffed cream walls. Some of these chairs partly conceal a portable electronic whiteboard, the surface of which is itself almost entirely obscured by boxes, arrows, and even what appear to be formulae, all in assorted colours. In the boxes, and beside the arrows, various phrases are written: 'beliefs and values clarification', 'CHD', 'tertiary prevention', 'self-empowerment', 'AIDS update', 'community development', 'models and values', and others too difficult to translate. One of the group – the oldest by a few years – begins to speak.

JAMES: As you requested Ms Grant, we have assembled the department for you – apart from Joan and Michael who are on study leave, and Alison who is off sick. We can give you about an hour. I'd like first to introduce everyone, then you can tell us a little about yourself and what you are after, and ask us questions. Okay?

DIANE: That sounds fine.

JAMES: Well then, starting from your left let me introduce John Barnes (a Health Education Officer), Carol Jones (another HEO), Ann Pryor (Deputy Director of Health Promotion), Ian Peterson (Senior Health Promotion Officer), you and I have already met, and Martin Miller (also a SHPO). With the others I mentioned we make up Willesville District Health Promotion Unit and, more broadly, we are all members of what has come to be known as the health promotion movement.

I won't ask each of the staff to introduce themselves personally – we do not have overlong and I'm sure you'll get to know us all better as you ask your questions. Now would you mind telling us a little about yourself, and your project?

DIANE: Sure. I'm Diane Grant. As you know, I work for the *Willesville Chronicle*. I've not been with the paper long – just a few months – I'm 'health and social services' – along with a few other things... To tell you the truth I seem to be more 'miscellaneous page filler' at the moment, but officially one of my main jobs is to report on health matters: a seeker after truth for a local rag in a small town. You can imagine what I require I'm sure.

ANN: Scandal and dirt if you can get it? A story you can flog to the nationals?

DIANE: Definitely the latter, since you ask. But I'll settle for a 'Day in the Life of a Health Promoter' for the moment. (*The group laughs loudly, as people tend to in the presence of strangers*) What I thought might be a good theme for my article would be if we pretended that I've come along as a punter. I'll act as if I've turned up out of the blue and want some advice about my health. I'll tell you where I feel I have a problem, and you can put me right. Will that be alright? (*Ann and James shuffle their chairs back an inch or so, virtually as one*) Oh, I think I forgot to mention, Colin will be along at 10 to take a few pictures.

ANN: Colin? Pictures?

DIANE: For the article, obviously. You won't mind posing in front of your posters and displays, will you?

IAN: Yeeess, it'll be okay so long as we can choose which ones to stand in front of.

DIANE: No reason why not, though I don't think any of you ought to be snapped in front of that (*she glances at the whiteboard*). Much too busy.

JAMES: Okay Diane, let's get cracking then.

DIANE: Excellent. I've got a drink problem and I want to know how to sort it out.

JAMES: Right . . . this is a role-play, right? (*Diane nods, smiling*) Okay. Over to you I think John.

JOHN: Hi Diane. I'm the alcohol person here. I co-ordinate the Drinkwise programme.

DIANE: Drinkwise?

JOHN: Surely you've heard of it. There are safe levels of drinking – 21 units and 14 units of alcohol per week for men and women respectively – and the Drinkwise programme aims to get this message across and to give people strategies for safe drinking. For example, if you are out in a crowd it's easy to drink more than you want so one way to keep things under control is to have a soft drink every other round . . . I'll give you some leaflets on it. If you like you can visit the Drinkwise website too. Here's the URL. (*John writes down* http://www.drinkwise.co.uk/about.htm *on a scrap of paper and hands it to Diane*)

DIANE: Thanks – I have heard of Drinkwise, now you explain it, but I've never been sure what these 'units' are. Is one drink one unit?

JOHN: No. A unit is a 'standard measure' of alcohol. A half pint of beer, a single whisky, a glass of wine – each of these is a unit.

DIANE: So how many units are in a bottle of wine?

JOHN: That depends on how big it is, naturally. And how strong. But, on average, about six or seven.

DIANE: So I can have two bottles of wine a week?

JOHN: I would advise less, and definitely no more. Or you could have 14 small whiskies or 7 pints of beer – though if you like stronger beer you must drink proportionately less, depending on the alcohol content.

DIANE: One pint of weak beer a day is all I can have? More than this isn't safe?

JOHN: I wouldn't recommend drinking every day, and fewer than 14 units would be a healthier target . . .

DIANE: Oh dear, I *do* have a drink problem . . .

JAMES: In fact you probably don't. And I feel I ought to mention that John is using old advice on safe drinking levels.

DIANE: What do you mean?

JAMES: The government advice on sensible drinking was revised in the mid-nineties. Safe levels were raised to 28 units for males and 21 for females, and the advice is now being offered a bit more subtly – the official view is that people should think in terms of daily benchmarks for their drinking, taking account of their tolerance, weight and general physical condition. And there is increased emphasis on personal responsibility and choice.

DIANE: I find that rather bizarre, actually. Why should I be confident of any advice you give if it can so easily be changed? Presumably the nature of alcohol itself has remained the same, so are you saying the previous guidelines were simply mistaken? And has it now become clearer that people are responsible for alcohol choices as a matter of fact, or is this just the fashionable way to think?

JAMES: These really are big issues, perhaps we could come back to them a bit later? (*Quickly*) And Diane, I hasten to add that an actual consultation wouldn't happen like this, we don't just pass on information, or just instruct. There are various educational strategies we might and do adopt. With a drinking problem there is much to be considered, and a lot would depend on how bad it is. If you were a confirmed alcoholic we would be looking at a medically managed programme, detoxification, time in a DDU and so on. But assuming you were not in that state but were just worried about the level of your drinking, then we would want first to establish what your attitude is, and how you behave. When do you drink? With whom? How much at one time? What do you know? How much are you in control of what you do? What decision-making skills do you have? How do you feel about yourself? How confident are you? How high is your self-esteem? – and so on. I'm sure John didn't mean to give you the impression that he merely passes on leaflets and website addresses – this is only a small part of good health education.

DIANE: Health education? I thought this was a health promotion department.

JAMES: It is, but we do health education as part of our health promotion.

DIANE: What's the difference then?

JAMES: It's not easy to say quickly. There's a fair bit of controversy about it as you'll find out if you look in our journals library. But shouldn't we finish dealing with your drink problem?

DIANE: I suppose so. But I'd like to come back to this question later. It may be important.

Anyhow, say John helps me sort out my knowledge and my confidence and the rest. What can he then do to actually help me stop drinking?

JAMES: John?

JOHN: Well, there are a number of things I could try. It depends what we find, but let's say you find it hard to say no to a drink when you are socialising. If you find yourself 'giving in', not wishing to be different from the crowd – am I right? – then we may need to give you some assertiveness skills – appropriate eye contact, facial expression, posture, the way you use your voice...

DIANE: I'm a journalist.

JAMES: Well maybe it will be that we find it is knowledge you are lacking, or will-power perhaps, or if your problem is severe you might need counselling, or a self-help group . . .

MARTIN: Or perhaps it's just a matter of Diane behaving more responsibly, don't you think John? To avoid cirrhosis of the liver, obesity, and heart disease it is imperative that she moderates her behaviour. (*Looking Diane in the eye*) Don't you know what you are doing to yourself?

ANN: Martin! It's really time you ditched that model. It's old-hat, healthist, and victim-blaming.

MARTIN: I don't accept that. It's a matter of fact that excessive alcohol consumption causes increased morbidity, and that prevention is basically a matter of self-control – you don't get drunk if you don't drink . . .

ANN: Diane, I'm sorry about this, but Martin's a bit of a traditionalist (*glaring at him*) to say the least. Most enlightened health promoters don't go along with this medical model stuff anymore. Sure it's where we *came* from, but it's far too rigid. There are lots of ways to promote health, and very many people from very many backgrounds are in a position to do it. Its not just a job for the doctors, or for the nurses, or even just a job for the health service come to that. Health promotion is not something that should be restricted to one or two professions. Health is more important than that.

I don't think it's really a question of you adjusting your behaviour to avoid disease, Diane – it's a question of you being *empowered* to make the choices that are right for you – and there are hundreds of ways to do that. In the end you've got to be able to think critically about your value system.

And Martin, for one thing Diane's a journalist – journalists tend to drink, you know? If that's her culture then you can't go round imposing the values of your culture onto her . . .

MARTIN: (*Abruptly*) She won't be able to do much journalism with advanced liver failure. What's more, if my model is inflexible then so is yours. When was the last time you changed your mind?

ANN: Don't be ridiculous.

MARTIN: I'm not being ridiculous actually Ann. Why do you think Diane consulted us? She wants to know what to do for the sake of her health. She doesn't want some New Age course on self-awareness and self-actualisation. She's the client, we're the professionals, and we can give her expert advice. My expert advice is that she will be a lot happier if she learns to drink moderately. Whether she can 'critically assess her value set' has nothing to do with it.

JAMES: (*Leaning forward, so as to put the increasingly frosty stares of Ann and Martin out of sight, as well as to get closer to Diane*) As you can see we do have some, um, healthy differences of opinion here, but we're hardly unusual in that.

DIANE: No?

JAMES: I think you'd find that there would be similar disagreements in most health promotion departments of any size.

CAROL: And that's not the whole story either! (*James leans back again, with a just audible sigh*)

Some of us are actually honest about health promotion. Unlike Ann we've gone past empowerment rhetoric. We aren't afraid to front up with the radical political model. Why do you think you drink Diane?

DIANE: I like to?

CAROL: Maybe, but it didn't just occur to you out of the blue did it? The reason you drink is because the brewers want you to. They spend millions on advertising so they can get fat on your hangover. Martin's part of their little game, would he but realise it . . .

MARTIN: Come off it Carol, that's a bit rich. You know I hate drink . . .

CAROL: I know, I know, but so long as you support a system which patches people up when they get into trouble the brewers are in clover. If you really want to free people from drink you have to get to the roots of the problem – and that means you've got to act politically. It's not Diane's fault that beer is brewed, that brewers sell it aggressively, or that journalists drink . . .

DIANE: Excuse me, but that *is* a bit of a cliché, if you don't mind me saying so.

CAROL: The point, Diane, is that we shouldn't blame you – you are the victim and we should attack the causes of your problem, which are well beyond your control.

DIANE: Can we take stock for a minute? If I really were a client of yours I think I'd be seriously confused by now.

JOHN: You'd be on your way back to the bar wouldn't you?

DIANE: I might, you know. Look, when you said you are all part of a health promotion movement I assumed – obviously naïvely – that you'd all be pulling in the same direction. But that doesn't seem to be so. Martin's telling me to get a grip on my habit before it's too late, Ann wants to expand my self-awareness so I can really and truly know whether I want to go on drinking and you, Carol, would close down the brewing industry if you could. Now does anyone want to tell me how I can make sense of this?

JAMES: I know it looks confusing but it's not actually so bad. There's no doubting that each of us wants to promote your health – everybody's health for that matter – it's just that we disagree about the *methods* we use. Martin favours one model of health promotion, Ann another, and Carol yet another, but we're all for your health.

DIANE: (*Sceptical*) So what model do you follow James?

JAMES: Well let's just say I mix 'n match.

DIANE: But *how* do you do that? How do you decide when to go with Martin's model, and when to be persuaded by Ann?

JAMES: I'm Head of Department here, Diane. I try to be diplomatic.

DIANE: But the problem's more than that, surely. I mean, apart from when you are trying to appease sensitive egos, what *reasons* do you have for choosing one model and not another?

JAMES: I go for the most effective approach.

CAROL: Which of course will prompt Diane to ask what you mean by 'effective' James. Effective to what *end*, she might ask.

DIANE: Actually I was going to ask something like that. You said each of you were 'for my health' but I don't see how you can be because each of these models seems, in one way or another, to be in conflict with the others. I haven't thought about this properly, of course, but from what you've said it is as if what counts as *success* is different for each of you. And I reckon this means that if you say that success for each of you is 'the state of my health after you've done your work' then you must all see health in *different* ways.

Tell me if I've got this wrong: on Martin's model I'm healthy if I've not got alcohol-related disease, and if my behaviour means I'm in no danger of becoming diseased I can drink if I want to, but not very much. On Ann's model I've got to be aware of all the pros and cons. Then I've got to decide, as free from pressure as possible, how I want to conduct my life. If being part of the crowd, going to the pub every night, having a laugh, getting drunk sometimes, is how I *prefer* to live, then I'm healthy (I can drink 'til the cows come home if I want – if I *really* want). On Carol's model, if she got her way, the breweries would be closed down because they cause illness, and I wouldn't be able to drink even if I felt like it. My choice would have been a 'false choice' but now – free from being coerced to make myself ill – I would be healthy. I think I see the point of all these models, at least a bit, but they don't fit together do they?

JAMES: This is getting very complicated, and I see that Colin's arrived. I assume you are the cameraman from the *Chronicle*?

(Colin, who has just been shown into the Meeting Room, confirms his identity) Perhaps if we could at least get the pictures out of the way that would be a help. Diane, may I make a suggestion? I have a few papers and extracts from books about definitions and models in health promotion you might find make useful background reading. How about if you take a look at these and then come back to see us next week?

DIANE: I'm not sure I can do that. I've a lot of deadlines. It would take too long.

JAMES: Then perhaps after work? I could spare you an hour if that suits you. You might not believe it but some of your concerns bother me too. It would be good to talk to an outsider about them.

DIANE: Alright then. That sounds good. I'll call you tomorrow to fix it up.

Where's the Beef?

SCENE ONE

Diane and James are seated at the lounge bar of the local public house. It is almost 5.30 p.m. and the room is slowly filling with customers – mostly local businessmen, and one or two women. Diane has a gin and tonic. James' orange juice sits on the bar, at his elbow.

DIANE: Is this your local?

JAMES: It's the nearest pub to the office, but I hardly ever come here. I don't drink much.

DIANE: Naturally.

JAMES: It's nothing to do with my job. I just don't drink much. Never have.

DIANE: But it would be difficult if you did, as a health promoter?

JAMES: Possibly, though as you found out last week it all depends which model I choose to adopt.

DIANE: Fair enough, but whatever trendy 'model' you 'adopt', the fact is that if you became ill through drinking too much you'd get the push, wouldn't you?

JAMES: I suppose you're right. In many settings health promotion is still dominated by medicine and medical values, which means disease and illness are usually taken to be the primary target of health promotion work. If I educate someone about the dangers of alcohol the expectation is One that they will drink less, Two that they won't get an alcohol-related illness, and Three that they won't therefore become a burden on the health service and so on other taxpayers... Yes, you're right in what I think you're implying. The prevalent view – despite changing fashions – is that there must be a practical health pay-off. It is assumed that there must be an 'outcome' from my professional 'input', which should be 'improved health status' – or some similar phrase.

DIANE: So you reckon the bottom line is still to keep people out of hospital. That's what I got from those extracts you gave me. Behind all the rhetoric and vague slogans – I was amazed by how much waffle there is by the way – what actually counts is how much sickness, or should I say morbidity, you have been able to prevent. There's all the leftish *talk* and then there's what health promoters actually have to *do* as part of their employment.

Health Promotion, Second Edition: David Seedhouse
© 2004 John Wiley & Sons, Ltd: ISBNs 0 470 84732 8 (HB); 0 470 84733 6 (PB)

Despite the 'right on' stuff the real authority – at least in the public sector – still rests in the hands of government which sees health promotion as part of efficient medical services. And if this is true – and I bet it is – it means that a lot of what goes on at the surface of health promotion is nothing more than middle-class Politically Correct angst – especially all that big bad capitalist industry stuff. Carol is hardly going to persuade Gordon's to stop selling this (*she holds up her drink*) but it makes her and her friends feel better to sound off (*she mimes quotation marks with her fingers*) at the political level. If she can actually get paid to indulge herself like this – well, why not? What does she do, exactly?

JAMES: She's our AIDS worker. But look, I don't want to get into a debate with you about whether we're somebody else's pawns, or just wasting our time. I might think that some of us are not as productive as we might be, but that's not for you to know on or off the record. Anyway, I would like to try to explain what was going on last week. To be honest this is more for my benefit than to help you write your story. I'd like to get it clearer myself and I rarely get the chance to talk about my work, out of the office, with such an intelligent person.

DIANE: (*Genuinely flattered*) It might turn out to be useful one way or another.

JAMES: Look, I'm not going to tell you this so you can print 'the confessions of a philosophically troubled civil servant' in some magazine.

DIANE: Don't worry. My editor isn't usually over-interested in controversies of a philosophical kind. In any case I've got a bag full of suitable literature from you already. I'll probably use a bit of this, and some photos from the Health Roadshow you did last month. People having their blood pressure and cholesterol checked, exercise bikes, lung-testing machines, no-smoking displays, free condoms – that's all.

JAMES: Good. Then I'll tell you what I think . . .

Health promotion is an awful mess. Most of the time I ignore the fact, and get on with whatever I have to do. But sometimes, whenever it rises to the surface of my mind, or whenever I witness my staff in such obvious conflict about what they are supposed to be doing at work, I have to face it: I'm a middle manager in a very confused profession.

(*He sips his drink*) When I do face up to the truth and sit down to try to sort the muddle out, I get so far and then it all becomes a mess again. Have you ever gone to night school, or used tapes, to learn a foreign language? (*Diane smiles ruefully*) Well, to me, trying to understand the point of health promotion is rather like beginning French or Spanish from scratch. You make progress with the basics, and you feel good about that. Then you switch on the radio, or foolishly decide to listen to the final lesson on your tape, and you hear native speakers in natural conversation. Pretty soon you learn not to do it any more. Why torture yourself unnecessarily? And then you think – why bother with the basics either? How often will I really need Spanish after all? You find yourself studying less and less, thinking about it less, and eventually you give up learning the language altogether. I can't sort it out so I switch off . . . but I don't suppose this is making any sense.

DIANE: No, no it is. I've read some of those papers, remember? And I'm beginning to become intrigued by the same problem as you – I want to work out what health promotion is all about . . . oh, by the way I don't mean to be rude and I do want to listen but I only have time for one more drink, OK? I've got a story to write up this evening, and it won't wait.

JAMES: Fair enough. (*To the barman*) Same again, please.

If it's alright with you I'll go through my usual train of thought – I can get the 'basics', up to about lesson three. When I get lost I'll ask you if you can see any way forward that I can't. It won't take long to get there, I'm sorry to say. The only place I can start is from the mess we're in at the moment. You've already seen some of that.

The way I see it there are three main features to the mess. These are the fact that health promoters disagree about what they ought to be doing, the lack of any half-decent definition of health promotion and health education, and the welter of terminology (a lot of which I reckon is virtually meaningless) used to cover up the mess – the rhetoric supposed to turn a pig's ear into a silk purse. Because health promotion is such a mess I can't even hold these three features above it, in my mind's eye, for very long. When I think about them they tangle around themselves, and then fall back into the muddle.

DIANE: A bit like IR and ER verbs in French?

JAMES: Yes. Quite a lot like that come to think of it. It just seems to be a never-ending circle, with no reason to it. Health promoters disagree about goals and methods because health promotion is not properly defined. Because health promotion is not properly defined health promoters are bound to disagree. Health promoters can be found in all sorts of organisations, they come from different social backgrounds, they have different political values, and they have received different sorts and standards of education, and so on. So if they don't have a useful definition they can hardly do anything other than fall back on their pre-existing biases and lay philosophies of life, and so they will inevitably fall out with each other. And yet if there is a health promotion *movement* or *profession* to which everyone belongs – and all the health promotion gurus say there is – then what I take to be fundamental disagreements simply cannot be fundamental. I must be wrong. They must only appear to be disagreements. It must be possible to reconcile them somehow or else there couldn't be a movement or a profession, could there?

But as far as I can see at the moment, all the disagreements are not resolved because they are not resolvable. They're just pushed aside either by sweeping generalities – health promotion is 'about empowerment', or all health promoters are 'working towards' 'Health for All' – or by baffling pseudo-technical terms like 'models', 'intermediate indicators', 'health status' and the like. And, as these terms distract attention from the fundamental disagreements, at the same time they contribute further confusions of their own. Health promoters *also* disagree about the meaning of 'empowerment', or the accuracy or relevance of the 'indicators', and so it goes on. It just gets worse – for me anyway. As time goes by more terms crop up, new issues emerge, fresh models are advocated – yet the basic differences, like those you saw within my team, are left behind and (conveniently?) forgotten. So they remain permanently unresolved. In fact it can even seem like they *have* been resolved because no one is particularly bothered about them any more – there are all the new 'how should we do this project?' and 'what method should we use to do that?' type of problem to worry about. (*He pauses to drink*)

DIANE: But surely there are health promotion text books which define health promotion?

JAMES: You'd think so, wouldn't you? But they mostly only raise the issue at the outset. Or far worse (*he grimaces, and he too mimes quotation marks in the air*) they explore the issues around the concept. Invariably there's some sub-heading in the first chapter of any book for students of health promotion which asks 'what is health promotion?' or something to that effect. Then, without bothering even to attempt a decent answer, the question is skipped. But I don't think you can skip this question because if you leave it it just hangs there and clouds everything else.

DIANE: How?

JAMES: For example, to say that 'health promotion is any planned measure which promotes health' isn't exactly illuminating is it?

DIANE: Is that an official definition?

JAMES: It's in most of the popular health promotion text books, and is endorsed by the World Health Organization.

DIANE: But how does a definition like that give any guidance? How is a health promoter to know *what* strategy to plan? Presumably there are all sorts of ways to promote health. How is she to choose?

JAMES: Ah well she often doesn't have much of a choice in fact. She certainly doesn't have an entirely free choice. I can at least see this part of the muddle clearly. The health promoter's choice is shaped, in part at least, by the history of health promotion. And when you begin to understand the history you begin to see how the mess has evolved.

As far as I can make out the idea of health education (a forerunner of health promotion) grew out of the belief that the incidence of disease could be reduced through teaching people – and especially school children – better hygiene and healthy living habits: cleaning teeth properly, bathing regularly, eating fresh greens and so on. Clearly the main reason for this health education was to prevent avoidable medical complaints. But over time (and especially during the last thirty years or so) the notion of health education has expanded to mean something *more than* the prevention of medical ills. For many people engaged in health education – Ann for instance – the promotion of *autonomy*, not disease prevention, is now their main purpose. They do still teach preventive measures but they consider this work part of a broader task to supply the *means* to a healthy or autonomous life, not only an end in itself. As a result – since they aim to 'empower' people, to offer better means of living – they add, to the more traditional forms of health education, learning programmes designed to raise self-esteem, increase assertiveness, improve 'decision-making skills' and so on.

DIANE: From personal hygiene to personal autonomy in thirty years. That's quite a switch.

JAMES: You're absolutely right. It *is* quite a switch, although I think a lot depends on how you look at it. To an educator it seems very natural to mix information-giving and instructing – the preventive bits – with the provision of the skills to sift through the information and instructions – the autonomy creating bits. This is simply what good teachers do. They impart what facts they can and at the same time they say to the pupils – here's how to be constructively critical of what you hear and read, here's how to think about this information for yourselves. To a medical person, on the other hand, this combination does not seem at all natural.

Say, for instance, a surgeon has seen the damage cigarettes have done to scores of his patients. He knows that smoking damages the body, and can cause appalling death – have you ever seen anyone suffocate over a period of months? (*Diane shakes her head slowly*) For such a surgeon it is very straightforward. It is a fact that smoking causes disease and distress, and disease and distress are bad (this is a fact too). Clearly, therefore, smoking is bad. And this is not something it is appropriate for a person to make up his mind about. There is nothing to decide. Facts are facts and from the doctor's perspective if they were widely appreciated in their proper tragic detail people would not smoke.

I'm sure this is one source of one of the parts of the muddle – people from different backgrounds tend to perceive health promotion very differently and – generally speaking – its history continues to show a growing divide between two main groups, the doctors and the teachers.

If there had been no further developments then I think we would have sorted the mess out by now. There would have been two sorts of health education, looking increasingly different from one another, and sooner or later one would have changed its name. Probably the original type – the hygiene version – would have become 'disease prevention studies' or 'disease protection', though admittedly this is a lot less appealing title than 'health education'.

Unfortunately, however, there is more to the confusion than this. Just as the educators became frustrated with the hygiene movement so there has been a growing dissatisfaction with health education itself. Many, like Carol, have come to feel that health education is only tinkering, and only tinkering with a secondary problem at that. If the main causes of ill-health are environmental, or work-related, or brought about by powerful business interests which are forcing people into unhealthy behaviours, then this is where efforts to improve health should be directed. Health education – teaching individuals healthy lifestyles – has come to be thought of as a poor relation to health promotion, which is said to include action to change *society* not just individuals' thinking and behaviours. In fact many health promoters disparage health education these days. Try calling Carol a health educator and see what happens!

DIANE: I can imagine. Look, I think I'm beginning to get a bit dizzy with this myself. Perhaps I will have just one more drink. Will you? (*To the barman*) Same again for me, and another for him thanks. So the health educator can be a modern hygienist *or* an autonomy creator...

JAMES: Or both...

DIANE: But the health promoter is only a modern hygienist.

JAMES: It's really interesting you should say that. Tell me why you think so.

DIANE: Because you said that health promoters see the social environment as causing ill-health, and I took this to mean that the reason health promoters are opposed to – say – industrial pollution is because this pollution makes people sick – and, like your surgeon said, this is obviously bad. The health promoter *doesn't* provide skills for the individual like the health educator. Therefore the health promoter is a modern hygienist – clean rivers, clean lungs, good nutrition etc.... through influencing broader policy-making not through empowering the individual.

JAMES: Fascinating. That's the way I see it too, but it isn't how most health promoters see it. For one thing they say that health promotion *incorporates* health education, and for another that creating a healthier environment will mean that people will have greater autonomy.

DIANE: But if Carol shuts down Gordon's gin factory, and the Rolling Rock Brewing Company, and all the other alcohol producers, then we couldn't choose to do what we're doing now. So how does that empower us?

JAMES: This is where I begin to hear the *advanced* foreign language. Perhaps you see? It seems to me that with questions like that we're getting right into ethics. Stopping people doing something in what *you* define as their best interests, when by their actions they obviously disagree with you, seems to me to require a strong moral justification. But we don't hear much at all about ethics in health promotion – apart from transparent attempts to convince ourselves that we are a profession by printing a 'Code of Ethics', that is. But ethics aside, just the down-to-earth stuff gets worse. There has been one further stage of historical development. This is known as 'Health For All', or the 'Health For All' movement.

DIANE: I've heard of that. But wasn't it 'Health For All 2000'?

JAMES: It used to be in the early '80s, but reference to '2000' or 'by the year 2000' has virtually disappeared now. It was never going to happen. Most of the targets the HFA lot set came to look more and more unrealistic the closer we got to the millennium, and nobody wants to look foolish if they can help it – so they changed the logo and Health for All 2000 simply faded away . . . I'm rather cynical about HFA actually, and one of the reasons is that they use such slippery slogans – one minute it's 'the right to health', the next 'prere-quisites for health' (one of which is global peace would you believe), the next 'equity', the next it's 'well-being', or 'quality of life', or 'belonging', or 'becoming' – the list goes on. But none of these terms and principles ever seem to be properly defined either.

DIANE: I think I've asked this question before, but in this case how does the HFA crowd decide what to do?

JAMES: That's yet another huge question – you see how quickly we slip into the tougher language sections? It seems to me that in Health For All there are all the earlier difficulties and inconsistencies, plus a whole lot of new ones brought on by all the talk of 'equity' and 'social justice' and the like. In fact the more principles the HFA movement claims to uphold the messier it gets.

How do *I* decide what to do? As a practical health promoter I do what I can. I mix 'n match as I said to you last week, though I confess that I don't always know *why* I choose one approach or target rather than another. I try to educate, I try to prevent disease, I go along with the campaigns and projects in the hope that they'll do some good, but I don't really see how it all fits together. I can't make sense of 'health promotion' overall, and this really does not satisfy me. I feel anxious about it, and sometimes I feel I'm rather a fraud. Perhaps I'm being too precious. Perhaps I'm not cut out for the job. Perhaps I'm just missing the point somewhere along the line. But I suppose what bothers me most of all is that many of my colleagues in the profession don't seem to share my anxiety. They are oblivious to the mess that I see, yet I know full well that they can't understand a word of the advanced language course either. They're all for 'Health For All' and that's all that matters.

DIANE: Four legs good, two legs bad.

JAMES: Pardon?

DIANE: It's a slogan the animals chanted in *Animal Farm*, whenever a contradiction between theory and reality threatened.

JAMES: Oh yes, I remember. Very good...and not far wrong about some of them I think...(*Seeing her empty glass*) But you'd better be going now, I've kept you far too long already...Thanks for listening, honestly. If you have any thoughts about all this later on...well, do let me know.

DIANE: I will. But if what you say is true then I'm not sure that you will ever be able to make sense of it – though isn't this just the way of the world James? It all seems crazy when you stop to think about it, which is why most people don't bother, and get on and live lives which make sense for them – and sod the rest.

JAMES: I know. I do do that in my life in general, but I feel it ought to be different at work, in my professional life. I need to be able to see the wood for the trees, to work out the basic set of reasons for my work, to be able to say *why* some of the terminology is empty – and why some of it is important. When I mix 'n match, when I side with Carol instead of John, or John instead of Martin, I need to know how to justify what I'm doing – I can always justify it *ad hoc* with one practical reason or another – but I need to know where I stand fundamentally as a health promoter. And if I can't find this rock then I think maybe I'd better give it up, don't you?

DIANE: No, actually, I don't...But thanks for the drink. I must be going now. If we don't meet again I promise I'll send you my article, though don't expect any answers will you?!

SCENE TWO

A few days later Diane 'phones James at work.

JAMES: Hello, James Campion.

DIANE: Hello James, Diane Grant here.

JAMES: Diane. Good to hear from you. How are you? How's the article coming on?

DIANE: I'm fine thanks. And the article's shaping up, though I don't think my editor will think so when he sees it. Anyway, I have an unusual favour to ask of you.

JAMES: Ask away.

DIANE: I'm really getting interested in this health promotion stuff, you know. At first it was just a throwaway story for the *Chronicle*, but now I've done some reading, and thought about it some more, I think there's something important here and I want to get to the bottom of it...(*She takes a breath*) So I've been thinking, could you arrange for me to be a health promoter for a month?

JAMES: That is unusual. I suppose it *could* be arranged...oh I don't see why not, in principle...there'd have to be rules, you wouldn't actually be allowed to do very much, and

I'd need to discuss it with colleagues of course. And what about your other reporting duties?

DIANE: I could manage and, well, to be honest I'd be looking to place this story else-where. One of the Sunday magazines, or the *Examiner* ... something like that. I don't intend to stay in Willesville forever. I might even get a book out of it.

JAMES: I see. If you did write an extensive piece I'd want to see it first, and I'd want you to change anything that might be damaging to us.

DIANE: I don't normally do that but, in the circumstances, I'll gladly let you vet anything. In any case what I'm thinking of, at the moment, is a very long way from an exposé of incompetence, corruption and the like. I studied Social Sciences and Humanities at Univer-sity and I know enough to see that there are some important social issues here which I'd like to tease out. I would have thought this would already have been done but, apart from a handful of interesting journal pieces, I can't find anything – and I know how to look. There's a gap here (*she laughs*), maybe even a gap in a market somewhere. I'd like to get below the surface crust of health promotion. You know, dig below all these 'messages' to 'eat less fat', 'wear a condom', 'stop smoking', 'drink moderately', and get to what is really going on, because what is really going on seems to me to be ultimately *ideological*. Do you know what I mean?

JAMES: I think so. I *feel* that health promotion is ideological, that it is to do with much more than preventing diseases, that it is to do with *shaping whole lives* in some way but – as we discussed – I can't put my finger on precisely how these things connect. Have you got it any clearer now?

DIANE: A bit, I think, but I want to check it out in practice. I want to see if what I do as a 'health promoter' really is inspired by social values, or if I'm reading too much in. I don't want to fall flat on my face.

JAMES: OK. I'll do my best to arrange it. But tell me what you are 'reading in' at the moment.

DIANE: Well ... not very much actually, but it's a start. I came to you to find out what health promoters do, and I stupidly expected that you'd all be trying to change my behav-iours, to stop me drinking, to get me to exercise, to give me diet sheets and so on. I found, as you know, that some of you wanted to do this but that some wanted to do other things which they consider to be more important (like trying to make me more politically aware), and that others went so far as to disagree about the behaviour change stuff entirely. What was going on? I wanted to know.

I discussed this with you and it turned out that you – one of the bosses – wanted to know too. You are clearly an intelligent person so I assumed that it was not just that *you* couldn't work this out but that the matter itself is confusing – and my reading and other inquiries have more than confirmed this. Then it struck me that health promotion students, and health promotion workers in the field, if they are at all thoughtful, must also have difficul-ties in grasping the rationale for their work (unless they are totally single-minded – evan-gelists of some kind). But surely, I thought, there must *be* a rationale somewhere. Then it occurred to me – why *a* rationale and not *several* rationales? And if so what are these rationales, how do they affect practice, and how are health promoters to decide between them?

Then there's the matter of *process* and *evidence*. How does health promotion work? Does it work as its advocates think it does? I found quite a lot of writing about this. In fact most books and papers supposedly on health promotion theory are actually not about basic theory at all but about how best to do it – about process – about which method or model to use if you want to change lifestyles, develop communities etc. But there's very much less about what a *desirable* lifestyle or community is, and less still on how to justify any such claim.

I also found a fair bit of discussion about how difficult it is to evaluate health promotion, and various papers and publicity material which says virtually everything on a continuum from health promotion is highly cost-effective to health promotion is practically useless. Some say it has dramatically reduced smoking and prevented a hetero HIV epidemic, others think it a complete waste of time and money. I hope to find out more about this for myself as I work as a health promoter but the way I see it, to answer the question 'does health promotion work?', you must first have decided what you mean by success and to do this must have some sort of social theory.

So I feel I've made some progress. But then it begins to get confusing – your foreign language again.

JAMES: So, apart from seeing what health promotion is like at first hand, how are you going to take things further?

DIANE: Well, I obviously can't do it by myself. As my day job permits I'll do more library research, and I'm going to take some professional advice too.

JAMES: In what way?

DIANE: I know a philosopher from a few years back. He was a promising postgrad. at the time. He went on to take a special interest in the philosophy of health. I've faxed him, explained my interest and how far I've got – i.e. virtually nowhere! – and asked him what he thinks. Anyway, he e-mailed back and I'm seeing him tomorrow. Apparently he's working on health promotion himself at the moment, believe it or not. He says that talking with me will probably help him too – so we're all set.

JAMES: You're certainly taking this seriously Diane. Let me know how you get on, and I'll be in touch as soon as I've fixed you up at this end.

Glad to be Vague

Let's try to get a few things clear. First and foremost you must appreciate that health promotion is a magpie profession. Over the years its theorists and practitioners have accumulated countless trinkets from other disciplines, and now possess a stockpile of adopted techniques, models and goals. A glance at the health promotion literature will show that health promoters use booklets (derived mainly from work in *medicine* and *education*) to educate patients in hospitals, surveys of people's beliefs about health, illness, well-being and quality of life (collected from *sociology*, *psychology* and *epidemiology*), miscellaneous morbidity and mortality figures (from *epidemiology* and *statistics*), behavioural change techniques (from *psychology*), legislative change (from *law* and *politics*), lobbying over the health effects of environmental pollutants (from *pressure group politics*), lectures and group work in schools (from *education*), 'look after yourself' exercise and nutrition programmes (from *physical education*), advertising campaigns (from *psychology*, *politics* and *propaganda*), opportunistic fitness testing (from *medicine*), joint programmes with food manufacturers to offer approved products and educational materials in supermarkets (from *marketing*), life skills teaching (from *education* and *psychology*), health belief models, health action models, theories of reasoned action (all from *sociology* and *psychology*) and a great deal more besides.

But why is health promotion like this? Why do health promoters behave like magpies? Why is health promotion so miscellaneous?

A LITTLE ANTHROPOLOGY

Viewed from a purely theoretical perspective the obvious answer to these questions is this: health promoters operate eclectically because health promotion does not possess a unifying rationale. However, if anthropological considerations are included, the questions may be answered in other ways.

Vagueness of purpose can bear strategic advantage. By not specifying the precise nature of health promotion the so-called health promotion movement[6] has been able to welcome – and to welcome quickly – a wide variety of interested and influential parties. As it has done so health promotion has rapidly gained status, inter-disciplinary credibility, and access to very considerable state and private funding.[7]

Health Promotion, Second Edition: David Seedhouse
© 2004 John Wiley & Sons, Ltd: ISBNs 0 470 84732 8 (HB); 0 470 84733 6 (PB)

If no one of influence in the 'movement' can see any practical merit in posing tough theoretical questions, why ask them?

> Everyone involved...wants to get something from health promotion and wants to contribute something, and all bring their own viewpoints to bear on it. Is it any wonder that the people engaged in this developmental venture have different opinions, and become uneasy when definitions seem to prescribe what should happen...?[8]

So long as the meaning of health promotion is allowed to remain fuzzy health promotion will continue to suggest many different things to many different people and, politically, this is a singular strength. Fuzziness can foster comradeship and can allow people to identify with an apparently consolidating, external idea (I am a health promoter – I belong to the health promotion movement – I am for health). Lack of precision about ends can also help make divergent practices seem harmonious.

The seemingly perpetual theoretical fog which envelopes the 'movement' reinforces the belief that health promotion is essentially a practical task. Where everything seems so philosophically murky it is very tempting to conclude that health promoters might just as well get on and do it. Some authors are so keen to 'go for it' that they decry theoretical analysis altogether:

> The question 'what is health and thereby health promotion?' continues to de-energise all those involved in this activity (sic). Debates about the meaning of health have led to more conflict and inaction than they have solved (sic). To clear a way through this morass, let us state quite clearly that health promotion is an activity whose basis resides in gaining change, change to promote health. The methods of change are its subject. It draws on the skills and practice of change that are well-established in politics, economics, the media, therapy, education, advocacy, legislation etc.

> The object of health promotion is the promotion of health. To shift gear and move away from this inward looking tautology we must take a pragmatic and commonsense approach to the meaning of health, an approach which asserts that health is gained and lost in the real world in almost every action we indulge in: in our work, at our leisure, with our family and friends. It is easy to recognise that all of these contribute to our health, to our being able to live socially and economically fulfilling lives.[9]

The appeal of such a down-to-earth approach is easy to see. Ashton and Seymour's apparent iconoclasm must feel like a blast of fresh air to practitioners fed up with rambling articles and debates about the meaning of it all. To paraphrase the duo:

> Everybody *knows* what health promotion is. It's simply commonsense. People should be as healthy as possible. We should all be able to live socially and economically fulfilling lives. Further talk is unnecessary. It just gets in the way of the action, which is all that counts in the end.

THE PROBLEM WITH ANTI-THEORY

As attractive as this straight talking may appear, it fails to stand up to intelligent scrutiny. Where does the purely pragmatic health promoter begin to promote health? How can she possibly sort out what to do first? Maybe she will decide to begin with the most urgent health problems. But unless she has some theoretical grasp of what a 'health problem' is, and unless she has some philosophically based system of ranking such problems as 'more urgent' and 'less urgent' she will – as a matter of fact – be unable to identify which problems to work on. Alternatively she might simply resolve to tackle whichever problem comes along first. Strictly speaking the **anti-theorist** may as well take this line. If the meaning of health promotion is of no importance then any starting point must be as good as any other. But of course unadulterated pragmatism can result only in unadulterated arbitrariness: either that or the down-to-earth health promoter must concede some theoretical preference after all.

ANYTHING IS POSSIBLE

Imagine that the health promoter takes a lucky dip and decides to begin by promoting health through legislation. Assume too that she has influence and a chance of successfully lobbying for a change in the law. An *inescapable* question then arises: which law reform will be most health promoting? To achieve most effect should she seek increased taxation on alcoholic drinks? Should she try to legalise cannabis (some research shows this might have health-enhancing effects)? Perhaps she should try to effect a bye-law that inner-city supermarkets should be permitted to stock only wholemeal breads (to ensure healthy eating habits in the least well-off citizens). Or perhaps she should campaign for a law to mandate attendance, for all people of 12 and over, on a health education course at least once every three years? Perhaps unemployment should be outlawed. Perhaps it should be made compulsory that everyone pursue socially and economically fulfilling work. Maybe National Military Service should be reintroduced for 18–20 year olds. Or perhaps she should work to have first-time offender drunk-drivers banned from driving for life.

In the absence of a substantial account of the meaning of health promotion each of these proposals *could* be said to be health promoting because each might conceivably bring about somebody's idea of better health. Equally, each of the proposals could be said *not* to be health promoting because each might be thought, by someone with different prejudices, to lead to less health. The **anti-theorists** assume that the habitual harvesting of ideas and techniques developed elsewhere automatically provides a rationale for their 'discipline'. But haphazard acquisitiveness can no more furnish a theoretical basis for coherent practice than a magpie can be a discriminating collector of fine art. To claim that health promotion is nothing more than 'commonsense' and 'well-established' practice is either hugely naïve or – if you happen to be in a position where you can implement your own preferences – is an effective means of deflecting dissent in order to pursue activities which may seem like commonsense to you – but with which not everyone agrees.

THE PROBLEM WITH INADEQUATE THEORY

Most health promotion theorists are less extreme than the **anti-theorists** and at least try to offer rudimentary accounts of health promotion's content. Typically a theorist will raise the question 'what is health promotion?', point out that it is controversial, and put forward a general answer (hardly ever an original one, and often merely a statement taken uncritically from World Health Organisation (WHO) literature). After this he will move quickly on to explain what must actually be *done* to bring more health into being and – like the **anti-theorist** – will concentrate on describing those methods *he* considers best suited to the practical challenge.

Here is one example of the first part of the above process:

> We accept the definition in the Ottawa Charter (1986) of health promotion as 'the process of enabling people to increase control over, and to improve, their health'. We believe this definition gives added scope and purpose to health promotion...[8]

It certainly does, and this is precisely the problem. Since the statement is circular and non-specific it adds *infinite* scope and purpose: it can mean anything anyone wants it to. This sort of 'definition' justifies nothing, yet offers an unconditional welcome to any target, any method and anybody.

In similar fashion, Keith Tones and Sylvia Tilford decline to offer a meaningful definition of health: '...detailed discussion of the nature of health has been considered outside the scope of this book'[10] yet nevertheless feel able to claim that:

> (a) semantically...more logical course [[]is to use[]] the term health promotion to refer to any measure designed to promote health. In such a guise, health education will form an integral part of health promotion. The World Health Organization adopts this perspective, viewing health promotion as a '...unifying concept for those who recognize the need for change in the ways and conditions of living, in order to promote health'...Health promotion in this sense is therefore concerned with all the factors which influence health...
>
> For present purposes, health is viewed as both a positive state of wellbeing and as absence of disease. Four major influences affect health status: (i) the health and medical services, (ii) genetic endowment, (iii) individual behaviours and (iv) the socio-economic and physical environment.[11]

But although this line of argument is virtually *de rigueur* amongst leading health promotion theorists, it is patently not up to scratch. These are its bones:

   i. we refuse to, or are unable to, discuss the nature of health
  ii. health promotion is that set of measures which promote health
 iii. health promotion has to do with all factors which influence health

(Note that so far nothing of any substance whatever has been said. Unless we are first told what 'health' is we cannot possibly know what the authors are trying to communicate.)

  iv. although we cannot even begin to offer a serious definition of the goal of health promotion (i.e. health), because the Lalonde Report, the Ottawa Charter and the WHO tell us to, we have decided to think of health both as 'a positive state of well-being' and as 'the absence of disease'
   v. even though neither we nor any other health promotion authority defines 'a positive state of well-being' we are sure that not only do the 'four major influences' affect people's 'disease status', but these (more than any other influence we might have listed) affect 'well-being' too.

Such reasoning tells the reader very little, if anything, about the nature of health promotion. Which individual behaviours affect health, for instance? All of them or only some of them? If all of them, then health promotion is surely an impossible task – how can any profession hope to work on all individual behaviours? If only some of them, how does Tones' account help the health promoter work out which they are? If we can agree on the nature of disease (which is by no means a straightforward matter itself[7]) and if we can agree that certain behaviours are likely to cause certain diseases (also a scientifically and ethically controversial issue[7]) then we may just be able to decide on a defensible strategy to promote 'health as absence of disease'. But how can we decide on a defensible strategy to promote 'positive well-being'? Which are the key individual behaviours in this case? How do we know unless we know what well-being is? And worse, unless we know what well-being is how can we be sure that by trying to change those individual behaviours which we believe cause disease, we will not at the same time *reduce* well-being? Without detailed explanation of health promotion's goals and of what is meant by each of the 'four major influences' we really cannot tell what best to do in the name of health promotion – it just *looks* like we can, until we start to think about it.

Of course, health promotion theorists offer numerous examples of what they take to be 'good practice'. But these examples by themselves do not provide the missing theory. They can appear to do so to workers so busy they do not have the apparent luxury of time to think, but without philosophical justification any coherence is bound to be either coincidental or illusory.

THE ILLUSION OF SHARED MEANING

In the absence of properly thought out definitions of 'health' and 'health promotion' it is inevitable that consensus-seeking health promotion theorists will concur that health promotion is basically about promoting health (what else could they say?). But unless health promoters explicitly agree about why they are doing what they are doing, it is likely that any accord they may *feel* will be illusory. And this is not a trivial matter. *The illusion of shared meaning* can have damaging consequences for both giver and receiver of health promotion.

By way of initial illustration of health promotion's many illusions, consider two cases where health promoters' feeling of shared meaning is false:

CASE ONE

Bill Murphy and Clarissa Rieley have been working together as health promoters for over five years. They both think health promotion is extremely important and seriously under-resourced. Bill and Clarissa have never discussed in depth what they mean by health promotion – each naturally assumes the other has the same basic understanding of its targets, even though they may sometimes disagree about which methods to use. However, whenever Bill thinks about the task of health promotion the image that remains longest in his mind is that of a doctor dispensing advice to a patient in a surgery. Clarissa, on the other hand, hardly ever thinks of clinicians in relation to health promotion. The dominant picture in Clarissa's 'mind's eye' is of a youth leader encouraging school children to try to formulate provisional life plans and goals.

This may seem only a subtle discrepancy, but it is certainly a difference that Bill and Clarissa would benefit from discussing in detail. The different images that spring to each health promoter's mind indicate that they do not share the same fundamental view of health promotion. Bill's unreflective belief is that health promotion is part of a movement which has medicine as its inspiration, but Clarissa sees education and behaviour change at its heart. Were it ever to fall to the two of them to decide where best to allocate scarce funds their illusions would be shattered.

CASE TWO

Ann Pryor and John Barnes, whom we met earlier at the Willesville Unit, *are* aware that they have conflicting ideas – Ann thinks health promotion means enabling people to make their own health decisions, and supporting them in those decisions even in those cases where she does not agree with their choices. John, on the other hand, thinks there is an objectively correct set of decisions which people are duty-bound to make if they are to improve their health. Yet despite this quite basic difference of view Ann and John work well together, and are both happy to think of themselves, and each other, as health promoters.

This second is the more serious case of the *illusion of shared meaning*. Bill and Clarissa do not realise that they have different ideas, but Ann and John *know* both that their views conflict *and* that they often lead to advocacy of conflicting policies, yet nevertheless still believe they are pursuing the same general end. In this second case the *illusion* would quickly dissipate if they had the tools to discuss their purposes in philosophical depth. But since they do not John and Ann can agree to differ over this particular conflict of view and rest assured that they agree about everything else in their work. But it is only if they are theoretically blind that they can do this. Their conflict is so central that it must affect everything they do in the name of health promotion. Undoubtedly Ann and John disagree about much more than they are prepared to recognise.

Hollow Words –
And How To Reveal Them

SECTION ONE

The *illusion of shared meaning* can persist only if health promoters are happy to leave their most important words ill-defined. Once it becomes the norm to insist on clarity, once the question 'but what precisely do you mean?' becomes thought of as a responsible inquiry rather than a mischievous irritation, then health promotion will begin to come of age.

But health promotion has a long way to go yet. Consider the 1986 Ottawa Charter 'definition', so frequently accepted by health promotion writers. Despite its popularity, a dispassionate reading shows that it asserts only the *banality* that health promotion is 'the process of enabling people to increase control over, and to improve, their health'. It is disturbingly easy to demonstrate – by means of a simple substitution technique – that this famous phrase is either so vague it could mean almost anything, or is simply meaningless.

Look what happens when alternative words are substituted for 'health' in the Ottawa mantra:

Substitution Type One   'Life promotion is the process of enabling people to increase control over, and to improve, their lives'

Substitution Type Two   'Crabble promotion is the process of enabling people to increase control over, and to improve, their crabble'

Substitution Type Three   'Scrabble-playing promotion is the process of enabling people to increase control over, and to improve, their Scrabble-playing'

TYPE ONE: STATEMENTS OF LIMITLESS MEANING

Reflect on the first change to the keyword in the Ottawa 'definition':

Health Promotion, Second Edition: David Seedhouse
© 2004 John Wiley & Sons, Ltd: ISBNs 0 470 84732 8 (HB); 0 470 84733 6 (PB)

> Life promotion is the process of enabling people to increase control over, and to improve, their lives

Without a more specific indication of what is meant by 'life promotion' the expression might mean anything, however strange. For example, if a 'life promotion' specialist were to be of the view that regularly eating raspberry jam enables people 'to increase control over and improve their lives' then the advocacy of daily raspberry jam consumption would – in the absence of any compelling argument why not – qualify as a legitimate 'life promotion' activity. So would teaching better lawn-mowing techniques, or enabling someone to improve her soccer skills. So long as meaning is left vague teaching 'advanced blackmail' to an embezzler, or demonstrating strict disciplinary techniques to parents who wish to keep their children subservient could be life promoting. The more nebulously a goal is stated the more legitimate means there will be to achieve it, and in the case of 'Ottawa life promotion' the goal is so loosely characterised as to permit unlimited practical possibilities.

Although the above examples may seem bizarre, they are clearly allowed by the above statement. It is very important to appreciate this because the substitution of 'life' for 'health' leaves the **type** of statement unchanged: whether the word 'health' or the word 'life' is used the statement has limitless meaning. 'Life promotion' can mean anything that 'promotes life' and 'health promotion' can mean anything that 'promotes health'. And in the absence of more detailed, theoretically grounded definitions, the nature of life and the nature of health remain open to the very widest interpretation. Of course, the 'life promotion' substitution *seems* to make some sense. Just as most people have an understanding of 'health' so the expression 'life promotion' is bound to have one meaning or another for most of us. We know that the word 'life' is important – and therefore do not tend to worry too much about specifics, assuming that most people see it the same way. But this is merely a product of the *illusion of shared meaning*. Only when we get down to detail can we find out whether we truly agree or not: do you think parents should raise subservient children? Do you think people should be compelled to consume uncontrolled doses of fluoridated tap water in the interest of their health? Do you believe public money should be invested in sports education for talented kids? Do you think parents should be forcefully persuaded to have their infants immunised? How important is raspberry jam to you?

TYPE TWO: MEANINGLESS STATEMENTS

The comforting *illusion of shared meaning* can be seen even more clearly when **Type Two** statements are considered. To use the **Type Two** example given earlier:

> Crabble promotion is the process of enabling people to increase control over, and to improve, their crabble

Every competent adult can offer an interpretation of 'life promotion', but this is not so with 'crabble promotion'. As it stands, without further explanation, the statement is meaningless. If we do not know what 'crabble' is, 'crabble promotion' is an empty expression. Perhaps a 'crabble' is a muscle in the human body. If this were so then the statement *would* make sense. But if a 'crabble' *is* a muscle then any potential 'crabble promoter' obviously needs to have this explained to her. Once the specifics have been clarified she might be able to do something to improve people's crabbles: she would have a target at which to aim and might be able to devise appropriate methods to achieve it.

It *may* be that the actual Ottawa statement is of **Type Two**, since it does not specify the meaning of 'health', and for all some of its readers know 'health' may indeed be a meaningless word. However, the Ottawa declaration is surely intended to refer to something identifiable, something meaningful – some thing, property, or state of being that a person might 'increase control over'. But in this case, if the authors of the Ottawa statement regard health as definite and bounded, then they really ought not to have kept this to themselves. If they wished to communicate with working health promoters they should have spelt out their thoughts, and explained where boundaries are to be drawn. In other words, if health promotion's leaders wish to converse fully and openly with practitioners they must do more than offer further vacuities about 'enabling', 'empowering' and the 'health field':[12] they must use **Type Three** statements instead.

TYPE THREE: STATEMENTS OF LIMITED MEANING

Unlike **Types One** and **Two**, statements of **Type Three** refer to something definite. Take the previous example of this **Type**:

> Scrabble-playing promotion is the process of enabling people to increase control over, and to improve, their Scrabble-playing

So long as he knows what Scrabble-playing is, the would-be Scrabble promoter has a clear and simple boundary within which to devise and test out strategies to improve it. Any Scrabble promoter worth his salt will know the difference between good and bad Scrabble-playing, and ought to be able to work out all manner of ways to promote the best tactics (Look After Your Scrabble-Playing classes; self-help Scrabble groups; Scrabblewise events; 38 Targets for Better Scrabble – all this and more, no doubt).

Unfortunately **Type Three** clarity about the purpose of health promotion is not offered by the Ottawa definition, nor does it occur anywhere else in the Ottawa Charter or in any other officially sponsored declaration. The WHO does make use of **Type Three** statements – notably in its 38 targets for health.[13] However, not all these targets are **Type Three** (see Exercise Six, Targets 2 and 24 for two examples of **Type One** targets). And where they are of **Type Three** (see Exercise Six, Target 5 for instance) they are offered as if they are self-explanatory. But **Type Three** statements cannot justify themselves. Sustained philosophical analysis – and ultimately a good theory of health – is required to do this.

EMPTY DEFINITIONS © WHO

A defender of the Ottawa Charter might object that the definition of health promotion as 'the process of enabling people to increase control over, and to improve, their health' is **Type Three** rather than **Type One** when it is read along with other official definitions. That is, it might be argued that the definition does make sense so long as the WHO's definition of health is itself understood. However, examination of the WHO's statements about health reveals further, very substantial conceptual difficulties. Things get worse, if anything.

As usual, the most debilitating problem is ambiguity. The WHO seems to want to have as broad a definition of health as possible, and seems also not to want to admit to any conceptual errors. This catch-all policy has two main implications. The first is that the organisation now boasts *two* definitions of health, which are either incompatible or incoherent when read together. And this, in turn, creates considerable and persisting confusion amongst the WHO's many sycophants. The following quote illustrates both these problems perfectly:

> As I probably don't need to remind you, the World Health Organization's definition of health, as shown in Figure 5 is 'a state of complete physical, mental and social well-being'. Although it has been criticised by many people, it is still the one which rolls off the tongues of people toiling in the vineyard of health when they are put up against the wall. As you also no doubt know, it was elaborated in 1986 in the Ottawa Charter for Health Promotion as shown in Figure 6.

A state of complete physical, mental and social well-being and not merely the absence of disease and infirmity
WHO Constitution, 1948

Figure 5   Original WHO Definition of Health

To reach a state of complete physical, mental and social well-being, an individual or group must be able to identify and to realize aspirations, to satisfy needs, and to change or cope with the environment. Health is therefore seen as a resource for everyday life, not the objective of living. Health is a positive concept emphasizing social and personal resources, as well as physical capacities.
Ottawa Charter for Health Promotion, 1986

Figure 6   Expanded WHO Definition of Health[14]

The author of this quote, Irving Rootman, is of the view – which the WHO seems not to wish to discourage – that the WHO has built on its 1948 definition to produce an expanded 1986 version. However, if this is what the WHO intended, they now offer a combined definition which just does not make sense. This really ought to be obvious, but since it is not clear to at least one health promotion expert it is worth using the substitution technique to elucidate further.

A Substitution Recipe

Take the 'Original WHO Definition of Health' and substitute 'bliss' for 'complete physical, mental and social well-being and not merely the absence of disease and infirmity' (this is surely not an unreasonable substitution). This gives:

> Health is a state of bliss.

Now carry this substitution into the 'Expanded WHO Definition of Health'. This gives:

> To reach a state of bliss (health) an individual or group must be able to identify and to realize aspirations, to satisfy needs, and to change or cope with the environment. Health (bliss) is therefore seen as a resource for everyday life, not the objective of living. Health (bliss) is a positive concept emphasizing social and personal resources, as well as physical capacities.

Obviously this does not add up. In short it says:

> To reach a state of bliss it is necessary to have bliss as a resource, but bliss is not the objective of living.

And this is nonsense, of course. One of the WHO's definitions of health has to go. Should the first be retained? Surely not, as the substitution of 'perfection' for 'well-being' shows. Read like this:

> Health is a state of complete physical, mental and social perfection and not merely the absence of disease and infirmity

the statement is even more obviously of **Type One** – of *limitless* meaning. What is social perfection? What is mental perfection? What is social well-being? What is mental well-being? Without more detail there is no end to the list of possible descriptions that might be made of these states. The original definition undoubtedly ought to be abandoned, and the WHO would do well to explain this – and the reasons why – in an official publication at the earliest opportunity (it is still not too late).

We are now left with the 1986 version, which is not an expanded definition at all. It is a different one. What does this latest definition actually say? In translation it claims:

1. A state of complete physical, mental and social well-being is possible.
2. Aspirations and needs must be satisfied to reach this state, and the environment must be changed or coped with.
3. (*Surprisingly, given the 1948 version*) health is merely a resource for everyday life, not a resource to achieve complete well-being.
4. Health is a positive concept (*whatever this means*) which is somehow to do with these social, personal and physical resource(s) for everyday life.

Points 1 and 2 are so different from points 3 and 4 that it is advisable to split the 1986 version in two. This gives:

A. To reach a state of complete physical, mental and social well-being, an individual or group must be able to identify and to realize aspirations, to satisfy needs, and to change or cope with the environment.

B. Health is therefore seen as a resource for everyday life, not the objective of living. Health is a positive concept emphasizing social and personal resources, as well as physical capacities.

Point A can now be seen to be utterly trivial. It says nothing more than this:

If individuals or groups are not already in a state of complete well-being, some things will need to change if they are to get there.

This is a **Type Two** statement, and so can be disregarded. This leaves two sentences, given as point B. The first makes a clear – and important – distinction: namely that health is not the objective of living but a resource for living. The second, which ought then to go on to make **Type Three** statements – so spelling out the nature and content of this resource – completely blows the opportunity. Ignoring the phrase 'positive concept emphasizing', which almost certainly means nothing, we are left with the **Type One** statement:

Health is social and personal resources, as well as physical capacities.

An ally of the WHO might argue that health is precisely those resources which realise aspirations, satisfy needs, and change or cope with the environment – in other words, that part A of the 1986 version must be included to make the statement meaningful. But this will not do either. Which needs, for instance, should health (as resources) satisfy? A need for a long life? A need for caffeine? A need for a dangerous life? A need to acquire material wealth? The questions could go on forever, and the WHO's 'definitions' will never be able to answer them because they are badly written and impossibly vague. Despite its claims to be defining health and health promotion for the world the WHO, in its most often quoted official writings, shows itself to be at the head of the **anti-theorist** pack. It suits the WHO to have health mean anything they want it to. But if their statements are to make sense, if health is to be a *useful* guiding idea, it cannot mean *anything*. It must have limited meaning, and this meaning must be fully explained and fully defended. Decent definitions can come only from decent theorising – they do not spring from thin air, nor from political compromise, and are never, ever worked out at feel-good conferences.

EXERCISE ONE

CONCEPTS, VISIONS OR ILLUSIONS?

In a paper entitled 'Concepts and Visions', published by the Department of Community Health, at the University of Liverpool in 1988, John Ashton sketched out five 'principles of health promotion', as follows:

The experience of those active in this field since 1974 has helped to define five principles of health promotion:

- Health promotion actively involves the population in the setting of everyday life rather than focusing on people who are at risk for specific conditions and in contact with medical services;

continues

continued

- Health promotion is directed towards action on the causes of ill-health;
- Health promotion uses many different approaches which combine to improve health; these include education and information, community development and organisation, health advocacy and legislation;
- Health promotion depends particularly on public participation;
- Health professionals – especially those in Primary Health Care – have an important part to play in nurturing health promotion and enabling it to take place.

If possible:

1. Categorise each of these statements into one of the three **Types** of statement.
2. Consider each **Type One** statement carefully, and attempt to convert it into a **Type Three** statement.
3. Briefly indicate any areas of controversy your translation has brought to light.

Teaching notes for: Concepts, Visions or Illusions?

John Ashton's 'principles' are actually descriptions, not principles. Whether or not they are *true* descriptions is arguable, though this could be discovered through empirical investigation if necessary. But this is by the way: the doctor's statements are ideal for this opening exercise simply because they are so vaguely expressed.

As a teacher, you might decide to encourage students to try out some substitutions on these statements, though most are written so idiosyncratically that it is probably better to concentrate on the existing ambiguities. For instance, you might ask students to try to work out what 'Health promotion is *directed toward* action...' is supposed to mean (they may well think it implies that health promotion itself is *not* active). Or you might ask them what meaning they think the phrase 'Health promotion *depends particularly* on public participation' is supposed to convey. Is health promotion bound to fail if the public do not participate? Is it essential that the public participate in the setting of health promotion goals and in choosing the methods to be used? Have students consider which they think the author intends. And then have them discuss whether either of these statements is correct as a description of actual practice.

If this is the first exercise you attempt, and if your students are unused to philosophical analysis, you may find the going tough. Students may not realise what is required of them, and will be unsure how best to proceed. But do not lose heart. Persevere with questioning. Even if the students feel they have dealt with all possible issues, show them they have not. For instance, ask them 'what is public participation?'; ask them to list different ways in which the public might participate in health promotion; ask them 'does health promotion depend upon democracy – and if so, why?', ask them 'what should health promoters do to/for people who do not wish to participate?', and so on.

continues

continued

THE EXERCISE QUESTIONS

1. Because the 'principles' are so general it is likely that students will decide they are *all* of limitless meaning (**Type One**). But if they don't you should try to pull out the meaning(s) students are *adding* without noticing they are doing so. This can be most instructive.

2. The aim here is to have students convert statements of limitless meaning (**Type One**) into expressions of limited meaning (**Type Three**) – and to show, as the students do this, how much more contestable these apparently run-of-the-mill statements have instantly become.

   For example, the 'second principle' might be converted as follows:

   > Health promotion is directed towards action on the causes of emphysema.

   You might then remind students that according to research papers X, Y and Z, one of the main causes of emphysema is cigarette smoking. Ask students, in the light of this evidence, what action they think health promoters should take. Action against smoking might, for example, take very different forms. For example:

   a. campaigning against tobacco companies

   and/or

   b. sabotaging packs of cigarettes so as to get particularly toxic brands withdrawn

   and/or

   c. forming radical medical groups which make it clear that doctors will discriminate in favour of non-smokers

   and/or

   d. stepping up non-smoking education amongst smokers.

   As you work on this exercise you should emphasise the practical importance of *always* aiming to move from **Type One** statements to more definite statements of policy as quickly as possible. You should also point out that by doing this the controversial nature of each claim becomes strikingly clearer. And that as things do become clearer, so open and meaningful debate becomes increasingly possible.

3. Finally, host an open discussion on the underlying disputes about goals and methods the conversions will inevitably have exposed. And in closing be sure to point out that the 'five principles', as they were, are a perfect illustration of the *illusion of shared meaning* in health promotion.

SECTION TWO

THE MODELS MUDDLE

It is not only 'health' and 'health promotion' that health promotion theorists have left up in the air. Despite much huffing and puffing in certain journals, there is little evidence of productive theorising about any of health promotion's key words. All the most important terms – 'community', 'education', 'enabling', 'empowerment', 'well-being', 'quality of life' and 'models' – remain frustratingly vague.

It *is* possible to select and pursue health promotion targets in the presence of ambiguity. Indeed, as we saw earlier, ambiguity tends to make the process of selection and justification less controversial, and also helps health promotion theorists avoid philosophical labour. But if health promotion is finally to become intellectually serious about what it is doing its theorists must confront indeterminacy, not hide behind it. In order to be clear about what success means, and to be able to properly express and fully justify the goals of the health promotion process, adequate definition is an indispensable first step. Partly to illustrate this point more fully, and partly to set the stage for an argument that the shape and content of any health promotion activity depends ultimately on human choosing, health promotion's use of the word 'model' is discussed below.

WHAT IS A MODEL?

Here is an extract from a mainstream paper which attempts an explanation of the meaning of 'models':

> Before we describe how to define the term conceptual model, we should note that the term *model* has many different uses and meanings. Included among these are: a conceptual framework for organizing and integrating information; a diagrammatic system of measure (i.e. mathematical and statistical models); and a conceptual structure successfully developed in one field and applied to some other field to guide research and practice (i.e. an analogy). Also, the term *model* often is used interchangeably with the term *theory* or is used to mean the visual representation of the elements of a theory.
>
> Our working definition of conceptual model derives primarily from the first usage. We define a conceptual model as a *diagram* of proposed *causal linkages* among a set of *concepts* believed to be related to a particular public health problem. By concept (also referred to as a factor or variable), we mean an abstract term able to be empirically observed or measured. Hence, a conceptual model, through concepts denoted by boxes and processes delineated by arrows, provides a visual picture that represents a research question under investigation or the present focus of a specific intervention effort. A conceptual model can be informed by more than one theory and conceptualized at multi-levels (from micro to macro). As importantly in an applied field, it allows the inclusion of processes or characteristics not grounded in formal theory, but that represent empirical findings or the experience of practising professionals.[15]

This is not an easy passage to swallow quickly, nor is the method by which to 'empirically observe or measure' an 'abstract term' immediately obvious. Nevertheless it seems, for these authors at least, that a 'conceptual model' is a 'visual' representation of 'linked concepts', and that the way in which the designer chooses to draw the model constitutes her 'proposal' about the relationship between the 'concepts'. On the printed page such a 'model' will typically appear as a collection of boxes with words inside (to indicate the 'concepts'), the boxes usually being joined together by lines or arrows (see the example in Exercise Two, below). The traditional general term for the authors' 'conceptual model' is a hypothesis, though most health promotion models are poor substitutes for carefully stated, testable conjectures.

In the above quote Earp and Ennett begin to distinguish different types of model. They explain that:

a. there are 'mathematical and statistical models', which are alternative descriptions – or specialised translations – of patterns and processes first observed in other ways. (For example, in order to clarify the most important features of population growth or decline, changes can be converted into numbers and these numbers, in turn, can be translated into representative graphs and charts.)[16]
b. 'models' can be guides to research and practice in the sense that examples of success can be taken from one area and applied to a different one.
(For example, automated car manufacturing was used as a model by one famous pop music producer who wanted consistently and repeatedly to turn 'raw materials' – voice, looks, mannerisms, agility – into a polished product – a pop star.)[17]
c. 'models' may represent the elements of theories, and are sometimes thought of as interchangeable with the theories.
(A simple set of directions, written by one person in order to help another find her way from one side of town to the other, is one example of this sort of model.)[18]

As we will see, it is possible to make further distinctions, and to draw wider conclusions. However, Earp and Ennett's paper is at least clear that a model is not a simple notion. Indeed, given that several articles on models have appeared in health promotion's periodicals[19–21] it ought by now to be taken as read – at least amongst those health promotion theorists who publish in these journals – that the word 'model' has a variety of meanings which are difficult to state clearly, and hard to disentangle. And given this, one might think that all experienced health promotion theorists would recognise the potential for confusion, and would therefore exercise appropriate caution when using or discussing models. Unfortunately this is not the case.

This is how models are explained at one point in an internationally recommended student textbook:

The Preventive Model

The first approach to be considered might be labelled a **Preventive Model**. While the term model is frequently misused, it is employed here because the meaning of Medical Model – from which the approach to health education currently under discussion is derived – is widely understood and accepted. The goal of the Preventive Model of Health Education is to persuade the individual to take responsible decisions, i.e. to adopt behaviours which will prevent disease at primary, secondary or tertiary levels. This is the traditional and orthodox approach which also incorporates the sub-goal of proper utilisation of health services (to prevent disease at primary, secondary and tertiary levels). Occasionally, in an attempt to refurbish a somewhat negative image, or as a deliberate marketing strategy, the Preventive Model may claim to be promoting positive health but its definition of success is unambiguous. It is concerned to produce behavioural outcomes.

> Health education will have been effective only to the extent that individuals or communities demonstrate that they have adopted a more healthy lifestyle. For instance, successful health education about heart disease would be able to show that there had been an increased level of exercise together with various medically approved dietary changes such as a reduction in the intake of saturated fats. People would also have stopped smoking.[11]

This brief extract is, at best, theoretically erratic. For instance the reader is informed that 'model' is a frequently misused term, from which it must follow that there is at least one correct use. Yet from everything else Tones and Tilford say in this and similar passages it is obvious that, whatever the correct use is, they are unaware of it.

Consider their opening gambit: 'The first approach to be considered might be labelled a Preventive Model'. Here they use two words – 'approach' and 'model' – as if they are interchangeable, which they are not. An 'approach' means, roughly, 'a route', 'a path', 'a way towards something'. I approach a building when I move toward it with the intention of arriving at it; I make an approach to you if I have an idea I want to put to you (my path is to put the idea clearly, my aim is to have it accepted by you); if I tackle a problem with a strategy to solve it this strategy might then be said to constitute my approach.

A certain form of model (see iv on p. 45 below) may be made to *represent* an approach – as a map can represent a road or other route. Another sort of model (see v on pp. 45–46 below) can be *used* as part of an approach, but a model cannot itself *be* an approach. Tones and Tilford should have said either:

> The first approach may be modelled in the following way

or,

> The preventive model is a basic representation of a complex approach, and here is what the model looks like.

In which case they would then have had to have offered a simplified representation of the key features of the approach. But what they certainly cannot say is that:

> The first approach to be considered might be labelled a preventive model

because this renders the 'approach' and the 'model' synonymous (and therefore the use of the word 'model' superfluous). This mistake would be paralleled if a Maritime Museum were to attach a label saying 'Model of HMS *Victory*' to the real HMS *Victory*, and announce 'this ship might be labelled the model of HMS *Victory*'.

Tones and Tilford press on in their book to outline the:

Radical-Political Model

> ...those who reject the victim-blaming ideology of the Preventive Model might be said to advocate a **Radical-Political Model** of health education. Its goal is to get to the roots of the problem of ill health or, to change the metaphor, 'refocus upstream'. It is concerned to achieve social and environmental change by triggering political action...

> It is apparent that measures of success for a Radical-Political Model of health education would require very different evaluative measures (*sic*) than the narrower preventive approach. Health educators would need to demonstrate at the very least a height℮ level of awareness or critical consciousness. Ideally a consciousness raising pr℮ would also lead to measurable action.[11]

The authors' view that the radical-political model of health education: '... is concerned to achieve social and environmental change by triggering political action' seems to imply that the radical-political model is a conscious being. But of course in none of its forms can a model of this sort be 'concerned' to achieve anything. What Tones and Tilford ought to have said is that:

> ... people who wish to bring about social and environmental change sometimes try to do so by initiating political processes. Their methods and goals may be represented (modelled) in the following simplified form ...

But they did not. Instead their unfortunate use of the English language merely helps to reify the idea and use of models further – even though the task of any educator should be to achieve precisely the opposite effect.

Many similar criticisms could be levelled at these, and other, sections in *Health Education: Effectiveness, Efficiency and Equity* (all editions). No doubt it will be said that these criticisms are pedantic, that everyone knows what the authors are on about just as everyone knows the meaning of 'medical model'. But the truth is that everyone does *not* know what 'the medical model' means (I have worked full-time in medical schools for well over a decade and it does not mean anything to me – it used to, until I discovered that the world of medicine is far too complex to be simplistically modelled). And nor can anyone know with any accuracy what the authors are trying to explain in these poorly conceived passages.

It is the *illusion of shared meaning* once again. If the words are quickly skated over it is easy to imagine that we know what 'getting to the roots of the problem of ill health' means. But only a little thought shows that the authors' meaning is obscure. Just what *is* 'the problem of ill health'? What exactly does the problem consist of? How could the problem be modelled, for instance? Could it be modelled in only one way, or might several models be offered? And if so, would these models be compatible or would they conflict? How would we be able to identify the *correct* model of the roots of the problem of ill-health if we were offered alternatives from which to choose? Just as soon as serious questions are asked Tones' and Tilford's words smudge into a blur.

THINKING CLEARLY ABOUT MODELS

Health promotion theorists get in a muddle about models because health promotion has not yet developed a tradition of critical analysis. Unlike the theoretical writings to be found in more established disciplines, those who write about health promotion tend to be concerned much more with 'getting a message across' than with establishing precise meanings and applicable theories. Consequently it is common to find general, theoretically unsupported 'position statements' ('this is what we believe health promoters should and shouldn't be doing') and extremely rare to discover analysed sets of distinctions. Yet it is not particularly hard to begin to categorise the different features of health promotion's key words, and it can be enormously clarifying and productive to do so – as the following brief analysis shows.

USES AND MEANINGS OF THE WORD MODEL

The word 'model', like the word 'health', has a range of meanings. Although some of these may seem trivial, their importance should not be pre-judged.

Here is a list of possible distinctions:

i. *Model as a type within a series*
   On this understanding the word 'model' refers to varieties of some thing or some idea which can be subsumed under a *general category*, and described as models *within* or *of* it.
   Motor-cars are often made in a variety of styles within a series. Each of these adaptations is known as a different model. Ford, for instance, has offered several models within the general categories *Cortina* and *Fiesta*.

ii. *Model as a means of display (as in 'to model')*
   Used in this sense a model shows off, or models, some other thing to a desired effect. Fashion models, for instance, are employed by dress designers to display clothes.

iii. *Model as an example from which to copy*
   Used to convey this meaning a model is a reality from which copies of some kind can be made. For example, models are employed by artists to offer a reality from which they can copy an image. Another instance of *model as example* occurs if a person, practice or institution is cast as worthy of imitation, and is therefore deemed to be a *role-model*.
   It is not necessary for exact copies to be made of the model. It is enough that the example is used as a guide – even a very rough guide – by the copier. An artist may, for instance, use his model to inspire an abstract painting, using only a very few of the model's features – though he must use some.

iv. *Model as a simplified representation of a more complex reality*
   Used in this sense a model is a less complicated depiction of reality. This sort of model is often used in education. For instance, Natural History Museums offer models of evolution (often in the form of pictorial 'family trees'), and sports coaches use diagrams and toy figures to depict the key elements of 'plays' or 'moves' they wish to get across to their players. Hobby kits or Airfix models (aeroplanes, ships and so on) are further examples of this type of model. They represent certain key features of the reality they are meant to mimic, but also omit some. They must, of course, or else they would not be *models as representations*, but the real thing.

v. *Model as a representation of a more complex reality used deliberately to throw light on a problem*
   Used with this meaning models can be employed as tools of investigation, in which case they will be guided by theory and hypothesis. It may be the modeller's belief that this sort of model represents reality – but she will not know for sure. The way in which the model is cast will, therefore, reflect the exploratory suggestions and insights of the inquirer who has developed them, in addition to (possibly) representing *some* features of reality. For example, it might be speculated that people who suffer from certain forms of psychosis react to audible stimuli in characteristic ways (and in ways different from non-psychotic people). Since the

physical reality of the brain is so complex, in order to investigate such an idea it will be necessary to isolate certain features of interest. Investigators might, for example, seek to detect electrical signals from areas of the brain thought to be significant, to convert these into readable patterns by the use of mathematical techniques (mathematical modelling), and then to use these models to further their research programme – that is, to use the results to prompt further questions and projects.[22]

The use of 'model' in the health promotion literature seems usually to be either i, iii or iv, or some combination of these three categories, vi. But unless the different categories are explained by the health promotion theorist or researcher, it can be very difficult to work out what is being said in any given context.

MODELS AS GIVING SHAPE

All words, if they are to convey a meaning, must have some limit beyond which it is incorrect to use them. It is not of central importance to the current discussion, but it may be of some interest, that the general limit to the meaning of the word model seems to be *giving or being given shape*. It appears to be essential to the notion that a model must in some way *conform* to a pattern, *impose a* pattern, or *reveal* a pattern. For instance, the model of car must *conform* to a pattern (it must have recognisable features of the general series) but may also, as new models are developed, add to the pattern, and *impress* new shapes on the general conception of the series. Indeed it is possible that investigation of a number of different models in the series might *reveal* patterns of which even the original designers were unaware.

The same pattern (and limitation) can be seen in each of the five categories listed above. Fashion models are shaped by their clothes but also lend their own shape and movement to the clothes. The artist is ultimately restricted by the shape and form of her model but does have some freedom of interpretation – and may indeed have her imagination fired much more creatively than if she had no model in front of her. A role-model is a template, though the imitator can also add further elements. A model as representation is shaped by reality, as is a model used more speculatively – the hope, in this last case, is that the theoretician's guesswork will ultimately reveal the true shape of reality.

It may also be interesting to note, in passing, that the limit to a model's shaping is always set by one or more theories. Fig. 2 is correct; Fig. 3 is incorrect.[23]

THE SIX DISTINCTIONS APPLIED TO A WELL-KNOWN MODEL OF HEALTH PROMOTION

Fig. 4 is a well-known model of health promotion. On the face of it, Tannahill's model (he developed it in earlier solo publications)[24] consists of nothing more than three overlapping circles, the numbers 1–7 and the terms 'health education', 'health

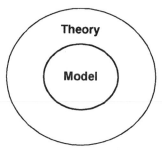

Figure 2   Models are shaped by theories

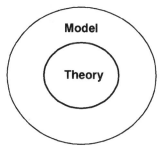

Figure 3   Theories are not shaped by models

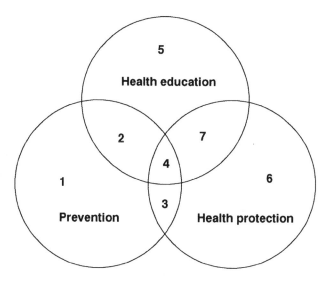

Figure 4   Tannahill's model of health promotion (taken with permission from R. S. Downie, C. Fyfe and A. Tannahill, *Health Promotion: Models and Values*, Oxford, 1990, Figs 4.I and 6.I)

protection' and 'prevention'. The numbers are meant to refer to different combinations of health promotion activities.

The question is: what *sort* of model is this? Although it is *never* asked in the health promotion literature, this is by no means a trivial question. It is, I believe, crucially important for any reflective health promoter to be able to work out both what she is being asked to accept, and what she is being asked to do to other people, by the authors of health promotion models.

There are always six possible answers to the question, as we have seen. Tannahill's model might be (i) *a type within a series*, (ii) *a means of display*, (iii) *an example from which to copy*, (iv) *a simplified representation of reality*, (v) *a representation used deliberately to throw new light on a problem*, or (vi) *some combination of these*. In order to find out which it is, it is necessary to study Tannahill's explanation of his model (some of which is quoted below), which he offers under separate headings, corresponding to the numbers in his figure:

1. *Preventive services, etc.* Examples such as immunization and cervical screening have already been touched upon...Hypertension case-finding, screening for handicapping congenital disorders, developmental surveillance, and the use of nicotine-containing chewing gum to aid smoking cessation are other examples.

2. *Preventive health education.* This includes educational efforts to influence lifestyle in the interests of preventing ill-health, as well as efforts to encourage the uptake of preventive services. In addition, the two-way nature of the educational process must not be forgotten: communication channels must be used to ensure that appropriate (wantable) preventive services are provided...

3. *Preventive health protection.* Numerous examples have already been mentioned... Fluoridation of water supplies to prevent dental caries (and possibly also osteoporosis) is another.

4. *Health education for preventive health protection.* One of the most notable successes in this category has been the intensive lobbying for seat-belt legislation (it having been shown that public health education alone was ineffective as a means of securing widespread use of belts in motor vehicles). Efforts to stimulate a social environment conducive to the success of preventive health protection measures are also important here.

   [So far, the emphasis has been on prevention. As can be seen from Tannahill's Fig. 4.1, the remaining domains lie outside the sphere of prevention. They are concerned with the enhancement of what he calls positive health.]

5. *Positive health education....* positive health education falls into two categories: health education aimed at influencing behaviour on positive health grounds (such as the encouragement of a productive use of leisure time in the interests of fitness and well-being); and that which seeks to help individuals, groups, or whole communities to develop positive health attributes (health-related lifeskills and a high level of self-esteem), which are central to the enhancement of true well-being...

6. *Positive health protection.* A positive dimension to health protection has already been mentioned...An example is the implementation of a workplace smoking policy in the interests of providing clean air. Another is the commitment of public funds to the provision of attractive and accessible leisure facilities in order to promote positive health.

7. *Health education aimed at positive health protection.* This involves raising awareness of, and securing support for, positive health protection measures, among the public and policy-makers...[6]

Under Section 1 Tannahill merely lists examples of conventional medical activities such as immunisation and cancer screening programmes. By indicating that this list is part of his model, it seems he must be presenting a model in sense (iv) – i.e. that he must be offering the model as *a simplified representation of a more complex reality*. Tannahill continues to describe existing provision under 2, claiming unsurprisingly that *preventive health education* includes education to prevent ill-health and to encourage the use of preventive services. However, he also goes on to make a *recommendation*. He says:

> In addition, the two-way nature of the educational process must not be forgotten: communication channels must be used to ensure that appropriate (wantable) preventive services are provided.

This is clearly a prescription rather than a description, which means that this part of Tannahill's model must be a model in sense (iii). That is, it is offered as **an example *from which to copy*.**

Sections 3 and 4 are descriptions, though 4 also seems to offer a recommendation:

> Efforts to stimulate a social environment conducive to the success of preventive health promotion measures are also important here.

What sort of 'social environment' is best for 'preventive health protection' is not specified at this point in the treatise. Later, though, it becomes much clearer that only a certain form of social order will do for Tannahill and his friends – and this confirms that the above quote is undoubtedly a prescription.

Sections 5, 6 and 7, though as thin on detail as the others, seem more like efforts to persuade than descriptions – though it might be said that they are also (very general) descriptions of certain sorts of practice (selected by Tannahill from a wider set). Thus we are told, for instance, that 'positive health education' is:

> ...health education aimed at influencing behaviour on positive health grounds (such as the encouragement of a productive use of leisure time in the interests of fitness and well-being)...

This version of health education is not universally held. Therefore its inclusion in the model is also a form of advocacy.

WHAT SORT OF MODEL IS THIS?

Given that the practices Tannahill describes actually happen, and given that Tannahill has chosen these from alternatives, his model must be a model in senses (iv) and (iii), and therefore also in sense (vi). Tannahill does not make it clear that this is a multiple model and, by mixing what *is* the case with what the author thinks *ought to be* the case, gives the impression that the model presented is the most desirable version of health promotion – or is even the only *genuine* account of health promotion available (it is surely revealing to see, that without any explanation, the model described as '**A**' model of health promotion (his Fig. 4.1) is magically transformed into '**The**' model of health promotion (his Fig. 6.1) 26 pages later in the book).

At best this is carelessness. At worst it is an attempt to convert the reader by stating deeply contestable assertions as if they are obvious. But they are not obvious at all – nothing is in health promotion. In fact Tannahill's model and explanatory section use several **Type One** statements, elide representation and recommendation, and combine this with conviction politics, apparently in an attempt to bombard the reader into submission.

And this is not the whole story. Tannahill's model is also a model in senses (i) and (ii), and this renders its matter of fact presentation insidious. The model is a *type within a general series* (i), and as such is one of many philosophically vacant models that have appeared in health promotion publications over the years.[25,26] It is not innovative. It poses no deliberate questions. Nor does its inventor offer any serious justification for it. The model merely reflects and perpetuates an already widely held impression that this is what health promotion is about. Its circles and words may be slightly different from those of other models, but it nevertheless sits firmly in the tried and trusted tradition.

YOU HAVE TO BE ALLOWED TO ASK QUESTIONS TO FIND OUT WHAT'S GOING ON

Read at face value, as Tannahill's model undoubtedly has been by very many trainee health promoters, things seem straightforward enough: here is an illustration of what good health promotion involves, it says. However, it is no minor matter that the reader accepts the legitimacy of this model, and if she is not encouraged to ask critical questions (as she certainly is not – Downie, Fyfe and Tannahill tell their readers what they ought to think) then the chances are that this is the picture of health promotion she will adopt and carry with her. And once she believes that this is the way things are and should be she is much more likely to accept a lot else besides. For instance, immediately following his description of his model Tannahill writes:

> The following summary definition of health promotion arises out of the model presented here. (Note the incorporation of the goal of health promotion as presented at the end of Chapter 2.)
>
> *Health promotion comprises efforts to enhance positive health and prevent ill-health, through the overlapping spheres of health education, prevention, and health protection.*
>
> The cardinal principle of health promotion thus defined is empowerment. Health education seeks to empower people by providing necessary information and helping people to develop skills...[6]

If you read this quickly it may seem a reasonable enough statement (particularly if you have had no difficulty in accepting the model). But read it carefully and you will see how manipulative and theoretically undefended it is. Most seriously, the 'summary definition' of health promotion is not argued for. Instead we are told that it 'arises' from the (philosophically vacant) model that has just been sketched out, plus 'the incorporation' of a goal 'presented' (again not argued for) earlier in the text. Tannahill does not explain why this goal is not part of his model of health promotion (surely it ought to be), nor does he explain the mechanism by which this goal fits with the methods he advocates, and nor does he attempt to justify his choice of goal at this important stage in his book. The reader is just asked to 'note' it, as if it were unproblematic.

The reader already knows from the model of health promotion offered on the previous page that health promotion *is*, according to Tannahill, no more and no less a combination of 'health education', 'prevention' and 'health protection'. Nevertheless, this is reconfirmed in the definition which offers no more *argument* than that:

Health promotion comprises efforts to promote health, through health promotion.

Of course the author means much more than this, as you will see in greater detail in Part Two, if you bear with me. An explicit and meaningful definition of Tannahill's idea of health promotion would spell his thoughts out very clearly (this is, after all, what definitions are supposed to do). Elsewhere in *Health Promotion: Models and Values* it emerges that 'positive health' is not just any sort of health, nor is it just anyone's view of health either – it turns out that some people's accounts of health are wrong. Readers learn that 'necessary information' means a certain restricted type of information, 'skills' are a particular set, and 'empowerment' is empowerment to achieve those behaviours and attitudes that happen to be valued by Tannahill and his associates.

There is really no need for tautology in health promotion. As we shall see in Chapter Five, a meaningful definition of health promotion – in line with Tannahill's beliefs – would go something like this:

> Health promotion comprises efforts to enhance ways of acting and believing based on conservative political values and to prevent disease and illness, through a co-ordinated plan to influence individual behaviour in specific ways (health education), providing and strongly promoting the uptake of medical surveillance (disease prevention), and by legislating to guarantee or firmly enforce some behaviours in order to reduce some morbidities (health protection).

Such a definition would have the advantage of being both informative and honest. It would also, of course, have the disadvantage (for Tannahill and his supporters) of being obviously open to question, so platitude is preferred in the hope that the 'summary definition' will prove amenable to as many parties as possible.

SYMPTOM AND CAUSE

Clearly not all the above arises from the careless use of the word model. There is a range of reasons and causes for Tannahill's disingenuity at this point in his account, though lack of precision about *what sort of model* is being put forward is one of the causes (it is also a symptom of health promotion's theoretical barrenness – such imprecision is unacceptable in serious academic disciplines). If it were to be common practice amongst health promotion crusaders to be as clear and explicit as possible about what they are doing then such fudging would not be possible. At the very least Tannahill would have had to have said something like:

> The figure entitled 'A model of health promotion' is a model in the following senses . . .

He would then have had to explain that the model incorporates both a *selective* account of practice and some of his own *opinions* about what should be done in health promotion's name. He would then have been obliged – or might even have wanted to – add a statement along these lines:

The model I offer you is therefore one illustration of my understanding of health promotion. It does not and cannot spontaneously generate a definition of health promotion, but is presented as it is because I *already have* certain ideas about what health promotion is. Readers should note that these ideas are based on certain values and preferences that I hold, and are by no means universally accepted . . .

If practitioners take it for granted either that the health promotion models they are told about really do exist, or that they always accurately represent reality (i.e. that health promotion models are always models in sense (iv)) then it becomes difficult if not impossible to see beyond them. And if reality is not as the models have it then health promoters are almost certainly going to miss it. It is only by fostering attitudes critical of conventional assumptions that it is possible to judge the extent to which models are real or are fiction, and it is only by learning this that substantial theoretical progress can come.

TO AVOID FALLING FOR AN ILLUSION ASK: WHAT IS MISSING FROM THIS MODEL?

Health promotion theorists are in continual danger of confusing superficial frameworks with actual reality. There is, at the moment, a strong tendency to discuss and apply either mistaken or highly naïve models as if they are all there is. To guard against this – and perhaps eventually to make philosophical and practical progress – health promoters should continually ask not only 'what sort of model is this?' but: what is *MISSING* from the model I have invented/borrowed/copied/am being told to use? Is it an accurate representation? Has every important feature of the model been simplified? Or have only the most *obvious* features been scaled down? If a version of the model were to be based solely on the details as represented – would the model be a blueprint for something that could actually work? In addition, independently minded health promoters should habitually ask: if certain features have been *selected* and others discarded, why has this been done? What is prescriptive about the model? And, whose values does it incorporate uncritically?

EXERCISE TWO

DIFFERENT SORTS OF MODEL?

Here is a discussion of a simple model which Earp and Ennett, the authors of the extract below, use in their teaching:

> As an example, we use a simple model of compliance that we have used in class (Fig. 1). The concepts of this model are the communication between a physician and patient, the patient's understanding of a treatment and the patient's compliance with a medical regimen. The arrows, by their directionality, indicate that the communication between a doctor and patient influences the patient's understanding of some recommended treatment which, in turn, influences the patient's compliance.

continues

continued

It is clear from the model that physician–patient communication is the predictor variable, or the 'cause', and that compliance is the dependent variable, or the 'outcome'. As the model is conceptualised, the patient's understanding of the regimen is a mediating variable (i.e. an intervening, explanatory variable or process between the predictor variable and the outcome).

Of course, as students are quick to point out, this is an incomplete and unrealistic model. There are other factors certain to affect compliance either directly or indirectly. For example, the degree of difficulty for the patient in carrying out the regimen, whether cost is covered by medical insurance, or particular characteristics of the condition, such as whether it is symptomless, could affect compliance. Also, compliance could be affected by factors that influence physician–patient communication. For example, does educational level of the patient or whether the doctor and patient are of the same gender affect communication and, in turn, compliance? Clearly, the model becomes more complex as variables are added that the investigator feels are needed to account for the outcome (Fig. 2).[15]

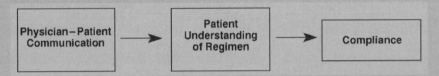

Figure 5   Simple three-variable conceptual model

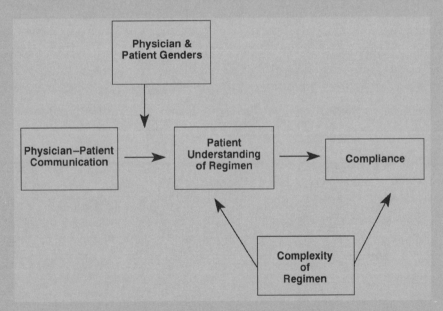

Figure 6   Five-variable conceptual model showing modifying and confounding variables

Study the passage and figures carefully, then read the section **Uses and Meanings of the Word Model** (pp. 45–46) in the main text of *Health Promotion: Philosophy, Prejudice and Practice*.

continues

continued

Now answer these questions:

1. In what sense(s) are Earp and Ennett's Figs 1 and 2 [Figs 5 and 6 above] models?
2. Choose any other model from the health promotion literature, and explain the sense(s) in which it is a model.
3. Discuss the health promotion implications of accepting this model as accurate and usable.

Teaching notes for: Different Sorts of Model?

The aims of this exercise are:

i. To show how pervasive the *illusion of shared meaning* is.
ii. To show how important it is to be clear about what is being said, even in the most apparently innocuous of passages.
iii. To allow students to practise their analytic skills on one of the most ubiquitous ideas in health promotion.

One of the most fruitful ways to conduct this exercise is to have students divide into groups (of 4–5 if possible). These groups should first review the six distinctions in the **Uses and Meanings of the Word Model** section in the above chapter, to make sure they understand them clearly (they may find it useful to come up with their own illustrations of each type). You should be on hand to deal with any questions and uncertainties.

Once the groups have the distinctions firmly in mind they should turn to Earp and Ennett's extract, and tease out the different meanings of 'model'.

1. For example, Earp and Ennett's Fig. 1 (Fig. 5 above) might be either:

   a. *a simplified representation of a more complex reality*

   or/and

   b. *an example from which to copy*

   If b. then it is a *recommendation* that physician–patient communication *ought* to lead to patient understanding and that this *ought* to lead to compliance. It instructs that to secure compliance you should act in this manner (taking into account the added factors included in Earp and Ennett's Fig. 2 [Fig. 6 above]).

   or

   c. *a representation of a more complex reality used deliberately to throw light on a problem.*

   In other words, it might be an explanation of what goes on in actual consultations.

continues

continued

Put these possibilities to the students. Are the authors suggesting that you accept their role-model uncritically (they do not seem to be encouraging reflection on the notion of 'compliance', for instance), are they simply showing you the basic bones of a more complex reality, are they wanting you to *reflect* upon their theory, or are they merely trying to show students how to use models?

2. If this is the first time students have attempted this exercise you should help them select simple models. It is possible that some of the students' choices will be models in only one of the six senses. If so, try to find more ambiguous examples, and encourage free discussion (you may wish to remind students of the six senses of model from time to time – perhaps have these on an overhead transparency).

3. This is an important part of the exercise. Have students re-read the criticism of Tannahill's model in the above chapter (pp. 46–52) and encourage them to discuss the various pressures which might be placed on them as health promoters were they to be asked to accept uncritically the model they have chosen to discuss.

Evidence and Ethics

THE ILLUSION OF SHARED ETHICS

The illusion of shared meaning naturally gives rise to a further worrying mirage – *the illusion of shared ethics*. At the heart of any health promotion project there will be very many ethical matters which ought to be aired, explained and discussed by all those affected (promoters and recipients alike).[27] Yet despite this there is, amongst health promoters, strikingly little serious debate about the ethics of what they are doing (the few discussions that do exist are not particularly penetrating).[28–30] Ethics is rarely thought to be an issue in standard health promotion work (Tones and Tilford,[11] for instance, fail even to list ethics in their subject index) even though it ought to be the first, last and integral concern of any project. The reason for such a gross oversight is most probably this: unless you possess a decent understanding of the reasons why you value health promotion it is extremely difficult to offer an ethical justification for your practice, and harder still to admit that alternative ethical positions are worthy of consideration.

In order to appreciate the extent to which ethics pervades health promotion – and therefore to see the full size of the discipline's theoretical crisis – it is necessary to be aware of the difference between facts and values: an extremely important distinction which, remarkably, remains almost entirely invisible in health promotion.

FACTS AND VALUES, EVIDENCE AND ETHICS – AN INITIAL EXAMPLE

If health promotion is associated with any one thing in the public eye, it is the campaign against smoking. Almost everyone, it seems, accepts that *as a matter of fact* smoking is bad for health, that it should be discouraged or even banned in some situations and that it is unquestionably ethical that health promoters do what they can to reduce smoking levels. But it is not, as the following illustration demonstrates beyond doubt.

Health Promotion, Second Edition: David Seedhouse
© 2004 John Wiley & Sons, Ltd: ISBNs 0 470 84732 8 (HB); 0 470 84733 6 (PB)

FOUR MORALLY CONTROVERSIAL HEALTH PROMOTION PLANS

Here is **Plan A**:

Health Promotion Plan A

HEALTH PROMOTERS SHOULD ENCOURAGE PEOPLE TO SMOKE

Because
- Smoking helps people cope with life
- Promoting smoking will help the tobacco industry employ more people (it is well known that unemployment is a cause of ill-health)
- Smoking raises taxes which governments can elect to spend on health services
- Smoking reduces the level of chronic sickness in the elderly population because smokers tend to die sooner than non-smokers. Promoting smoking will lower the cost to the state of geriatric care
- Young people think smoking is cool – it makes them feel they belong, and a sense of belonging is very important for health
- Smoking is enjoyable – most smokers get pleasure out of smoking

HEALTH PROMOTERS SHOULD ENCOURAGE PEOPLE TO SMOKE BY MEANS OF ONE OR MORE OF THE FOLLOWING METHODS

- *Campaigning for unrestricted advertising* – in a capitalist country it ought to be legal to advertise any product that it is legal to sell
- *Comprehensive advice on how to get the very most enjoyment from cigarette smoking* – what to smoke, what strength cigarette is best in which circumstances, when to use a filter and when not, how to roll your own, what the optimum frequency should be (this advice should be based on detailed scientific research undertaken by health promoters)
- *Advertising widely the many mental and social benefits that smoking offers*

It is highly unlikely that anyone would be so bold as to put forward **Plan A** as a *health promotion* strategy (there are a handful of organisations[31] which argue that individuals have a right to smoke if that is what they choose to do, just as they have a right to engage in other behaviours which carry personal risks, but not even these groups dare claim that smoking is actually *good* for health). By contrast, variations on **Plan B** abound. However, even though this deluge of **Plan B** material makes it look as if anti-smoking policies are factually desirable, closer study shows this just is not so. Just like **Plan A**, **Plan B** is not based only on matters of fact, nor is it *obviously* the right thing to do. **Plan B** is a combination of evidence *and* supposition, and is therefore open to challenge.

Here is **Plan B**:

Health Promotion Plan B

HEALTH PROMOTERS SHOULD TRY TO STOP PEOPLE SMOKING

Because
- Smoking causes sickness and shortens lives
- Smoking makes people unfit
- The medical treatment of smoking-related disease is expensive. Where such disease is treated by publicly funded medical services smoking incurs financial cost to the state
- Smoking leads to absenteeism and loss of productivity, and so incurs further cost to the state
- Smoking damages non-smokers, physically (through passive smoking) and economically (because of its cost to the state – a cost which is ultimately borne by the individual taxpayer)
- Smoking is unaesthetic (it stains) and unhygienic (it smells)

HEALTH PROMOTERS SHOULD TRY TO STOP PEOPLE SMOKING BY MEANS OF ONE OR MORE OF THE FOLLOWING METHODS

- *Education* – smokers should be presented with comprehensive evidence about the damage they do to themselves and others, and enabled to make fully informed choices
- *Training* – stop-smoking techniques should be freely and liberally available wherever people smoke. People should be given every opportunity to change their behaviours
- *Indoctrination* – anti-smoking propaganda should be widely distributed to counteract the marketing campaigns of the tobacco companies. It should be made plain that tobacco-related disease is to be feared (scary real life images should be used), and the huge profits that tobacco companies make as a result of their trade should be given maximum publicity – as black a picture as possible should be painted about the undesirable effects of smoking and the immorality of the tobacco industry
- *Legislation* – tobacco advertising should be banned, tobacco products should be taxed at a very high rate, smoking in public should be forbidden, smokers should be forced to bear the cost of all medical treatments made necessary by their smoking, smokers should be separated from non-smokers wherever possible
- *Prohibition* – smoking should be outlawed altogether

Both **Plans A** and **B** originate in alternative interpretations of the merits of smoking – neither plan is a neutral response to evidence, rather each is constructed according to this general formula:

Various pieces of evidence + Various sorts of opinion = A health promotion plan

Therefore *both* **Plan A** and **Plan B** are morally controversial. Any plan based on the above formula must be. No doubt **Plan A** will appear manifestly problematic – perhaps even shocking to some people – while initially only parts (if anything) of **Plan B** will seem to require ethical justification. But even though the plans may seem to be in completely different moral dimensions, appearances can be deceptive.

Because late twentieth-century Westerners have become so accustomed to the unremitting association of the words 'smoking' and 'bad for your health' this may not be easy to digest. If so, the following illustration should dispel any residual illusion: **Plan B** is *just as arguable* as **Plan A**.

ANTI-RUGBY HEALTH PROMOTION

New Zealanders are passionate about Rugby Union. In a nation of close on 4 million people there are approximately 300,000 regular rugby players.[32] Looked at from one point of view so much regular exercise undertaken on such a large scale seems to be just what the (health promotion) doctor ordered. However rugby is a dangerous game, injuries are common, and cost the New Zealand nation approaching NZ$30 million each year – or the equivalent of about NZ$1 million every playing Saturday (this money is paid through a 'no-fault' national injury and accident compensation scheme, administered by the Accident Compensation Corporation, and known as 'the ACC').[33,34]

There is greater risk of injury the higher the grade, but across all levels 13% of injuries result from foul play, 42% of players start each season with either a current injury and/ or a chronic injury, and countless players place themselves at risk of various harms not during the match itself, but because (in keeping with hallowed tradition) they drink so much alcohol afterwards.

Now suppose that someone in government with responsibility for health promotion takes a hard look at these statistics and decides that rugby is an *unhealthy* activity. Suppose that this member of government believes it would be far better for the health of all New Zealanders if those presently addicted to playing rugby could be persuaded to stop. And suppose further that this government health promoter were to want to inaugurate a major campaign against rugby playing. Suppose she wanted to initiate **Plan C**:

Rugby is New Zealand's most important national institution. New Zealand's rugby players know the risks, they know the pleasures, and they are prepared to take their chances. It is, therefore, safe to say that the great majority of New Zealanders would not approve of **Plan C**, though its reasoning would be influential in some quarters, and a minority of the population would welcome it.

If **Plan C** were to be implemented (Kiwi readers: please try your best to suspend disbelief at this point) the value tensions and moral questions would be plain to see. It would be obvious that **Plan C** is *not purely factual*. Alternative evidence would be advanced in favour of rugby in response to the health promotion initiative. The plan would be attacked for exaggerating the risks and underplaying the benefits, there would be complaints about the insensitivity of the hard-hitting advertisements and protests that – because of raised anxiety – some rugby players could no longer take the same pleasure out of their game. No doubt there would be talk of rights, of the importance of people being free to choose, of the dangers of 'healthism' – it is easy to imagine the outcry. Yet this hypothetical proposal is very close to the reality of current anti-smoking health promotion and indeed virtually parallels the apparently unobjectionable **Plan B**.

Health Promotion Plan C

HEALTH PROMOTERS SHOULD TRY TO STOP PEOPLE PLAYING RUGBY

Because
- Rugby causes serious injury and shortens lives
- Rugby makes people unfit
- The medical treatment of rugby-related injury incurs considerable cost to the state
- Rugby leads to absenteeism and loss of productivity, and so incurs further cost to the state
- Rugby damages non-rugby players economically
- Rugby is unaesthetic, it promotes aggression, venerates brawn over brain, and presents a negative image of New Zealand to the world's more cerebral societies

HEALTH PROMOTERS SHOULD TRY TO STOP PEOPLE PLAYING RUGBY BY MEANS OF ONE OR MORE OF THE FOLLOWING METHODS

- *Education* – rugby players should be presented with evidence of the damage they do to themselves and others, should be shown alternative leisure activities, and enabled to make fully informed choices about their behaviours free from social pressures
- *Indoctrination* – anti-rugby propaganda should be widely distributed to counteract the marketing campaigns of the sportswear companies and brewers (who currently promote rugby very aggressively in New Zealand), glossy 'Stop Rugby' brochures should be sent to all New Zealanders, there should be a 'National No-Rugby Day' each year on a Saturday in July (mid-winter in New Zealand), and terrifying advertisements showing ex-rugby players paralysed as a result of neck injury should be repeatedly aired on TV
- *Legislation* – there should be a ban on the advertising of rugby games, admission to rugby matches should be highly taxed, and so on

EXERCISE THREE

EVIDENCE OR OPINION?

Take any of the **Plans A**, **B** and **C** and, if possible, distinguish:

1. Indisputable evidence
2. Disputable evidence
3. Statements of opinion

Then:

4. Identify those statements which most obviously have moral content
5. From this set extract two statements – one with which you most agree, the other with which you most disagree
6. Offer the strongest possible justification for your selection

continues

continued

Then:

7. Argue against your preferred statement
8. Argue in support of your least preferred statement
9. Finally, argue in favour of your most preferred statement

Teaching notes for: Evidence or Opinion?

The three **Health Promotion Plans** have deliberately been presented without *painstaking* attention to detail, both to represent the way such plans actually tend to be written in practice, and to allow thoughtful students to begin to spot flaws and to raise issues for discussion.

Exercise Three is fairly advanced, and is not easy to do well. It requires patience on behalf of both teacher and students, but if it works it can be of great value in increasing students' appreciation of how very important it is for health promotion advocates to be careful about what they say.

There is also a tendency for this exercise (and perhaps for some of the others in the book) to appear negative. Some students may consider it to be 'nit-picking'. In order to counter this view it is important to emphasise that if something is not clear then it can be misleading – and it is surely important for health promotion material not to be misleading. Furthermore, criticism of something that is open to criticism is not an end in itself but part of a process which must be undergone if a better theory (or a more defensible **Plan** in this case) is to be constructed.

STARTING OFF

To begin with, unless the class or group is already very experienced in this sort of analysis, it is advisable for you to lead the whole group and to start with an apparently simple task. Before you discuss *disputable* and *indisputable* evidence, ask the students to identify those statements that are based on evidence and those statements that are based upon opinions or values. By way of example, in the case of **Plan B**, one might anticipate the following reactions.

Taking the first six statements in turn:

> **Smoking causes sickness and shortens lives**

Possible Student Response

The first reaction may be that this is either a statement of fact or (from more sophisticated students) that it is based on evidence that is *almost certainly* true – students might claim that 'everyone knows this is true these days' or that there is

continues

continued

a 'great body of scientific evidence' which supports it. It is also possible that someone will point out that this is not so with all people. Such a student might argue that it may be the case that a smoker has a shorter life due to other reasons, or she might point out that a combination of reasons is always necessary to explain mortality (for example, she might point out that more 'working class' people smoke and that 'working-class' people live shorter lives anyway). This sort of conversation is to be encouraged, and if you have research material available then this ought to be brought fully into the debate.

It is possible that students will wish to amend the statement to 'smoking makes *some* people sick and shortens the lives of *some* people'. Indeed, thoughtful students may insist on many further qualifying statements before they are satisfied. Nevertheless, it is almost certain that the majority view will be, taking the complexities into account, that this statement is either true or at least based on very strong evidence.

Smoking makes people unfit

Possible Student Response

Once again you should anticipate that thoughtful students will question this statement, most probably on the same or similar grounds to those they have raised in the case of the first statement. I have found that some classes also want to make a distinction between physical and mental fitness (possibly prompted by what they have read of **Plan A**). When presented with the statement in question, one of my students with a background in psychology pointed out that there is research to show that smoking can improve short-term memory retention, and other students have commented that smoking can relieve stress. If this is the way the discussion develops it is almost inevitable that someone will say 'ah yes, but is the relief of stress through the use of an addictive habit *really* stress relief?' or 'surely there are better ways to relieve stress' – in which case the conversation should be allowed to develop for a brief time. But then you should pose the main question again: *is this a factual or an evaluative statement?* Insist that students address it, if you can.

Further discussion may then follow. 'What is meant by fitness?' 'Is physical fitness a good thing?' 'It depends how the fitness comes about, surely', and this too should be encouraged. Ultimately a good group might conclude something along these lines:

We think there is evidence that smoking X no. of cigarettes regularly over a period of at least Y causes the physical fitness (measured in ways a, b, c, d, e, etc...) of some or most people to drop (depending on what else they are doing – if they also increase their exercising they may conceivably become fitter). This much is true. However, there is an element of value-judgement here in that there is not a *necessary* connection between high physical fitness and health.

continues

continued

If you do generate such an interesting answer, continue to press students to explain further.

> **The medical treatment of smoking-related disease is expensive. Where such disease is treated by publicly funded medical services smoking incurs financial cost to the state**

Possible Student Response

Very good student groups might decide that it is useful to split the two sentences. The second sentence:

> **Where such disease is treated by publicly funded medical services smoking incurs financial cost to the state**

might be seen (correctly) to be circular and therefore analytically true – or true by definition. That is, it really says nothing more than 'where the state treats smoking-caused disease in a medical system it funds, the state incurs the financial costs'. Of course, it may be that – inspired by **Plan A** – students will challenge the notion of 'cost' in various ways. However, such a challenge is best done with reference to the first sentence:

> **The medical treatment of smoking-related disease is expensive**

where the use of the word 'expensive' *could* be said to have evaluative content, or at least to be relative to the goal the medical treatment is aimed at. Students may raise such issues as: 'can a cost be put on human life and happiness?', 'is the cost of smoking-related disease markedly more expensive than the cost of treating non-smoking-related disease?', 'what is the factual difference between expensive and inexpensive treatment?', 'can such a difference be maintained without referring to values?'

If these issues are raised then further discussion should most certainly be encouraged.

> **Smoking leads to absenteeism and loss of productivity, and so incurs further cost to the state**

Possible Student Response

There are, of course, many possible responses to this statement, but the best one probably is that it is too woolly. How do we know that smoking leads to absenteeism? Perhaps if smoking helps people cope with stress, it makes a contribution to keeping absenteeism lower than it might otherwise be? Students may argue that it is a very sweeping claim to associate smoking with loss of productivity, and that considerable and complex research is required to assess the truth of an assertion such as this. They might continue in this vein to point out

continues

continued

that because no one knows the statement to be certainly true, the fact that it is included in **Plan B** means that it must have an evaluative element since it is being used in an attempt to *persuade* people not to smoke. If this happens you might see value in pointing out that the entire **Plan** is persuasive, and ask if that places the **Plan** *entirely* within the realm of ethics.

> **Smoking damages non-smokers, physically (through 'passive smoking') and economically (because of its cost to the state – a cost which is ultimately borne by the individual taxpayer)**

Possible Student Response

This statement is likely to generate a combination of at least some of the reactions listed to the previous four. Students will probably wonder how many, and in what ways, non-smokers are affected by smoking, will again want clarification of the meaning of 'cost', and may query the relationship between 'cost' and the burden on the individual taxpayer (for instance, it is argued by some that smokers bear a level of taxation disproportionate to the fiscal damage their habit causes to the state's coffers).[35]

> **Smoking is unaesthetic (it stains) and unhygienic (it smells)**

Possible Student Response

This can be a very useful statement at which to pause and take stock of the exercise. Arguably there are at least one and possibly two straight fact/value splits here. The most obvious, again with added provisos about how the smoking is done and for how long, is that smoking does indeed stain (this is demonstrable) but whether this is 'unaesthetic' depends upon what one values. If it is regarded as a sign of strength or beauty to have yellow fingers, and if smoking achieves this, then smoking *can* be said to have a welcome aesthetic effect. More broadly, smoking advertisements often portray smokers as elegant and sophisticated – to say that this is *not* so is not a statement built from evidence but one that stems from a particular point of view about what is attractive.

Dependent upon how one defines 'unhygienic' a similar discussion might ensue.

THE REMAINDER OF THE PLANS

Clearly there is much else to discuss with the plans. What is education? How does it differ from indoctrination? Is the most effective method (of trying to stop or trying to promote) smoking necessarily the most moral? Do teenagers really think smoking is cool – or are they forced into the habit through peer and advertisers' pressure? Is smoking enjoyable? Can smoking be enjoyable if the smoker is made to feel guilty about her behaviour? What exactly are the mental and social benefits of smoking?

Whichever direction the conversation goes it is unlikely that the class will quickly exhaust the material that might be discussed.

SMOKING TRUTHS?

Now consider one real example of anti-smoking health promotion. Here is a typical UK Health Education Authority (HEA) claim.[36,37] For the sake of balance let's call this (part of) **Plan D**:

(Part of) Health Promotion Plan D

Smoking
Giving up smoking is the most important step people can take to improve their health...

Smoking Facts
A smoker runs two or three times the risk of having a heart attack as a non-smoker...

Smoking can lead to bad breath, staining and yellowing of teeth, shortness of breath, and addiction to nicotine...

Smoking is anti-social. As well as causing annoyance by making hair and clothes smell unpleasant, exposure to other people's smoke can cause eyes to hurt, headaches, coughs, sore throat, dizziness and nausea.

DIFFERENT TYPES OF FACT

Each of the statements in **Plan D** is presented as an uncomplicated and unarguable fact: the only problem being to convince those who do not know these facts, or who are too addicted, or who have too little will-power, to quit. Some of the statements are certainly factual: smoking can stain teeth, exposure to smoke can cause coughs and – given that certain additional conditions apply – a smoker does run two or three times the risk of having a heart attack as a non-smoker.[7] However, to get a more complete picture of the smoking facts it is essential to be aware that there are different types of fact, and that the statements announced as **Plan D** actually make different levels of claim.

Consider, for instance, the statement 'smoking can stain teeth'. This is a straightforward assertion of a cumulative tendency of one action to cause one effect; it is testable, and it is certainly true (it is also true that 'smoker's toothpaste' will remove most stains – but this smoking fact is deliberately not mentioned). However, the statement 'a smoker runs two to three times the risk of having a heart attack as a non-smoker' is a far more complex assertion and – if understood in the same way as the previous statement, as a statement that one action (smoking) can directly and consistently cause a specific effect (a heart attack) – it is false, and therefore its inclusion as a 'fact' is deeply ethically controversial. While there are many studies which show that smoking does indeed increase some people's risk of suffering a heart attack, there is no simple causal relationship. There are very many variables to take into account (diet, exercise, weight, genetic make-up), and it is not certain that any individual smoker's smoking will cause her to suffer a heart attack. Data from 'the Framingham study'[38] for instance: '...suggest that the effect of smoking seen in younger men disappears in older men and is largely absent in women'.[39]

Thus there are at least two different sorts of 'smoking fact' in *The Health Guide*. The one commonplace and virtually certain, the other complex and only very generally true. Yet as they are presented both facts look (and no doubt are meant to look) exactly the same.

OPINIONS DRESSED AS FACTS

Some of the statements in *The Health Guide* are not facts in any sense, they are opinions (particular *interpretations* of the evidence). For instance, consider two non-factual statements about smoking (both presented as facts) contained in the booklet:

> Giving up smoking is the most important step people can take to improve their health...
> Smoking is anti-social.

Expand them just a little and it is possible to detect the way in which the authors of *The Health Guide* have merged together evidence and points of view to produce statements they mistakenly describe as factual:

> Giving up smoking is the most important step people can take to improve their health (**this is opinion**) because smoking is – as far as current research is able to establish – the greatest cause of preventable morbidity in individuals (**fact – if this is true**). The more disease a person has the less healthy he is (**opinion – it depends what is meant by health**) and the more morbidity there is in society the less healthy that society is (**opinion again**).

> Smoking can be unpleasant for others (**fact**) and there is evidence that it can cause disease in non-smokers through passive smoking (**fact – if this is true**). For these reasons smoking is anti-social (**opinion**).

EXCESSIVE ADVOCACY?

There is a great deal of evidence that health promoters have been remarkably successful in getting 'the anti-smoking message' across – so successful in fact that: '...the USA public now perceives the risks from smoking to be much higher than the actual risk'.[35]

Possibly the truth looks like this:[40]

	Perceived by smokers	Perceived by everyone	Actual
Lifet... ...ung cancer to smoker	37%	43%	6–13%
Lifetime mortality risk to smoker	47%	54%	18–36%
Lifetime mortality risk to someone (smoker and others)			23–46%
Average years of life lost	7.0–18.8**	11.5	3.6–7.2

** Variations with age: older smokers, presumably less affected over the years by recent information campaigns, perceive their average loss to be less than do younger smokers who have been more affected by that information.[35]

Although Viscusi's is only one study, and his results may be inaccurate, it is interesting to note that:

> Extrapolating from other facts about the relationship between risk perception and actual choice to smoke, Viscusi shockingly estimates that if people had accurate rather than inflated risk perceptions, another 8% of the USA population would smoke![35]

Now, given that 'giving up smoking is the most important step people can take to improve their health' the fact that this 8% do not now smoke must, presumably, be regarded as a success by health promoters. But, assuming that Viscusi's data are true, this success rests upon the American public being collectively *deceived* (albeit unintentionally, perhaps) about the actual physical risks they face or would face as smokers. Thanks to health promotion campaigners the USA public does not know the truth about smoking. Perhaps the end justifies the means in this case (a debatable point which, of course, cannot actually be publicly debated if the deception is to be kept up). However it is highly likely that such deception in other walks of life (even in *commercial* advertising)[41] would be widely condemned as unethical.

Imagine if the aforementioned government health promoter were to continue with her anti-rugby campaign when there was already evidence that New Zealanders greatly overestimated the risks. And imagine the reaction of most of today's Western bioethicists if they discovered that doctors had deliberately been grossly over-simplifying (as in the HEA guide) and even distorting information (as in Viscusi's data) in order to gain individuals' consent to surgery. Even if the doctors had a genuine altruistic concern for their patients, and had the future welfare of the human race at heart, it is hard to imagine (in today's ethical climate) that their actions could possibly be condoned.[42,43] Even if it turned out that the patients benefited, even if they were cured as a direct result of the intervention, we hold *not being deceived* in such high regard (in individualistic cultures at least) that the doctors' behaviour would be widely considered to be unacceptable.

But it is apparently alright for health promoters to deceive. Either that or systematic deception by official health promotion continues to proceed largely unnoticed. Health promotion is seen as mainstream, conventional, traditional – and so non-problematic. But once it is recognised that convention is not *automatically* morally superior (and it is very easy to see this – just consider the European colonists' continuing treatment of indigenous peoples,[44] or Western society's constant discrimination against homosexuals[45] – both of which are profoundly conventional *and* deeply questionable), and once it is seen that convention is *one* option amongst a host of others, then it is obvious that health promotion's generally uncontroversial appearance is just that – appearance.

Since matters of what to promote in the name of health, and how to do it, are quite clearly *not* finally decidable *purely* by appeal to the facts then continuing, in-depth discussion about values and social priorities is obviously required in a democratic society. To make such sustained discussion about matters of ethics possible health promotion's theoretical side patently requires considerable development.

EXERCISE FOUR

REAL LIVES

Think about the following residents of *Pakeha Street*:

Jane

Jane Smith is not happy, but she is getting by. She is 26, and works at home, caring for her two children (who are 2 and 3 years old) and the house. Jane has decided that she does not like her husband, John, very much – never mind love him. He is selfish, overbearing and, when they disagree, he must always get his way – or else he will lose his temper and sulk until he does.

Despite her feelings (and situation) Jane has decided to stay with John, at least until the children have left school. She hopes that she will be able to find some sort of employment when they are attending junior school. To cope with her life Jane smokes a few cigarettes a day, and has taken to drinking about half of a quarter bottle of vodka a day (John doesn't know she drinks).

Michael

Michael Jones (31) loves to be fit. He has been in training since his early twenties and has an excellent, sinewy physique. He particularly enjoys running, and regularly competes in long-distance events as an individual entrant. Michael is an administrator at the local government offices, but this is a means to an end only (he finds the work very tedious). He uses his wages to pay off a large loan he took out to build a fully equipped private gym at his house, to travel to running events, and to buy the latest gear and magazines.

Michael is single, has no close friends, and over the past few months has found that he has become increasingly tired and does not find it as easy to concentrate as he used to. Worse than this, from Michael's point of view, he has found that the muscles beneath his right calf are becoming stiff and sore, and that he is getting stabbing pains in his left knee as he begins each run.

continues

continued

Andrea

Andrea Barlow (42) used to be a secondary school teacher but lost her permanent post after a year-long virus infection, which she suffered in her mid-thirties. Since then Andrea has been a supply teacher, taking temporary work whenever she could. She has applied for dozens of full-time posts, but has had only one unsuccessful (and demoralising) interview.

Andrea's stints as a supply teacher have become shorter and shorter, and she suspects that certain people locally – who have influence in teaching circles – dislike her. She has had three temporary jobs in the past year and each time she has complained to the Head, after only a few weeks, that she is being picked on by other teachers. She claims always to get the most unruly classes and her notes go missing regularly.

Andrea lives with her elderly mother, Dorothy, who is becoming noticeably confused.

Now explain:

1. The health promotion priorities in each of these cases.
2. Which methods you believe to be most effective and/or most moral to employ in order to achieve these priorities.
3. If with others who have offered different answers to 1 and 2 attempt to persuade them that your priorities and methods are *truly* health promoting (take careful note, in so doing, of the extent to which values, ethics and prejudice must play a part, and the extent to which other people's prejudices become very difficult to counteract unless you have a developed theory to help you).

   If attempting this exercise independently imagine, in detail, how you would respond to a sceptic.

Teaching notes for: Real Lives

The point of this exercise is to emphasise the role of values, ethics, and prejudice in health promotion; to suggest to students that isolated opinions about how best to promote health are not enough (more extensive justifications are necessary); and also to give students an opportunity to discuss how to set health promotion priorities to help people who have life problems which defy simply categorisation.

The exercise is probably best done in small groups – ideally in three groups of 5 or 6, with each group taking a different example (although the characters are described only briefly you will find that there is much to discuss in each case). You should explain to students that before they begin to tackle the questions they should add any further information they deem necessary. A *reporter* should be chosen, and he or she should be prepared to note both agreements and disagreements as they arise during the group's deliberations.

continues

continued

Ideally students will find their task frustrating. It *ought* to be simple to decide to encourage Jane into social hobbies and wider networks, to determine to advise Michael to see a good physiotherapist and to suggest that he considers taking up other interests, and to persuade Andrea to visit a psychiatrist (and also to encourage her to ask for help from social services to enable her to cope with her ageing mother). But it is not so simple because:

a. each of these solutions carries a heavy price of its own
b. it is far from clear that all these ideas are legitimate health promotion work

and

c. it is likely that different health promoters will disagree about what to do.

Encourage students to bring these issues out into the open, and to discuss *what they need to do* to resolve them.

Some students like to have fun with this sort of exercise. You will, sooner or later, almost certainly hear the suggestion that Michael should have an affair with Jane while Andrea looks after the kids – or some other imaginative social arrangement. In my experience this is all to the good – light relief seems to help drive the more serious points home.

Progress So Far

From: **"D.Grant"** <**D.Grant@Willesvillehp.net**>
To: **David Seedhouse** <**david.seedhouse@aut.ac.nz**>
Date sent: **Fri, 3 November 2002 12:12:41**
Subject: **Re: Progress?**
Priority: **Normal**

Hello again,

Thank you for sending me so many of your thoughts on health promotion. You've been able to go into much more detail than I have, and I've found your observations really helpful. If you don't mind I'll briefly let you know where I'm up to, and then I've got a few questions for you.

I've started as a temporary health promoter at the Willesville Unit, and I'm finding it fascinating. I'm only there for a short while – and I'm very clear that my _main_ purpose is to write some good stuff about health promotion – but I also want to do some practical good if I can. So, I'm quickly getting up to speed on drugs and alcohol, and I'm looking to do preventive work with young people – if only for a few days. This means I'm running a couple of meetings with concerned parents, I'll be doing a bit of outreach with an experienced colleague in pubs and clubs, and helping to prepare a grant application for a new advice centre in town. Perhaps you know the sort of thing?

I reckon you'll be more interested to hear what I _think_ about what I'm doing, though. I've read a bit about the history of mind-altering substances and appreciate that different societies make very different responses to the problem – if they see it as a problem at all that is. In fact, if you had to ask me to make a judgement from right outside health promotion I'd probably say that much of the present approach to drug and alcohol abuse is rather irrational and sometimes even hysterical. However, as a health promoter – as someone who has chosen to enter this field – I think it would be pointless, unfair and irresponsible to try to subvert it and therefore I have decided to make some compromises. Your arguments make a great deal of sense to me but even though I don't entirely agree that what I'm doing is the best possible approach to take I have decided to do it nevertheless – so long as I think it can do _some_ good.

I believe you will disagree with my decision, and that you wouldn't be prepared to be part of a project which didn't make sense on _your_ terms – I wonder if I'm right?

And this brings me to my questions. I do appreciate you giving me so much of your time so I won't bombard you with all the things I'd like to. However I would like your thoughts on these two points:

1. **You are very critical of some of the other people who have written about health promotion. Sometimes you come across quite harshly. Do you mean to do this, and do you think it is a constructive thing to do?**

Health Promotion, Second Edition: David Seedhouse
© 2004 John Wiley & Sons, Ltd: ISBNs 0 470 84732 8 (HB); 0 470 84733 6 (PB)

2. **Everything you've told me so far has been – well – negative. You've gone out of your way to show what is wrong with health promotion but you've said nothing about what is good about it, and nothing about how it could be improved. I understand the sense of what you write but I want to know the way forward – I want to read what _good_ practice is.**

What do you say?

Thanks again,

Diane Grant

From: **David Seedhouse** <david.seedhouse@aut.ac.nz>
To: **"D.Grant"** <D.Grant@Willesvillehp.net>
Date sent: **Sat, 4 November 2002 10:10:27**
Subject: **Re: Progress?**
Priority: **normal**

Dear Diane
Thanks for your message. Believe it or not I understand your frustration. I'd ask exactly the same questions if I were you and – if I were a health promoter – I would have to make some compromises too, though I don't suppose I'd find it easy. But I'm _not_ a health promoter. I'm a philosopher whose job it is to criticise bad thinking, bad arguments and bad ethics. Lasting progress is not possible without this sort of critique – as I hope you'll come to see.

Can I ask you to be patient? I feel I've made a _necessary_ start on a construction programme. I have to begin by demolition because there is a lot of intellectual rubble in health promotion – an accumulation of _silt_ which really slows up the thought processes – and that just has to be got rid of first. And I haven't finished yet I'm afraid. There's more bad reasoning to expose before I can begin to build for you – but I assure you that I will build and that a positive theory of health promotion is possible.

◆

SUMMARY OF PROGRESS

Let me summarise where we are up to, by way of answering your second question. Basically I have argued that:

1. **Even though health promotion is deemed to be of considerable importance in many societies, and even though it is widely practised, it lacks a theory of purpose.**
2. **Health promotion does not have a theory of purpose because it does not have a tradition of critical analysis.**
3. **Without a theory of what it is for health promotion (like nursing) must remain a Magpie Profession.**
4. **So long as it is acceptable for health promotion to be a Magpie Profession sloppy thinking will prevail: weak definitions, assertions rather than arguments, and failure to confront the hard moral questions are a product of, and a vital support to, a Magpie Profession.**

5. **So long as it remains acceptable for health promotion to be a Magpie Profession it is bound to be a confusing field in which to work.**
6. **Contradictory beliefs and practices are allowed to co-exist under the health promotion 'banner'. Unless and until these conflicts are seriously analysed and understood for what they are, health promotion will never mature.**
7. **Health promotion is thought, by many theorists and practitioners, to be based primarily, or even entirely, on evidence and facts. But this is a crucial mistake. Health promotion is much more to do with values (and politics) than even the most radical health promoters realise.**
8. **In order to achieve a thorough understanding of health promotion it is vital to examine the world of values more deeply. This is what I propose to do next, and it is from this analysis that I will build a substantial theory of health promotion.**

----------------◆----------------

So I am, I promise, going to answer your second question Diane – which leaves your first. I'm pleased you brought this up because I do not wish to appear discourteous, though I suppose I'm bound to. Why am I so harsh in my criticisms of other health promotion writers? And isn't this destructive? Let me answer this by saying a little more about health promotion's lack of an analytic tradition.

I don't think there can be any argument about this. Health promotion is rarely debated philosophically and so the really tough questions are not asked: they are not asked of one health promoter by another, and they are rarely asked consistently by individual health promoters about their own practices. And in those cases where health promoters – like James Campion – do try to ask tough questions it is very hard for them to find the philosophical support they need to get decent answers: there are no courses to attend, and no good books to read on the philosophy of health promotion.

If you look at health promotion books and journals, with only very minor exceptions those writers who are interested in health promotion theory do not debate between themselves, rather they _cite_ numerous references which they assume support their own ideas, or which they believe their work adds to. It is almost as if it is subconsciously agreed that the health promotion edifice _needs_ a coat of theoretical harmony. So author X refers to author A's models of this, author B's approach to that, author C's method of doing this, and does not look for inconsistencies because he has faith that since they are all health promoting they must somehow be in tune. But I think I have shown clearly enough that this isn't so. Indeed, many health promotion writers agree with me up to a point. They worry about health promotion being diverse and 'ideological'. Yet in the end they still write as if there is a single field called health promotion. But obviously there isn't.

Such _false consensus_ can only happen in a field that does not have a culture of analysis. And without a reflective culture it seems to me that there also develops a strength-sapping tendency to defer to other people's ideas – however half-baked they are. And this, in my view, must change if progress is to come. I can see no other way forward.

If health promotion is to become a theoretically informed profession, criticism must flourish. And this means that _bad_ theories and _bad_ thinking must be exposed. This is hardly something to be ashamed of – it is expected and encouraged in other academic disciplines – in science, in philosophy, in mathematics – in these fields people put forward the best ideas they can in the best form they can and they expect to be criticised. Some (admittedly a minority) openly welcome criticism because they know they will learn from it. Some, of course, take criticisms personally – and sometimes it _is_ true that criticisms are meant _both_ professionally and personally – academia seems to attract more than its share of small-minded people. However, inquiry done in the proper spirit offers _and_ invites criticisms which are not even the slightest _ad hominem_. And this is the spirit in which I make my criticisms of some of the ideas of some contemporary health promotion writers. I do so knowing that it is frowned upon in this field, but I do it in the conviction that this is the only honest route to the development of a subject area. If people put forward untenable thoughts they should expect to have them scrutinised and criticised – I certainly do. Nothing I write is intended to cause personal offence.

But all this is by the way. The demolition is only the first part of the process, and not the most interesting either. Bear with me a little longer. Let me explain some more about prejudice, values and political philosophy in health promotion, and then the stage will be set for the construction of a sustained and practical _theory_ of health promotion.

———————— ◆ ————————

Message Ends

Prejudice First, Evidence Second

What Drives Health Promotion?

Health promotion theorists continue to skirt around one of the most fundamental questions of all: *what drives health promotion – evidence or values?* Because they fail to address this central issue head on, they remain deeply ambivalent about health promotion's inspiration.

At first sight such ambiguity is surprising, since there are really only two possible answers:

1. **Evidence drives health promotion** – some conditions and behaviours are *as a matter of fact* unhealthy; therefore health promoters must be opposed to them.
2. **Values drive health promotion** – people's values *determine* what is taken to be good or bad health; health promoters' values set health promotion priorities, health priorities do not set themselves.

There is a third alternative – that evidence and values drive health promotion simultaneously – but this is an incoherent position, as Chapter Six will explain in detail.

It should already be plain enough from the health promotion plans discussed in the previous chapter that the correct answer is 2: *values drive health promotion*. But, as study of almost all health promotion literature – official and 'radical' – makes painfully clear, this is hardly ever thought to be so. Of course all health promotion theorists and authorities, apart from those directly in State employ, acknowledge that health promotion involves values *to some extent*. But most of them *also* want to say that health promotion is not necessarily driven by values, and that there are factual health problems which all health promoters *must* see as problems.

Until this pervasive ambiguity is dispelled – until health promotion answers the *evidence or values?* question unequivocally – health promotion's essentially political nature will remain at least partially hidden. Part Two of *Health Promotion: Philosophy, Prejudice and Practice* attempts to show – step-by-step – what ought to be obvious already: health promotion is simply not possible unless its advocates hold deep political prejudices. All health promotion – even the most routine and mundane – is based on one political philosophy or another.

EXPOSING PREJUDICE STEP BY STEP

Consider the first answer to the *evidence or values?* question:

Health Promotion, Second Edition: David Seedhouse
© 2004 John Wiley & Sons, Ltd: ISBNs 0 470 84732 8 (HB); 0 470 84733 6 (PB)

EVIDENCE DRIVES HEALTH PROMOTION   ᠎

This point of view tends to be held by five main groups:

a. Government and other official health promoters
b. The news-media
c. The general public
d. Health promotion theorists (note, however, that virtually every member of this group gives this answer only *sometimes* and *inconsistently* – they also want to hold that *values drive health promotion*)
e. Many (though not all) health promotion practitioners.

Those who hold that *evidence drives health promotion* are likely to regard disease and illness as *objectively* bad, and to believe that health promotion's main supporting roots have grown out of basic public health measures – out of nineteenth- and twentieth-century battles against polluted food and water, poor hygiene and sanitation. To these groups health promotion looks straightforward enough. It seems to be an adjunct to good medicine – its army of workers dedicated to ensuring, by good preventive work, that the least possible number of patients present themselves at the doors of the medical profession. If there are any theoretical questions to be asked about health promotion, they concern the extent to which its various techniques are effective and efficient.[46]

Some of these groups (particularly a and b) may also be of the view that while there are activists on the margins of health promotion who make use of the obvious links between poor living conditions and high levels of morbidity to fuel political campaigns against social injustice, health promotion is only *circumstantially* political. That is, they think *it just so happens* that a disproportionate amount of preventable disease occurs in areas of greatest poverty, but the ultimate point of health promotion is to be against disease and illness wherever – and in whatever context – it occurs. Some methods may be more overtly political than others, but these are superficial differences. In the end, these groups believe that all health promotion techniques are directed first toward a *common* end: the reduction of morbidity and mortality.

Those who think *evidence drives health promotion* see the general picture of health promotion shown in Fig. 7.

More specifically still, those who believe *evidence drives health promotion* see the task of health promotion as in Fig. 8.

It is believed that health promotion has a core subject matter that just *is* a problem. The only choices are about which part of the core a particular health promoter tries to tackle, and which method she adopts to tackle it. Evidence of ill-health always comes first, values are secondary. It is only in the choice of method where the political element enters (encourage more exercise? encourage sensible eating? lobby super-markets? campaign against manufacturers who use saturated fats and salt excessively? encourage vegetarianism? expose corruption and cruelty amongst meat producers?).

Health Promotion's Tasks Are Generated In This Order

First: There is evidence of preventable health problems (this evidence is either factual or highly probable – and it is health promotion's main drive)

Second: There are strategies designed to deal with the preventable problems (there is usually a *choice* of strategy, and values may be *one of* the factors influencing the choice)

And in recent years, but still of secondary interest to most working health promoters

Third: There are additional strategies meant to promote the greatest possible health (sometimes described as 'positive health' or 'well-being') even where there are no existing problems

---

Figure 7 The (mistaken) perception that health promotion is driven by evidence

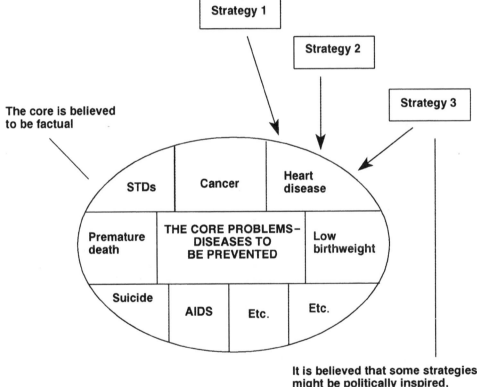

Figure 8 Health promotion's task as it looks to those who think it is evidence-driven

Reinforcement

This perception has been reinforced in mainstream health promotion literature over the years, even as the so-called movement has become more aware of its political influences. Tones and Tilford, for example, devote over 40 pages to 'the ideology of health promotion' in the opening section of their book, observing that different ideologies have underpinned different forms of health education over the years. They explain: 'It is clear...from even a cursory glance at models of health education that choice of model reflects underlying ideology'.[11] They even go so far as to quote openly left-wing writers who have accused the whole health promotion enterprise of supporting the capitalist social system. Yet they nevertheless fail to see the implication that health promotion cannot therefore be 'evidence-driven'. Rather they affirm – with convention – that what counts in the end is the prevention of *morbidity*, however politically radical the model. It is in this vein, for example, that they offer examples of successful health promotion they believe proponents of 'the radical model' might offer:

> The first example concerns healthy diet.
>
> A standard preventive model would seek to persuade individuals to adopt a prudent diet in order to minimize the likelihood of their falling prey to a number of dietary related diseases. The classic victim blaming approach would, in exhorting people to eat wisely, ignore the environmental circumstances which either promoted the consumption of unhealthy food or prevented people from adopting a healthy diet. A radical approach would set out to tackle those unhealthy environmental determinants of poor nutritional status. As Charles and Kerr (1986) have demonstrated in their research into the experience of 200 British women acting as nutritional gatekeepers for their families, ignorance of what constitutes healthy food is not the problem. Real barriers to choice included one or more of the following: accessibility and cost of healthy food; problems with food labelling or lack of it; relegation of the importance of providing healthy foods in the context of other social and domestic pressures; feelings of powerlessness.
>
> Effective radical nutrition education would, therefore, be judged by such measures as (in descending order of radicalism): decrease in poverty; successful battle with food manufacturers seeking to promote junk food and empty calories in western countries and formula baby milk and diarrhoea medicines in developing countries; providing a full range of healthy foods (preferably subsidized) at retail outlets and in the context of institutional catering; proper food labelling.[11]

They also offer other examples, including 'consciousness raising' about child cancer, teaching workers to monitor dust levels in textile factories, and women's health pressure-group work to allow women time to deliberate over whether or not they wish to be sterilised. What is most interesting about all these examples is not the rather bizarre idea that nutrition education can decrease poverty and the rest, but that the pay-off is *not* seen as ultimately political (even though the means used might bring about some desired social changes along the way). The final profit, even for the most radical model, is seen by those who think evidence comes first as being to do with nutrition, disease and the concerns of medicine (a decrease in poverty is not of itself seen to be to do with health but is thought of as a *means* to the end of better nutrition, and this in turn is seen as a means to better 'medical health').

VALUES DRIVE HEALTH PROMOTION

A few theorists consistently offer the second answer: *values drive health promotion*. Yet despite the fact that they are obviously right, their articles read as pleas from the wilderness, and mainstream health promotion goes steadily on, hardly ever pausing to consider that its work might be seen as controversial by those who disagree with its aims.[47]

Russell Caplan has recently argued that unless we try to understand the link between health promotion and political processes we will:

> ...remain forever lost in that mire of illusory technique which leads nowhere, and simply confirms and perpetuates the dominance of the status quo in health education/promotion and related concerns.[48]

Quite so. It is democratically unacceptable for governments to use public money without consultation to fund politically inspired projects which they claim to be value-neutral. But of course they do it, and will continue to do it unless health promotion gets its theoretical act together.

The main reason conventional health promotion gets away with its claim to be driven by evidence is that we are so accustomed to think of diseases and illnesses as objective. But there are other reasons too – one of which is that there are two very different versions of the *values drive health promotion* position. These may be called the *Stacey version* (after the sociologist most responsible for its spread in recent years) and the *fundamentalist version*.

The Stacey Version of 'Values First'

It is received wisdom, in many fields of social science, that we human beings do not perceive the world neutrally. Rather what we see is shaped by our social values. For example:

> *The social construction of medical reality*
>
> ...our basic concepts about the world – including those of medicine – are socially derived.
>
> ...seeing, experiencing or knowing the world is not a passive process. If the average layman is asked to describe a chair he will describe a structure with a seat, four legs and a back. A scientist interested in ergonomics or in mechanical engineering might describe a totally different perception. The structure described depends on preconceived ideas built up from knowledge and life experience in a particular social context.
>
> A middle-class child of a stable marriage might describe marriage in terms of a union between one man and one woman characterized by human exchanges which reflect consideration, compassion and endearment. The child of a broken marriage in the slums of Glasgow might describe the same phenomenon in terms of drunkenness, argument and physical violence. In both these examples the individual concerned perceives the physical structure or personal relationship in terms that reflect his own personal experiences in the social setting in which he is brought up. When he looks at chairs or at marriages he has already defined both subjects in the light of his experience and relates what he sees to his preconceived ideas.
>
> This point is of crucial importance for it means that what we see or know of the world is in part a product of how we organize or classify it. Furthermore, how we organize our sense data is not immutably fixed by some biological parameters, as we can observe other societies with other patterns or see differences within our own cultures over a period of time. It seems that in various ways – from parents, from schools, from our social environment – we learn how to see the world. Our knowledge, attitudes and beliefs, though they might seem to be very personal and individual, in fact derive from society. In this way our reality is 'socially constructed' and this construction forms the basis of one aspect of sociological study.[49]

In other words, most social scientists believe that ideas specific to one culture at one time (say to Western science in the eighteenth century or to Chinese medicine in the thirteenth century) 'convert' the physical and social world into what *seems* to be objective truth, but is not: as we interpret what we observe from *particular* scientific and moral points of view so we create a *particular* form of reality. If we were to interpret from different points of view then we would create a different reality.

Here is a quote from a standard textbook, illustrative of this sociological perspective:

> Taussig[50] argued that biomedicine, as practised in the West, 'reproduce[s] a political ideology in the guise of a science of (apparently) "real things". This process of turning 'ideas' into 'real things' within the language that we use (both for thought and communication with others) is termed 'reification'. Reification is the process of taking a complex and amorphous mixture of observed events, experiences, accounts and ideas, conceptually turning them...into a 'thing', and then giving that 'thing' a name (e.g. anorexia, pre-menstrual tension and post-traumatic shock syndrome). (Reification does not)...happen randomly or in a neutral fashion – they are not mere practical solutions to practical problems (such as finding a convenient name for a new phenomenon). While they may seem commonsensical... they (construct) and then (promote) a particular version of reality. In other words they are *ideological* in their impact, not just 'naming names' but...constraining people to see the world in a particular way.

> Young[51] used the illustration of the concept of 'stress' to argue that ideas like this allow the medical establishment to emphasize and highlight certain features of our social world. By treating 'stress' as a *personal* problem (requiring individual solutions), it becomes possible to deny and cover up other possibilities – such as being exploited in the workplace or in one's relationships. By believing themselves and presenting to others an image of their own explanatory system as 'incontrovertible fact', the dominant healers in a society can marginalize rival systems, treating them not just as inferior, but 'not really medicine at all'.[52]

Margaret Stacey argues that because we know the world can be 'constructed' in alternative ways it is essential that we do not study it only from *particular* perspectives:

> In order both to get as detached a view as possible upon our own health-care arrangements and to understand the nature of health and healing in a general way, it is essential to avoid ethnocentricity.[53]

If we see things only from one ethnic bias this will inevitably lead to the 'reification' Taussig talks of. To avoid this Stacey recommends that we should try to achieve impartiality by assuming that:

> ...the beliefs and practices of all peoples, formally trained or not, scientific or not, [are] of equal value and should be judged in the first instance by their own internal logic...Members of a group are liable to imagine that the way things are done by them is 'natural' and 'right' and perhaps even the 'best'...When, however, we come to study our institutions and those of others systematically, we have to suspend this belief, for otherwise we would work with an 'absolutism' which is inimical to proper scholarship.[53]

Now this is certainly an appropriate caution to those health promotion writers who see no difficulty in stating that their own preferences are obviously the best,[6] but if Stacey's view is maintained consistently (as it must be if it is to be worth anything) then it is self-defeating.[54] The problem is this. Stacey's point is that we are all biased and must try not to be. However, to be consistent, the belief that all beliefs and practices should be thought of as being of equal value must be just as biased as any other. Since there is, according to Stacey and her disciples, no way to know whether the statement:

> ...the beliefs and practices of all peoples, formally trained or not, scientific or not, [are] of equal value and should be judged in the first instance by their own internal logic...

is true or not, why assume it to be correct? Why assume that the beliefs and practices of all peoples are of *equal* value? Why not, for instance, start with the assumption that all beliefs and practices outside your culture are *better* than your own? Or why not assume they are worse?

If you say that there is such a thing as 'proper scholarship' then you are committed to the view that there is necessarily also 'improper scholarship' – presumably the sort of scholarship that does *not* regard all beliefs and practices as *prima facie* equal. But it is logically impossible (even 'in the first instance') to hold both that all beliefs and practices are of equal value *and* that there is 'improper' and 'proper' scholarship.

Health Promotion and the Stacey Line

In those health promotion circles which take the Stacey line it is frequently said to be inappropriate to hold *any* prejudice. The thinking is that a prejudiced health promoter will not be able to appreciate other points of view, and that this is a major problem in a profession which intervenes in the lives of people who may not share the professional's prejudices. Not only will the prejudiced health promoter cut herself off from potentially enriching experiences offered by alternative perspectives, but she will never be able to understand the thinking and actions of those clients who do not have the same values as she does, and might even damage clients through her inflexibility. She might even insist that a certain behaviour – one which is important to her client in ways that the health promoter cannot comprehend – is *definitely* 'bad for health'.

Linda Ewles and Ina Simnett worry about this possibility, and so seek to justify an anti-prejudice stance. Notice how theirs is essentially the Stacey position:

> ...the imposition of medical values on the client [frequently]...means the imposition of middle-class values on working-class people, and the ethical justification for this is doubtful. For example, losing weight and lowering blood pressure may be the most important thing to a doctor, but drinking beer in the pub with friends may be far more important to his overweight, middle-aged, unemployed patient. Who is to say which set of values is 'right' – the doctor or his patient? Whose life is it anyway?[55]

The Fundamentalist Version of 'Values First'

Those who believe that health promotion is sometimes driven by values *and* that it is morally right to hold at least some of them – object strongly to the idea that the task of the health promoter is simply to allow people to decide for themselves what is healthy. *Fundamentalists* fret that some people will decide inappropriately. Downie et al., for instance, criticise Ewles and Simnett as follows. They first quote them as saying:

> Traditional teaching operates in the hope that the 'right' attitudes and values will be 'caught' by learners. In contrast, we suggest that health education requires people to think critically about their values and build up their own value system.[6,51]

And then roundly condemn them:

> Social work literature in a similar vein suggests that in dealing with clients it is important to be 'non-judgemental'. Now, if the assumption here is that any set of values is as good as any other then it is not an assumption which is consistent with health education or promotion, or indeed any sort of education whatsoever. Certainly, it is important that people should be encouraged to think critically about their values, and although our predecessors in health education did not have such imaginative methods as are nowadays recommended for values-clarification there is no reason to think that the encouragement of critical appraisal has not always been part of health education. What does need to be questioned however is the phrase 'build up their own value system' and the correlative idea of the non-judgemental attitude.

> ...health education and other aspects of health promotion are activities committed to certain views on the nature of the self and what makes it flourish, and to views of a well-ordered society. No doubt there are a large number of acceptable ways of living one's life, all of which lead to the flourishing of human personality, but not *every* way is acceptable. Similarly, there are no doubt several acceptable forms of social and political organization, but not *every* way is acceptable to those involved in health promotion. If these positions are not shared by health educators and health promoters, then why adopt slogans such as 'Be all you can be', or why deplore the 'health divide'? In other words, health promoters cannot consistently accept the 'sneer' quotes in Ewles and Simnett's phrase ' "right" attitudes', for health promoters must believe that there are right attitudes to the individual and to society, or go out of business.[6]

Downie's view is the very opposite of Stacey's position – even though both *at times* argue that values come before the evidence. Where Stacey argues (sometimes) that any value (and indeed any practice) is in principle as good as any other, Downie believes that health is a 'positive value'. Proper health promotion, for Downie: '...is strongly normative; it endeavours to persuade people to adopt certain lifestyles, and is committed to furthering certain values'.[6] In other words, health is a better value than most (and possibly all) other values.

PREJUDICE CAN BE GOOD

Thus far we have a rather confusing picture. There is a key question: *what drives health promotion, evidence or values?* and several different answers to it. In sum, these are:

A. *evidence drives health promotion*: behaviours such as smoking cigarettes and never taking exercise are *objectively* bad
B. *values drive health promotion version 1*: health promotion strategies are driven by values but there are no objective values – only alternative sets of beliefs and practices. Therefore health promotion must not impose alien values on other people but empower those people to work out and act on their own values
C. *values drive health promotion version 2*: health promotion strategies are, and should be, driven by values. Some sets of values are better than others. What's more, there are objective values – values that are fundamental to health promotion. Health promoters must be committed to furthering these values even if this means overriding the values of some other people
D. *both evidence and values drive health promotion*: this view, in practice, is held both by those who take the *Stacey line* and by those who take the *fundamentalist line*. Study the work of any of these groups of writers (Ewles and Simnett's book[55] is a good

example) and in places you will see – in addition to their 'values first' stance – an *unquestioning* acceptance that some behaviours and some conditions are – as a matter of evidence – unhealthy. These behaviours and conditions are taken to be obviously bad – no argument is thought necessary to establish this.

THE WRONG ANSWERS

Answer A is false, B, if taken seriously, renders health promotion pointless, C is opinion dressed up to be absolute truth and D is incoherent. So what is going wrong, and is there a more plausible way forward?

The way ahead lies in *prejudice*, a feature of health promotion which none of the alternative positions A–D properly understands. For answer A prejudice does not come into the picture – one cannot be prejudiced about the truth, it says. One can be prejudiced only if one fails to perceive the truth. According to answer B prejudice is bad if it is allowed to overrule a different prejudice. For answer C prejudices are good if they are held by the group that gives the answer, bad if they are not. And for answer D evidence somehow either negates prejudice (Ewles and Simnett, for instance, accept that some evidence can compel health promotion activities) or justifies it (as we shall see, Downie et al. argue – erroneously – that the professional goals of health promotion *inspire* its political position).

But prejudice is more than good or bad, and much more than a matter of opinion. There are different sorts of prejudice, only two of which have a place in health promotion.

TYPES OF PREJUDICE

The rather hopeless situation described above persists because of a failure to distinguish three different types of prejudice:

1. **Necessary Prejudice**. A *necessary prejudice* is any belief on which a person grounds her reasoning and/or actions. Prejudice, in this sense, is a prerequisite for any thoughtful action (for anything other than instinctive or intuitive behaviour). In this sense prejudice is a 'pre-judgement' without which it is impossible to think about anything. Thus my belief that the sun will rise tomorrow is a prejudice, it is a prejudice that my friends are trustworthy, and a prejudice of mine that fire burns wood. Unless I judge these things to be true I cannot act in some of the ways I do. I might be wrong, but my pre-judgement, as I listen to my friend's advice not to build a north-facing log cabin in drought-stricken bush, is that I am right.

   A *necessary prejudice* may be either inescapable (for instance, in the sense that in everyday life it is simply absurd not to assume that heavy objects will fall to earth) or chosen (I choose to believe in the fidelity of my friends). Whatever the case, a prejudice should be considered necessary if it appears to be just not possible to act without recourse to it.

2. **Blinkered Prejudice**. A *blinkered prejudice* is a belief which is held to be objectively true. The person who holds a *blinkered prejudice* will not alter or abandon it whatever the evidence or whatever the argument he hears against it. Such a prejudice can be about physical matters – for instance, a person might believe absolutely that wood always burns when exposed to flame – or about matters of value – for instance, a person might believe absolutely that smoking cigarettes is always an unhealthy behaviour.

It is possible to make a further distinction in this category: a *blinkered prejudice* can be held either unknowingly or knowingly. Without realising it, most of us hold countless unexamined and *not necessary* prejudices (a common example is the belief that other races and cultures are inferior to our own). We also hold countless prejudices which we *have* deliberated over at one time or another, but which we have decided need no further reflection (a health promotion example might be the belief that 'the medical model is inadequate').

Necessary and *blinkered prejudices* can be identical. For example, the prejudice that it is not normally possible to walk up a smooth vertical surface can be necessary to the safe negotiation of the physical environment, and can be held in a blinkered fashion, as an incontrovertible fact, without ever causing any practical or moral difficulties.

What is most important, though, is not the *content* of the prejudices but *how* they are held. Those who have open minds will hold at least some of their prejudices (certainly those which are obviously based on values) tentatively, while those with firmly closed minds and fixed opinions will be entirely happy with *blinkered prejudice* of either sort.

3. **Reasoned Prejudice**. A *reasoned prejudice* is a position arrived at through reflection on either evidence or values or both, is open to revision, and is a prejudice which the holder is continually prepared to question and to defend if he believes it to be defensible.

Only the first and third forms ought to be countenanced by health promoters.

THE PATH BETWEEN THE DEAD-END ANSWERS

There is a view of social reality between the two 'values first' and 'evidence first' extremes which I believe to be true. My thinking is this. Firstly, there is no doubt that if we are to make sense of the world human beings must always interpret the evidence we receive in one way or another. There is also no doubt that not all interpretations are equal. It is possible to identify better or worse interpretations, and *sometimes* it is possible to say that our interpretations are completely right or completely wrong.

We interpret sound, for instance, through our physical auditory mechanisms – which means we can hear only certain sounds and only in certain ways – and we may also interpret what these sounds mean (if we hear breaking glass we tend to think that there has been an accident, if we hear laughter we tend to think someone is happy – though we may find out that we are mistaken on either count). Furthermore, we do not interpret only raw data, we also interpret the *content* of what people say to us. For example, we commonly interpret another person's point of view about something against our own point of view about it. If someone thinks in exactly the same way as I do about a cricket match I am inclined to think of him as a good judge: equally, if someone believes the British or American social systems to be the embodiment of all that is just then I would regard her with deep suspicion.

However, despite the fact that we are bound physically and psychologically to interpret the evidence we encounter, certain things are *indisputable* – both about cricket matches and in the observation of physical and social conditions – and certain other things are always *open to debate* because they are points of view. For instance, it is an *indisputable fact* that Chris Cairns hit a six off the bowling of Shane Warne during a cricket match in 2001, and it is also a *plain fact* that some people in the UK, the USA, India and elsewhere, live in considerable luxury while others have no choice but to sleep on the streets. To deny these things makes no sense at all. However, whether Cairns was lucky, whether Warne bowled a bad ball, whether it is right to award people very high wages for their special talents or knowledge, whether some people deserve to suffer poor living conditions: sooner or later this sort of consideration boils down to disagreement *beyond* the evidence. To illustrate some more: that persistent heavy drinking is likely to cause disease has been established by epidemiological research as firmly as that particular science can establish anything, but whether such drinking is bad for a person's health depends upon one's interpretation of health, and this in turn depends upon how one thinks life ought to be lived. If a person chooses a 'hard living' lifestyle, even if that person becomes diseased as a result, this does not automatically mean that his was a bad choice (not if this is the life he genuinely wanted to live). The *causation* of the disease is a matter of evidence or even fact, the *interpretation* of the behaviour that caused the disease depends upon what the interpreter values – that is, it depends on her prejudice.

And so it is that facts and values, evidence and moral beliefs intertwine. *Sometimes they can be separated out completely; other times, as in judgements about a person's health, they can never be fully separated because a judgement about a person's health necessarily depends upon evidence* **and** *the interpretation of that evidence.*

Sooner or later prejudice just has to enter any deliberation about health care policy, therefore prejudice is necessary in health promotion and therefore the *point* of health promotion will always be open to dispute. Ask yourself: how could anyone seek to promote health without holding a prejudice of some kind? Can anyone promote health without having an opinion about whether one way of living is better than another? It is not possible. The evidence is not mute – but it never speaks entirely for itself.

BACK-TO-FRONT HEALTH PROMOTION: HEALTH PROMOTION'S BIG MISTAKE

The health promotion 'movement's' biggest theoretical mistake is to misunderstand its basic inspiration. As we have seen, almost everyone – for at least part of the time – believes this to be the case (Fig. 7).

Health Promotion's Tasks Are Generated In This Order

First: There is evidence of preventable health problems (this evidence is either factual or highly probable – and it is health promotion's main drive)

Second: There are strategies designed to deal with the preventable problems (there is usually a *choice* of strategy, and values may be *one of* the factors influencing the choice)

And in recent years, but still of secondary interest to most working health promoters

Third: There are additional strategies meant to promote the greatest possible health (sometimes described as 'positive health' or 'well-being') even where there are no existing problems

---

Figure 7   The (mistaken) perception that health promotion is driven by evidence

But in fact this (Fig. 9) is the case.

Health Promotion's Tasks Are Generated In This Order

First: Health promoters hold particular values and political philosophies

Second: There is evidence of preventable health problems (this evidence is selected *according to* values and political philosophy – even the decision to call something a health problem or not is thus inspired[56] though this is not to say that the evidence is entirely shaped by prejudice – there can be better and worse reasons to intervene)

Third: Strategies designed to deal with preventable health problems are selected according to values, political philosophy and evidence – the key questions are: do we think this ought to be done *and* will it work?

And in recent years, but still of secondary interest to most working health promoters

Fourth: There are additional strategies to promote the greatest possible health (sometimes described as 'positive health' or 'well-being'), even where there are no existing problems

---

Figure 9   Health promotion is driven by values

Note that this fourth task (in Fig. 9), when perceived with values in the right place as in Fig. 6, can be seen to be unarguably politically inspired. As we shall see in Chapter Six, there has recently been a move to talk of 'positive health promotion' or 'well-being promotion', in an effort to break free of 'disease models'. However, once the grounding in disease is lost, *all that remains* as health promotion's inspiration are points of view about how people should behave, associate and act toward each other: and this is exactly the stuff of political philosophy.

More specifically, health promotion's strategies are generated by values (Fig. 10).

Figure 10 Health promotion's strategies are generated by values

The core of health promotion is not factual, but essentially prejudiced. Different health promoters hold different sets of prejudices. But whatever the set, it is this which inspires both the target and the strategy of health promotion work. Sometimes this is obviously so (in the case of 'consciousness-raising' about social injustice, for instance), sometimes less obviously (non-smoking strategies), but in all cases it is political philosophy (however implicit) which fires health promotion. It is only by understanding this that it is truly possibly to see the point of health promotion, and only by understanding this that one can construct an honest and workable theory of health promotion.

It is not really so difficult:

1. (Against the *Stacey line*) Not all values are equal – some can be more thoroughly justified than others (this is what moral philosophy is all about) and some – when applied – produce better practical results than others
2. It is necessary to hold at least some values in order to promote anything
3. It is necessary to take the fullest possible account of the evidence to work effectively
4. (Against the *fundamentalist line*) Health promotion does *not* have a necessary core set of values
5. Health promotion cannot be equally driven by both evidence and values
6. Health promotion is essentially political – the only honest and open way forward is to admit this – to embrace it, and so see the *correct* generation of health promotion's tasks.

The question now is this: *which* values should drive health promotion? What are the choices, and how can the health promoter decide between them?

The Political Tap Roots of Health Promotion

EXERCISE FIVE

HEALTHY CITIES OR POLITICAL CITIES?

Think about what a 'healthy city' would look like.

1. How would it be organised? Who would organise it? What could its citizens do? What would they not be able to do?

Now:

2. Explain the practical steps which, in your opinion, would be required to convert your own city, as it presently is, into a healthy city.
   As you think this through, notice the many practical obstacles that emerge, and which must be overcome if your plan is to succeed.
   (Note: do not try to convert an entire city – choose between 5 to 10 key features only.)
3. List possible objections to your plan that might be given by people who do not share your 'vision'. In other words, clearly identify the values that inform your plan, contrast these with the values of at least one group of people who would design a different sort of healthy city, and then explain how your opponents might draw on their values (and on evidence, probabilities and hearsay too) to argue against you.

By these means you will come to gain a more realistic picture of what might be involved in a genuine enterprise to develop a healthy city, and you will have laid bare the essentially political nature of the task.

Teaching notes for: Healthy Cities or Political Cities?

This exercise can be used for a variety of educational purposes. You might use it to draw out students' basic values; or to discover – by examining their practical

continues

Health Promotion, Second Edition: David Seedhouse
© 2004 John Wiley & Sons, Ltd: ISBNs 0 470 84732 8 (HB); 0 470 84733 6 (PB)

continued

proposals – the extent to which students believe health promoters have a role in improving cities and city life; or you might use it as an additional exercise to help students learn to disentangle evidence from values. For instance, you might ask students to identify desirable goals and then to say which aspects of these goals are to do with evidence, and which are *preferences* no evidence will ever shake. Essentially though, this exercise comes at this particular point in the book specifically to help you highlight the fact that health promotion is driven first by political values and only secondly by evidence.

The exercise has three main parts. The first two are practical. Only the third is meant to address questions of political philosophy directly. This is quite deliberate. These are not easy exercises for student or teacher, and the practical elements can be a welcome relief from intellectual puzzling. In any case, the practical challenge is a prerequisite. The practical steps need at least to have been outlined in order to begin to demonstrate that any imaginary healthy city must be fundamentally politically inspired.

The suggested use of the exercise is as follows:

Dependent on time available, after you have explained the general intent of the session, have students discuss the good and bad aspects of the city or cities most familiar to them (if you have a two-hour session, which would be ideal, devote around 10 minutes to this preliminary task). Following this, and without pointing the students in any particular direction, have them spend time (around 20 minutes in a two-hour session) either individually or in small groups, working out the practical steps required to convert their city (or nearest city) into a healthy city, or at least into a healthier city. Then allow some time (perhaps another 20 minutes or so in a two-hour session) for a free discussion about why one city can be said to be healthier than another, why certain practical goals have been chosen before others, about the extent to which a healthy city has to be a compromise between the alternative visions of different citizens (alternatives will inevitably emerge in anything other than the smallest groups), about the balance between medical services and other enabling services, and so on.

Next – and preferably after a break – comes the hardest part. In this section of the session your aim should be to draw out students' political values by encouraging objections, based on values, to the ideas they have generated. Individual students could be encouraged (and supported if necessary) to criticise their own schemes as if through the eyes of others. Students in groups could criticise the plans of their colleagues. Whatever the case, your role is to focus attention on the way in which the students' practical suggestions do not simply come out of the blue, but are inspired by deep-seated understandings of how people should live together in communities (i.e. to show that their suggestions are based on their own political philosophies, even if these are not articulated in the way a political philosopher might articulate them).

continues

continued

AN EXAMPLE

It is obviously impossible to predict the responses you will get from your students. What is predictable, however, is that these will depend on their political prejudices. If you know your students well you will probably already have an idea of how their cities will look.

In order to demonstrate the sorts of teaching tactic you might employ, here is an edited transcript of a response from one of my own students, and an indication of the way I chose to use it to point out the source of her ideas.

———————— ◆ ————————

STUDENT: I live in Auckland, New Zealand. I don't think my city is particularly healthy even though a lot of people find it a very desirable place to live. In fact I think Auckland has got a lot less healthy over the last ten years.

What do I think is most wrong with it, with health in mind? Well that depends what you mean by health, doesn't it?...OK, for the sake of argument I decided to think of health basically as the opposite of disease and illness (not very fashionable I know, but there you are). With *this* in mind I'd say the following things are most wrong with Auckland at the moment:

- There are too many cars
- People drive irresponsibly and there are too many road accidents
- There is traffic pollution
- Far too many youngsters are idle – they smoke, drink and don't exercise
- The hospitals are seriously under-funded
- In some areas of Auckland there are soup kitchens, and some kids go to school with no shoes
- The people who get sickest quickest and die youngest are the Maori and Pacific Islanders
- Mentally ill people wander the streets these days, and many live rough under Grafton Bridge (*a large road bridge crossing a deep valley, under which it is possible to find some sort of shelter*)
- Women's health issues are given insufficient attention...

How would I convert Auckland into a healthy city? Right. Taking the problems in turn I'd ban private cars from entering a 2 km radius of the Aotea Centre (*the opera house*); I'd invest heavily in efficient electrical (pollution-free) public transport; I'd increase the traffic police and penalise dangerous driving heavily; I'd offer much better job opportunities to young people, to keep them off the streets and to give them something to do – maybe I'd even insist that they got jobs; I'd tax private health care heavily and rebuild the public hospital system so as to guarantee the best care NZ can offer to all kiwis; I'd abolish soup kitchens and ensure that everyone had enough good food to eat as a social right – and I'd give free shoes to all needy kids; I'd offer special support to

continues

continued

under-privileged ethnic groups – positive discrimination if you like; I'd provide properly managed integrated care for the mentally ill and no one would be discharged if they were at risk, and no one would have to, or be allowed to, live beneath Grafton Bridge; and I'd discriminate positively in favour of women's health too.

———————— ◆ ————————

In order to expose the political source of students' ideas for healthier cities, it is suggested that you encourage objections to their thoughts, and that you raise objections yourself if necessary. For example, if faced with my Auckland student, you might decide, as I did, to pose the following questions:

TEACHER: First of all, what have you got against the car? Surely private transport is one of the most liberating features of modern life. This, more than anything else, has enabled people to explore their environment in a way previously available only to the very rich. Surely the private car allows individual freedom and choice.

It's very authoritarian to ban cars from cities. Who are you to say that public transport is a good thing? What's so good about people being *forced* into close personal proximity if that's not what they want? How is that healthy?

. . . And what of the hospitals? They were public in the past and they weren't efficient. Now Aucklanders have much more choice. They can take out comprehensive private insurance plans and they'll get world class care in the best environments whenever they need it. It should be up to them to decide to take out insurance or not . . .

And why would you shut the soup kitchens? Your healthy city sounds like the 'City of Spongers' rather than the 'City of Sails' to me. You'd offer so many handouts that people would have no need to do anything – then they'd be even idler and have more time to drink and get fat, and get diabetes . . .

And the same goes for the mentally ill. Mental illness has always been used as an excuse for irresponsibility, for wastefulness, for ineptitude – you'd mollycoddle people so much that it would be seen as a good thing to be mentally ill – they'd get a warm bed, recreation, three meals a day . . .

———————— ◆ ————————

You may not choose to be so deliberately provocative as this, but you should aim to counter the student's suggestions about how to create a healthy city with objections that are *even more obviously politically inspired* than the student's. Then, when the student reacts, as she is bound to, it will be quite obvious that she must react at the political level too.

The picture of a healthy city my Auckland student had in mind was plainly *not* evidence driven. For a start she had to *select* the problems she chose from a great range of alternatives she could have chosen, she had to *interpret* this evidence as

continues

continued

indicative of an unhealthy city (and there is of course no *necessary* connection), and as she put forward her constructive position she had to make clear decisions about those things she would insist on if she had the power and those things she would not (and these decisions undoubtedly sprung *first* from her wishes, not from the external evidence). Thus, as our conversation developed, I was able to pull out at least the basis of the student's political philosophy, and to argue that without this she would not even have known where to *begin* to create a healthier Auckland. Her outlook, I said (and she agreed, in the end) was basically socialist and communitarian, and would require considerable state power and will to intervene in order to reduce the health inequalities (or just plain social inequalities) between citizens – and this would mean reducing the freedom of choice of certain sectors of the city's population in order to benefit the least well-off. This, and not a neutral view of bad health, would be necessary to change the organisation of her city for the better, according to her prejudices.

Whatever suggestions your students make for change in their chosen cities, they will be politically based. You should, therefore, be able to demonstrate this on each occasion.

TYPES OF HEALTH PROMOTION, AND THEIR BASES IN POLITICAL PHILOSOPHY

Once you understand that *values drive health promotion* it becomes possible to see the discipline's full depth. Despite appearances – despite the muddled models, despite the foreground processes, and despite the rhetoric – health promotion is essentially inspired by political values. But can any values underlie health promotion, or are there reasons to favour some ahead of others? Again, the answer to this question depends upon theory. If you have a specific theory of health promotion not any values can inspire your version of the discipline, and your theory will clearly explain the reasons for this. However, without a theory, advocates of any particular set of values can offer no better account of their choices than that they prefer them – and this is hardly a sufficient level of justification for the work of such an influential profession.

Partly to explain this further, and also to offer a guide to practising health promoters who wish to work out the political sources of what they do, there follows a discussion of different types of health promotion and their political bases.

FROM A DISTANCE

Speaking very generally, there are five alternative forms of health promotion, only three of which are particularly significant. These three may be called **medical health promotion**, **social health promotion** and **good life promotion** (Fig. 11). Of these **medical health promotion** is, as we have seen, often considered to be objective (or

```
┌─────────────────────────────────┐      ┌─────────────────────────────────┐
│ (1)  Medical Health Promotion   │      │ (2) Social Health Promotion     │
│                                 │      │                                 │
│      Health promotion should    │      │     Health promotion should     │
│      work against disease,      │      │     change the social world - it│
│      illness and injury         │      │     should challenge those      │
│                                 │      │     social injustices which     │
│                                 │      │     cause ill-health            │
└─────────────────────────────────┘      └─────────────────────────────────┘

           ┌─────────────────────────────────┐
           │ (3)  Good Life Promotion        │
           │                                 │
           │      Health promotion should    │
           │      seek to bring about        │
           │      'positive health' or       │
           │      'well-being': it should    │
           │      create 'good lives'        │
           └─────────────────────────────────┘

┌─────────────────────────────────┐      ┌─────────────────────────────────┐
│ (4) Go For It Health Promotion  │      │ (5) Mix 'n Match Health         │
│                                 │      │     Promotion                   │
│     Health promotion is         │      │                                 │
│     commonsense: it is a matter │      │     Health promotion is a matter│
│     of doing what obviously     │      │     of being theoretically      │
│     needs doing - too much      │      │     flexible in order to make   │
│     thinking gets in the way of │      │     the most of practical       │
│     the action                  │      │     opportunities               │
└─────────────────────────────────┘      └─────────────────────────────────┘
```

Figure II   Different forms of general health promotion

evidence-driven) because it aims to improve measurable aspects of people's lives – it seeks less disease, greater fitness, longer life and so on. However, while there *is* evidence to suggest that not smoking, eating less fat, and taking regular exercise may help prevent some clinical conditions, no evidence can ever demonstrate that such a lifestyle is the *best* way for a human being to live. Most varieties of **social health promotion** hope to 'reduce inequalities in health' by improving the lives of the least well-off members of society. Like the advocates of the more narrowly medical version, **social health promoters** often assume that work against disease is objectively desirable, and so requires no further justification: the epidemiology (the evidence) is frequently thought to 'speak for itself'. But again, although such work may seem unarguably moral to many[57] it does not seem this way to everyone[58] and is, therefore, *not* unarguably moral. **Social health promotion** is value-driven too.

The activities undertaken by both the **medical** and **social health promotion** forms imply – and their advocates sometimes openly express – the moral claim 'this is how people ought to live'. The third approach, however, is more consistently forthright. It is overtly driven by prejudice. **Good life promotion** takes health to be more than the absence of disease, and consequently sometimes recommends health promotion activities which do not have to have the primary goal of preventing or eliminating maladies. **Good life promoters** think that health promotion should enable the achievement of 'vital goals', promote 'fulfilling existence', create 'well-being' – that health promotion should go beyond work against disease to bring about 'good lives'.

The two other minor forms miscellaneously combine the other three. Devotees of the **mix 'n match** approach usually favour one of the forms over the others but will, where it seems prudent, adopt policies and prejudices from elsewhere, even when this is theoretically inconsistent (James Campion is a **mix 'n matcher**). Those who use the **go for it** (or **anti-theory**) approach *seem* not to care where their ideas come from so long as health (whatever they think this is) is promoted in some way, however most versions of **go for it** health promotion can readily be traced to one political outlook or another.

Some health promoters may regard the different types of health promotion as a reader of Fig. 11 sees them: as separate and simple. Seen like this, the health promoter who wants to combat health problems that are traditionally the concern of clinical science will want exclusively to pursue **medical health promotion**, the health promoter concerned with health problems he understands to be caused by social factors will want single-mindedly to pursue **social health promotion**, and so on. However, the boxes are very rough representations only. Combinations are possible: for instance 1 and 3, 2 and 4, 4 and 5, and 1 and 2 are often seen together.

Elsewhere in the health promotion literature different distinctions, combinations and labels can be found,[48,55,59] though they all seem to conform to the general pattern shown in Fig. 10. Indeed they must, since each is based ultimately in a political philosophy, and there seem to be only a limited number of political positions open to the human race.[60]

The true picture of health promotion and its politics is far more complex than Fig. 11 depicts. The philosophy of health promotion is as complicated as the philosophy of politics, and is therefore impossible to illustrate simply and quickly. Nevertheless, the following section is an attempt to 'map out' the key elements of health promotion's political foundations, at least in an elementary fashion.

THE POLITICAL BASES OF HEALTH PROMOTION

Fig. 11 might be thought of as a bird's eye view of health promotion: it shows the subject as if its various forms were displayed on the rooftops of tall, separate buildings. But, as one might expect, things look very different (and more substantial) when viewed from the side. Fig. 12, though grossly simplified, is meant to indicate that each apparently free-standing form must rest ultimately upon some set of political beliefs.

The links between sets of health promotion activities and various political outlooks are enormously varied and complex. Furthermore, the nature of the links, the precise content of each type of political philosophy, and the extent to which each form of health promotion is *meant* to be based on a particular philosophy, are all open to wide interpretation. To do them proper justice these matters require sustained academic discussion of an intensity beyond the scope of this book. The aim here is merely to demonstrate the basic connections and to show that *some* connections are inevitable. It is enough to establish an outline of health promotion's political philosophy, for once it is conceded that there must be some such outline health promotion will never be the

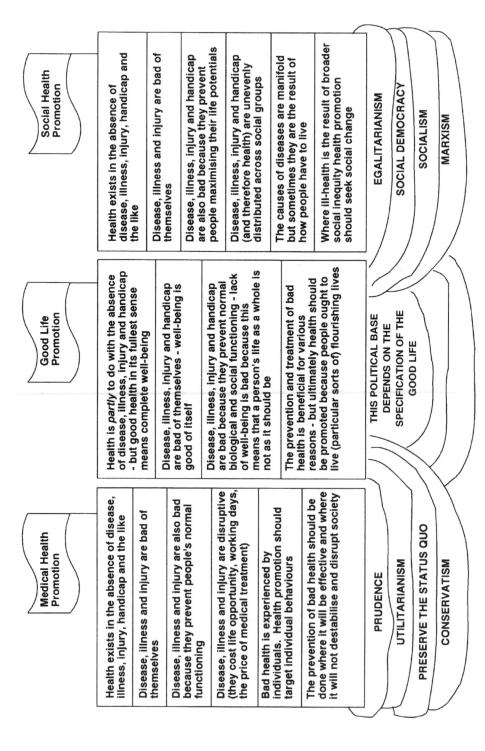

Figure 12   An elementary illustration of possible political bases of health promotion (only three forms depicted, for simplicity): on which base should the health promoter stand?

same again. And it is surely much more difficult to *deny* that the different forms are politically inspired than it is to assert it. If the inspiration of each type of health promotion is not broadly political then what is it?

SOME POLITICAL CONTENT

Although the details are perennially arguable, here is the possible content of each of the three main types of health promotion seen from the side (as depicted in Fig. 12). The nearer to ground, the more political they become. Indeed, if they did not stand on the ground of political philosophy none of them could stand at all.

MEDICAL HEALTH PROMOTION

Health exists in the absence of disease, illness, injury, handicap, and the like
Disease, illness and injury are bad in themselves
Disease, illness and injury are also bad because they prevent people's normal functioning
Disease, illness and injury are disruptive (they cost people normal life opportunities, and they cost nations both working days lost and the price of treatment and prevention)
Bad health is experienced by individuals. Therefore the basic target of strategies to improve people's health should be behavioural change/lifestyle change, in order to minimise social disruption
Prevention of bad health should be undertaken where it is shown to work and where it poses no threat to the stability of a society

The full nature of the underlying political philosophy of **medical health promotion** is clearly debatable, though the possible inspirations are by no means unlimited. The effects of **medical health promotion** in developed societies, for instance, are undoubtedly *not* revolutionary. This form of health promotion does not pose a challenge to the status quo in rich and stable societies, rather it supports it. Thus a plausible case could be made for the view that **medical health promotion** essentially emanates from a political philosophy of PRUDENCE, UTILITARIANISM, and the PRESERVATION OF THE STATUS QUO. In other words, it could be argued that **medical health promotion** is basically inspired by CONSERVATISM.

Of course, if a society did not offer medical care to all its population, and **medical health promoters** used the idea of health promotion to argue that it should, then **medical health promotion** could be more radical. It could, for instance, be inspired by, and try to foster, egalitarian ideals. Much depends upon the contexts in which the various forms are undertaken.

———————————— ◆ ————————————

ONE ILLUSTRATION OF MEDICAL HEALTH PROMOTION: THE HEALTH OF THE NATION

The upper levels (see Fig. 12) of the conservative version of this type of health promotion can be seen in almost any government-sponsored health promotion literature from almost any part of the Western world, and beyond (clear evidence of the usefulness of health promotion to reinforce existing social situations). The levels are very plainly displayed in the UK Government publication *The Health of the Nation*.[61] To discover its priorities it is enough to dip into the document at random.

Here, for instance, is the then UK government's idea of health:

Death

5.9 The commonest and most comprehensive measure of 'health' is that of life and death. National mortality data have been collected systematically since the first half of the 19th century. As well as 'crude' measures of numbers dying, health can be measured in terms of premature mortality, either by numbers of deaths below a certain age (typically 65 or 75), or else in terms of 'life years' lost...[61] [see Fig. 13]

A Health Strategy for England

Key Areas
5.4 The strategy will focus on key areas, judged against the following criteria:

First, the area should be a major cause of premature death or avoidable ill health (sickness and/or disability) either in the population as a whole or amongst specific groups of people;

and

Second, the area should be one where effective interventions are possible, offering significant scope for improvement in health;

and

Third, it should be possible to set *objectives* and *targets* in the chosen area and monitor progress towards achievement through indicators.[61]

The government thinks health is the opposite of disease, that interventions should be made only in those areas where they have already proven effective, and that improvements in health must be measurable (a stipulation which excludes – at a stroke – innumerable forms of improved health and life which the official line refuses to entertain).[62]

The government's health strategy: '...does not propose...to address every health...issue...(since)...little real progress would be likely to result...'.[61] and has

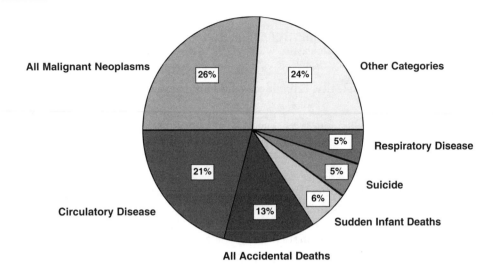

Figure 13   Distribution of years of life lost up to age 65 years*. By cause of death, England and Wales. All persons. 1988. *Death under 28 days excluded. Source: Office of Population Censuses and Surveys

identified 'four targets' only.[62] Given this, and despite the avowed intent to reduce 'health inequalities', it is difficult to imagine a more explicit statement of conservatism in the guise of health promotion. Governments and their statisticians know very well the extent and types of morbidity that result from poor housing and unemployment,[63] and how many road deaths and injuries are caused through excessive speed,[64] to give just two examples. Governments also know perfectly well that many people regard these as health issues, and they know too that these are matters about which much could be done to effect 'real progress' – given the will. But these concerns are not *seriously* discussed because the political philosophy on which this version of this form of health promotion is based simply does not allow it. In the 1991 document, the effects of unemployment are not monitored at all, and as for road accidents there are no specific targets (why not? this is a quantifiable area), only a section where the government says it will welcome *views* on targets:

> G.21 The Government would welcome views on a target or targets that might usefully be set:
> • should they look only as far as 2000, or would long-term development be better served by looking beyond that date? (*sic*)...
> • should targets be for the population generally, or for specific population groups (e.g. children, elderly people), or should both approaches be used?[61]

Such daft questions leave no doubt that the UK government is earnest only about (what it defines as) those key areas – death, sickness, disability – which are anyway the focus of (largely NHS) attention.

Given this reverence for conventional practice and the maintenance of existing priorities, it is no surprise that a major justification for **medical health promotion** in the UK is to reduce financial cost to the NHS:

Cost

5.12 A third measure of the burden of ill-health is cost, mainly cost to the NHS, although attempts are often made to measure wider social and economic costs (e.g. including lost production, social security etc.).[61]

And that the role of the Health Education Authority (now the Health Development Agency[65]) is to:

…provide direct public education, including the UK-wide mass media campaigns on HIV/AIDS. It fosters and supports other activities both nationally and locally. It can provide a framework for co-ordinated action, as with the Look After Your Heart programme.[61]

In other words the Health Education Authority does **medical health promotion** (and only **medical health promotion**), because (medical) ill-health can be costly and disruptive. Of course there are other reasons for trying to reduce disease and premature mortality, and presumably many of those who formulated this 'health strategy for England' will see their work as good for individuals – or just as good all round. However, in its cumulative effects on the population as a whole, **medical health promotion** is clearly done in order to preserve the present functions of society – both to ensure that as many people as possible can contribute to the system (in their place in the hierarchy) without being a burden on it, and also to ensure the stability of the system itself. (Note that I do not wish to argue here that this is a good or a bad thing – I am concerned only to show that it cannot be a *neutral* position.)

SOCIAL HEALTH PROMOTION

Health exists in the absence of disease, illness, injury, handicap, and the like
Disease, illness, injury and handicap are bad in themselves
Disease, illness, injury and handicap are also bad because they prevent people maximising their life potentials
Disease, illness, injury and handicap (and therefore health) are unevenly distributed across differently privileged social groups
The causes of disease, illness, injury and handicap are manifold. Sometimes, however, it can be shown that they are the result of how people either choose to or have to live
Where disease, illness, injury and handicap are the result of broader social inequities health promotion ought to attempt to change these social conditions (be they bad housing, poor community amenities, inadequate education, debilitating employment or whatever). Behavioural change is not necessarily out of the question but it is inappropriate to attempt behavioural change without at the same time attempting to remedy socially caused health inequalities, and therefore without at the same time attempting to empower the most unfortunate members of society to live healthier lives

The above is an illustration of the basic components of *one* possible variety of **social health promotion**. Different versions of social health promotion can be inspired by different varieties of ANARCHY,[66] SOCIAL DEMOCRACY, SOCIALISM, MARXISM and EGALITARIANISM,[67] and may have different bases dependent on their practical emphases, level of radicalism, and the context in which they are advocated. However, any form of **social health promotion** must have some grounding in a political outlook which begins by acknowledging that people are essentially *equal*, and can be understood not only as individuals but also as *communities*.

ONE ILLUSTRATION OF SOCIAL HEALTH PROMOTION: COMMUNITY DEVELOPMENT

Given an eye to see them, the connections between **social health promotion** and political philosophy are, if anything, even more obvious than those between **medical health promotion** and political philosophy. For example, since the early eighties many **social health promoters** have been very keen to 'develop communities'. This venture is justified either as being first good for the community's health (conceived of as the opposite of disease) and *in addition* being one remedy for perceived social injustice, or as being *both* good for health and for justice simultaneously, or occasionally as being *first* good for justice. In the end, though, the ultimate justification for any form of **social health promotion** turns out to be less morbidity and mortality.

HEALTH AND JUSTICE ENTWINED

Concern for people's health (as the opposite of disease) and general concern to improve social conditions tend to be entwined in most varieties of **social health promotion**. The following extract shows how this can happen – perceptions of social malaise can inspire both practical work against disease and work to create more power for the people:

> In 1981, in Liverpool, it seemed to be time to translate these ideas into reality. I developed the idea of a Neighbourhood Health Group, which was to combine campaigning on issues of public policy with practical organising in the local community. It seemed important to root it in the official NHS structure, so that it would have some chance of exerting real influence over the problems it tackled. The opportunity came in May, with the publication of 'Primary Health Care in Inner London' (London Health Planning Consortium, 1981). Known as the Acheson Report this was a wide-ranging study of the health care needs of inner London. It had potential implications for all deprived areas of cities in the UK. Among its most interesting comments (buried deep in the body of the report, and – sadly – not mentioned among its recommendations) were the following:
>
> > The identification of the needs of particular communities is essentially a local activity. For each neighbourhood – which may comprise a housing estate, a group of streets, a complex of flats – those responsible for providing health and related social services should meet together on a regular basis. In collaboration with neighbourhood groups and associations, voluntary organisations and representatives of the local community, the professional teams should identify the needs of the population they serve, assess to what extent those needs are being met by existing services, where there are duplications/gaps, or where the introduction of special programmes is required. We believe that effective local planning of this kind will maximise resources available to the community and – in times of severe economic constraints – minimise the effects of a standstill or in some cases cuts in allocated

> expenditure. It is particularly important, however, both to harness the resources of the community to the full and at the same time provide sufficient professional support so that the demands on local populations do not become burdensome resulting ultimately in complete withdrawal of cooperation (London Health Planning Consortium, 1981, p. 78).[68]

Thus armed Scott-Samuel went ahead and set up a Neighbourhood Health Group in a particularly impoverished area of Liverpool, for these officially sanctioned reasons:

Establishing the Group

Why had we chosen Speke in which to establish the Neighbourhood Health Group? Speke is a postwar council estate of 18[#]000 people (1981 census), isolated beyond Liverpool's airport at the south-eastern tip of the city. Unemployment had increased in the decade 1971–1981 from 12 to 30 per cent (compared with a doubling from 10 to 20 per cent in the whole of Liverpool) as many of the purpose-built factories on the Speke Industrial Estate closed down. There are many of the housing types, the environmental neglect and the vandalism which characterise the council estates built in many cities in the 1950s and 1960s that are now, prematurely, being rebuilt or demolished. In addition, there was a well-established local concern about health services, focused on the demand for a health centre and minor injuries unit. The estate was remote from the city's major hospitals, the ambulance service was said to be poor and local GPs were reluctant to commit themselves to entering a health centre. The Community Health Council had for some years been co-ordinating and representing these views to the Area Health Authority (AHA) and to the area's MP.[68]

But Scott-Samuel was not only concerned with problems '... root[ed] ... in the official NHS structure'. He also sought to develop the health of the community in the following more obviously politically contestable ways:

> ... two meetings were mainly concerned with issues relating to housing and the physical environment (both of which the group came to see as crucially important to the local public health) and to health care facilities. However, during its existence the group discussed a much broader range of issues than these; issues that related to the concerns and agencies of every one of its members listed ...

> One aspect of the group's functioning that was particularly satisfying was the readiness with which its members accepted, understood and expounded a wide-ranging concept of the public health. They did not need to be told (or to have it 'scientifically proved' to them) that poor nutrition, poverty, lack of education, social isolation or unemployment prevent people living healthy lives. *This was most apparent with those working closely with, or suffering the effects of, these conditions. It was equally the norm for all discussions in the group to feature a high level of participation. People far from the health area, who would not have had much to say on medical matters (like our community policewoman or social security officer), shared an instinctive understanding of the determinants of the public health.*

> *The NHG succeeded in generating participant community action in an area which had seen a wealth of 'community initiatives' come and go. However, given the nature of the group, such success could be achieved only at the expense of creating some controversy in 'establishment' circles. As far as the local authority was concerned, the group's activities and recommendations could be seen as challenging the role of the area's elected representatives. The health authority's lack of enthusiasm was more a function of its orthodox, bureaucratic practice of the 'medical model' of health care. This is a model based essentially on treating diseases in buildings, as compared with a social model of preventing disease – and promoting health – in neighbourhoods.*[68] (My italics)

The connections between political philosophy and **social health promotion** are surely blatant in this and similar cases. Those, like Scott-Samuel, who think of health promotion in this light are committed to the view that it is unjust (usually regardless of considerations of desert or blame) that people suffer deprivation in an otherwise plentiful world. Their political philosophy can often be described as socialist, and naturally they choose health promotion projects that will fit with this political philosophy – ideally they establish projects which will ameliorate social deprivation and improve people's health narrowly conceived at the same time (though sometimes – as in Scott-Samuel's case – the 'medical health outcome' is almost a camouflage, a secondary consideration, or something which will automatically follow once the basic problem is addressed).

GOOD LIFE PROMOTION

Health is partly to do with the absence of disease, illness, injury and handicap, but is more than just the opposite of these negative factors. Good health, in its fullest sense, means complete well-being
Disease, illness, injury and handicap are bad in themselves, and well-being is good in itself
Disease, illness, injury and handicap are bad because they prevent normal biological and social functioning. Lack of well-being is bad because this means that a person's life as a whole (including his thoughts, beliefs, attitudes, and values) is not as it should be
The prevention and treatment of bad health, and the promotion of well-being, are beneficial for many reasons (cost-effectiveness, less pain, a happier world, and so on). Primarily, though, these things should be done simply because it is important that people live flourishing lives

The philosophical foundation of this form depends essentially upon the way in which 'the good life' is characterised. In the example used in the following section the philosophy is deeply conservative (in Burke's sense).[69] It seeks to protect the status quo as the best possible social organisation, supports capitalism, and claims that many social inequalities are unavoidable – indeed acceptable. However, the range of alternative founding philosophies of **good life promotion** is as broad as the range of possible descriptions of the good life itself.

ONE ILLUSTRATION OF GOOD LIFE PROMOTION: THE OBJECTIVE GOOD LIFE?

In recent times some theorists have argued that health promotion means the promotion of good lives or well-being (these words are used so vaguely in the writings of these theorists, and in the health promotion literature in general, that they may be considered to be interchangeable – which is the policy I have adopted here). The most widely read proponents of this move to extend health promotion are Robin Downie, Carol Fyfe and Andrew Tannahill, whose book *Health Promotion: Models and*

Values[6] is a perfect illustration of the overwhelming problems associated with **good life promotion**.

FUNDAMENTAL DIFFERENCES – FUNDAMENTAL CONFUSIONS

Health Promotion: Models and Values is notoriously difficult to understand. Many students confess to being completely flummoxed by it, and give up trying to work out what it is getting at. The book seems incomprehensible because although its authors:

> ...tried to integrate [their] various perspectives into a unified philosophy of health promotion, pulling together threads from medicine, education, social sciences, philosophy, and health promotion research and practice... (p. vii)[6]

they were destined to fail because they were hoping to unite fundamentally different goals and approaches. The book's comprehensive ambivalence over the question: *what drives health promotion?* is part cause and part result of this failure. Sometimes it seems that the evidence is the driving force (especially where the authors talk of preventing 'negative health') and sometimes it seems to be values (where they talk of promoting 'good lives'). The effect is that the book's essentially political nature – which the authors do openly acknowledge in some sections – tends to be dissipated and sometimes wholly obscured by its reference to apparently *neutral* 'health promotion models', and its use of the supposedly objective language of **medical health promotion**.

Health Promotion Is Not About Promoting Good Lives

The basic point of *Health Promotion: Models and Values* is to argue that health promoters must have a clear vision of the good life, and that this good life must be based on particular political values. *But this is not what health promotion should, or can, be about.* Health promotion is about promoting health – not about promoting good lives, even though these may be *indirect* products of its activities. **Good life promotion** is an *illegitimate* extension of health promotion.

It is important to explain this as clearly as possible: thus what follows (in the sections below and in Chapter Six) is both an illustration of the thinking behind one form of **good life promotion** and final ground-clearing for the *theory* of health promotion to come in Part Three.

IT IS IMPOSSIBLE TO SYNTHESISE THE UNSYNTHESISABLE

Health Promotion: Models and Values is a Magpie's nest in which its authors try to synthesise the unsynthesisable. They aim to:

a. unite (what they call) negative and positive health
b. unite mental, social and physical aspects of health
c. unite health and well-being
d. unite the idea of health as *enabling* (i.e. as instrumental towards some further end) and as a *good in itself*

e. unite different models of health promotion (especially models of health education, of the prevention of medical problems, and of legislation for health).

Incompatible Ideas

Inevitably, the hoped for unifications do not succeed. They can seem to work only if the philosophical problems are rapidly skated over. Substantial analysis shows that any apparent unity is illusory. For instance, the authors claim that: 'Health promotion must seek to prevent ill-health in such a way as simultaneously to enhance positive health' (p. 25).[6] And that since the prevention of ill-health is an objectively good thing to do, so the promotion of 'positive health' must be equally objectively justifiable:

> ...it might be counter-productive to preach too much about giving up smoking or going to the pub every night; but, all the same, a health promoter is committed to the view that smoking and heavy drinking are objectively bad. (p. 143)[6]

Furthermore: '...there can be no doubt that taking regular exercise is objectively a good form of activity and should be part of a good life' (p. 143).[6]

But the authors are *not* privy to objective knowledge about the ideal type of health promotion. They do not have objective knowledge of the good life because this is not something that anyone can have objective knowledge about. Indeed they argue this themselves:

> In the area of political values, there can be room for difference of opinion about the relative importance of values such as liberty and equality but health promoters are surely committed to the view that a large health divide between rich and poor is wrong. (p. 143)[6]

What are they saying? They would have readers believe that health promoters who *know* what the 'objective good life' is can nevertheless *disagree* about the balance between liberty and equality in this good life. So they are in effect arguing that some health promoters can *know objectively* that people ought to be at liberty to pursue their interests while other health promoters can *know objectively* that people's freedom to pursue their interests should be restricted by a belief in equality.

Assuming that 'objective' means 'universally true' (which is clearly how it is supposed to be read in several parts of the book) the authors' reasoning collapses into contradiction as they begin to admit that there might possibly be reasons why a person might think some things in life are more important than avoiding negative health. They seem slowly to realise that positive and negative health are different – and wish to allow that positive health can sometimes override negative health – but they also see that this has disconcerting implications. The most disconcerting of all – from their particular political point of view – is that a person might seek positive health by doing things which will *cause* negative health. And they cannot permit this because of their commitment to **medical health promotion** so – bizarrely – they state that: '...positive health is a value, not the supreme value' (p. 149).[6] But if this is so how can it be that smoking is *objectively* bad *and* that a person could decide *to* smoke on the ground of *some other* supreme value? The only way anyone could do this would be to decide to do something objectively good by doing something objectively bad – which would be ludicrous. Apparently:

> It makes perfectly good sense to weigh health against other values, and sometimes it will be reasonable to give precedence to health and sometimes not. For example, someone with

a stressful lifestyle might give up his job – perhaps at some personal economic cost or even to the detriment of service to others – on the ground that his or her health was suffering. Equally, someone might reasonably sacrifice health for another value, such as dedication to a life of scholarship or service to others. (p. 149)[6]

But why are these sacrifices reasonable? Why, for instance, would a person choose to sacrifice health for a life of scholarship or service to others? The only possible reason he might do so would be to be more fulfilled or happier – in order, that is, to have more positive health (well-being) (a good life). So he does not sacrifice health for some *extra supreme value*, he sacrifices negative health for positive health – which leaves the authors arguing that negative health can sometimes be a good thing if it is in the interest of positive health. But then this commits them to the absurdity that, for instance, it is alright for a person *not* to exercise (which, they have previously explained, is an objective good) if this will obstruct her life of scholarship.

Downie et al. believe that:

It is not immediately clear that questions of social justice are raised by health and its distribution, as distinct from health care, health determinants, and their distribution. Moreover, even if we suppose that questions of social justice do arise over health, we must not immediately conclude that it is entirely the fault of a government if there is social injustice, or even that social injustice in health, if it exists, can always be rectified by government intervention. The relationships between these ideas of health, health care, health determinants, and social justice are of importance to health promotion, since a clarification will help to clarify the political stance of health promotion. Our argument will be that the political stance of health promotion *derives from* its own professional concerns. (p. 157)[6] (My italics)

But they have things entirely the wrong way around. They would like to think it possible to move from the objective knowledge that smoking is bad, for instance, to the objective knowledge that a life of non-smoking – and other moderate behaviours – is objectively good. But the move is really this: the authors *believe* that a life of moderation is best and have chosen to call this the objective good life – that's all. Unless they had such a firm set of political values in the first place they would be unable to put forward this particular account of health promotion. It is not objective health concerns which shape their account of the good life; it is their understanding of the good life which shapes what they see as health concerns.

ONE SORT OF GOOD LIFE BASED IN ONE SORT OF POLITICAL THEORY

Downie et al. characterise liberalism in relation to health like this:

The liberal position on the pursuit of health assumes the following:

1. A view of health as an instrumental or enabling value, and as not making a claim as a positive value in its own right.
2. The view that people have a right to pursue their own health but no duty to do so unless their ill-health is harming others, this view being thought to be an expression of autonomy, or the 'harm principle'.
3. The connected view that the government has no duty to safeguard or enhance health other than through the prevention of harm.
4. A negative view of health legislation, as restricting autonomy in the interests of health.

5. A negative view of autonomy, that you have it to the extent that you are not prevented from doing what you want to do.
6. An atomistic view of society, that it consists of associations of individuals linked by a common geography, system of government, and economic ties.

> Some of these assumptions are definitive of liberalism, and others are views which tend to go along with it in the context of health care. Together they constitute the bare bones of a coherent philosophy of health care and much besides. (p. 145)[6]

Having made up this strange list of statements (they do not give a single reference to any thinker who has stated these 'liberal assumptions on the pursuit of health') they: '...go on to criticise or at least to modify them in the light of the values of health promotion' (p. 145).[6] But this is extremely disingenuous. According to the authors, the values of health promotion *derive from* professional concerns and are therefore prior to political values: since they are partly embodied in medical practice, and are against disease and so on, they are presumably supposed somehow to be superior to, or more objective than, political values. Thus – and here's the trick – if the authors can show that their political values are in fact supported by or – even better – are the *same as* 'health promotion values' they will have shown that their political values are objectively the best, and will then be able to use them to criticise any other sets of values applied to health promotion! But of course this is a circular position. The authors tell us *both* what health promotion values and the best political values are and – unsurprisingly – these turn out to be one and the same. All that is really being put forward is **firstly** one particular set of political prejudices and **secondly** those reasons (why health promotion ought to be done) which fit with them: only the book's argument is not presented in this order. If it were it would be a lot easier for students to see it for what it really is.

A MATTER OF OPINION – NOT OBJECTIVITY

For the liberal (as the authors depict him), if good general enabling conditions are present then it is up to the individual to pursue his own life (whatever form this may take, and however much this way of living is disapproved of by the mainstream of society – so long as serious harm is not caused to others). But for Downie et al. the 'autonomous' individual must be enabled in only a certain range of ways, and must pursue only those goals this particular range is capable of causing (that is, she must pursue only that *form* of the good life which the recommended behaviours and social institutions can bring about). For the authors the autonomous person eats a balanced diet, does not smoke, if he drinks alcohol at all he drinks it in moderation, exercises regularly, goes to self-help groups if he has a problem (p. 169), and sees himself as a citizen in a 'responsible society':

> ...for wholeness or well-being we require (*sic*) that we should all see ourselves as members of a collectively responsible society. In other words, the members of the health care professions must be assisted by our own striving to become (in the words of St Paul) members of one another. (p. 169)[6]

Indeed. But perhaps it is not too uncharitable to suggest that it is all very well to say this if you have a happy and useful life. Given this it is not hard (perhaps it is even psychologically necessary for some well-off people) to urge everyone to support each other. But by urging this one is obviously seeking to maintain the status quo. And when the status quo is patently uneven – when not everyone has the opportunities open to professional people in secure and fulfilling employment – and when some people have no meaningful opportunities at all, then what, precisely, are you asking people to do? Is it really fair to ask us *all* to join together to preserve those conditions which are partly responsible for both negative health *and* for lack of (what you call) positive health?

THE GOOD LIFE?

Are these all *truly* components of the good life and the good society? They are each consistent with the prejudices expressed in *Health Promotion: Models and Values*:

a. Although it has a too-limited focus on negative health, **medical health promotion** is unequivocally a good thing, and is almost always supported by clear evidence (see Chapter 4 in *Health Promotion: Models and Values*, for instance).
b. That people have a duty to make sure they do not become sick:

> ...it does not follow from the fact that there is a human right to health and a correlative duty on governments to do what they can to improve health that there is not also a moral duty on people to do what they can to improve their own health. The parallel is with education. Governments have a duty to create facilities for education, but people have a duty to make the best use of these facilities. (p. 155)[6]

c. That if they fail in this duty they are irresponsible:

> ...no amount of improvement in social conditions is a substitute for people themselves taking responsibility for their own health and their own neighbourhood. (p. 167)[6]

d. That preventive and protective health promotion measures are necessary because not everyone can be trusted to look after their own health.
e. That prevailing social conditions are generally acceptable:

> Does it then constitute a social injustice that health determinants, the social and economic conditions for health, are much poorer in some than in other areas of society? It may do, but no one should underestimate the consequences, economic and political, of attempting to remedy this state of affairs. When the Black Report was published in 1980 the Secretary of State for Social Services pointed out in a Foreword that the additional expenditure was upward of 2 billion pounds sterling per year at 1980 prices. He therefore did not endorse the recommendations. Now it is easy to blame governments for failing to improve social conditions, and the evidence is that the social divide has increased since 1980. But in a democratic society a government can do only what its electorate shows a political will for it to do, and there is no evidence that the electorate is willing to countenance the massive redistribution of resources which would be involved...[6]

f. That good lives can be objectively defined by health promoters.
g. That alternative views of health promotion (including the liberal view) are objectively wrong.

Establishment Health Promotion

Though much of the political philosophy of *Health Promotion: Models and Values* must be assumed from what it says about other matters, it seems the authors are against unfettered market-liberalism (see their p. 158, for instance), and for state intervention (though the justification for this is very vague indeed):

> ...we argue...that if there is a causal link between furthering positive health and preventing ill-health, then there is a duty on governments to further the positive health of individuals as a means of preventing ill-health. (p. 155)[6]

(For some reason positive health here is not given the status of a value in its own right, but is considered a means to prevent ill-health only.)

However, there is a limit to state intervention. The rule of government must be balanced against the 'moral duty' of individuals to improve 'their own health'. Thus it seems that sometimes social conditions cause poor health, but governments cannot change social conditions very much because the people do not want them to. It would cost too much. Therefore the job of the health promoter is not to challenge those factors which *may* be unjust and which *may sometimes* cause ill-health, but to empower people to accept their lot, to do the best they can even in the poorest social conditions, and sometimes to hold them responsible if they fail. And this, the reader is asked to believe, is immeasurably better than 'the liberal' position which is an 'atomistic view of society', and which apparently sees society as a 'convenient fiction'. Downie, Fyfe and Tannahill's interpretation of the good life *may* be the good life in some people's eyes – indeed it clearly is, but it is not, by any stretch of the imagination, objectively so.

The authors' political philosophy – and so their good life – is, as far as it is possible to tell from such a contradictory book, in line with the state of affairs which persisted in the UK (where they wrote it) when they wrote it. The British government in the late 1980s did not espouse an unfettered free-market, and did not want an interventionist welfare state either, and the authors' version of health promotion mirrors these policies. The confused form of health promotion they put forward is, in truth, nothing more than a product of the pluralistic and ambiguous social values which existed in Britain at that time.

EXERCISE SIX

PRACTICAL OR POLITICAL ROOTS?

Consider the following **Targets** selected from the WHO's 38 **Targets** for the European Region:[11,61]

1. By the year 2000, the actual differences in health status between countries and between groups within countries should be reduced by at least 25%, by improving the levels of health of disadvantaged nations and groups.

continues

continued

2. By the year 2000, people should have the basic opportunity to develop and use their health potential to live socially and economically fulfilling lives.

4. By the year 2000, the average number of years that people live free from major disease and disability should be increased by at least 10%.

5. By the year 2000, there should be no indigenous measles, poliomyelitis, neonatal tetanus, congenital rubella, diphtheria, congenital syphilis or indigenous malaria in the Region.

9. By the year 2000, mortality in the Region from diseases of the circulatory system in people under 65 should be reduced by at least 15%.

11. By the year 2000, deaths from accidents in the Region should be reduced by at least 25% through an intensified effort to reduce traffic, home and occupational accidents.

12. By the year 2000, the current rising trends in suicides and attempted suicides in the Region should be reversed.

13. By 1990, national policies in all member states should ensure that legislative, administrative and economic mechanisms provide broad intersectoral support and resources for the promotion of healthy lifestyles and ensure effective participation of the people at all levels of such policy-making.

14. By 1990, all member states should have specific programmes which enhance the major roles of the family and other social groups in developing and supporting healthy lifestyles.

16. By 1995, in all member states, there should be significant increases in positive health behaviour, such as balanced nutrition, non-smoking, appropriate physical activity and good stress management.

17. By 1995, in all member states, there should be significant decreases in health-damaging behaviour, such as overuse of alcohol and pharmaceutical products; use of illicit drugs, and dangerous chemical substances; dangerous driving and violent social behaviour.

20. By 1990, all people of the Region should have adequate supplies of safe drinking water, and by the year 1995 pollution of rivers, lakes and seas should no longer pose a threat to human health.

21. By 1995, all people of the Region should be effectively protected against recognised health risks from air pollution.

24. By the year 2000, all people of the Region should have a better opportunity of living in houses and settlements which provide a healthy and safe environment.

29. By 1990, in all member states, primary health care systems should be based on co-operation and teamwork between health care personnel, individuals, families and community groups.

———————— ◆ ————————

Although the WHO does not explain them in detail, enough information is given to indicate that the targets are of different *kinds*. This may not be immediately

continues

continued

obvious, however. In order to demonstrate that the WHO's targets are not homogeneous, take the following steps. For each target (or a sample of targets):

Step 1: Spell out, in as much practical detail as you can, what you think the precise goals are.

Step 2: Spell out, as fully as possible, the practical steps necessary, in your own country, to achieve these goals.

Step 3: Whether you agree with the targets and methods or not, try to offer justifications for them (why are they worth doing? who will benefit the most? will anyone be disadvantaged? what vision of society informs them?).

Step 4: If possible, try to explain, in general terms, the political philosophy which inspires each target.

Step 5: Imagine you are a policy-maker working for the WHO. Briefly describe up to four **Targets** you would recommend for 2010, and explain the political philosophy which informs them.

Teaching notes for: Practical or Political Roots?

Like most of the exercises in this book, Exercise Six is not easy to do well, and is best conducted by *you* within a thoughtful group of students who have already successfully completed other exercises (at least Exercises One, Three and Five).

The aim of the exercise is:

i. To show how broad, ambitious and *debatable* the WHO targets are.

ii. To show that there are at least two different sorts of target being set: one sort expressing an intent to reduce the incidence of disease and illness, the other stating the importance of increasing people's social and economic opportunities.

It seems to be taken as read by the WHO that these things are both (a) unarguably part of health promotion and (b) necessarily related. Neither of these claims is correct, and this exercise should go some way toward demonstrating this.

iii. To show that even when they are so generally cast the WHO's targets are nevertheless political in nature.

AN EXAMPLE

As an example of how you might best achieve these three aims consider **Targets 2, 5, 16 and 24.**

──────────── ◆ ────────────

2. **By the year 2000, people should have the basic opportunity to develop and use their health potential to live socially and economically fulfilling lives.**

continues

continued

5. **By the year 2000, there should be no indigenous measles, poliomyelitis, neonatal tetanus, congenital rubella, diphtheria, congenital syphilis or indigenous malaria in the Region.**

16. **By 1995, in all member states, there should be significant increases in positive health behaviour, such as balanced nutrition, non-smoking, appropriate physical activity and good stress management.**

24. **By the year 2000, all people of the Region should have a better opportunity of living in houses and settlements which provide a healthy and safe environment.**

——————— ◆ ———————

Taking each in turn, here (in summary form) are some ways in which students might carry out the exercise's four steps.

TARGET 2

2. **By the year 2000, people should have the basic opportunity to develop and use their health potential to live socially and economically fulfilling lives.**

Step 1

Students will most likely be overwhelmed by this task, in the case of **Target 2**. Typically they might ask 'what does "basic opportunity" mean?', 'is "health potential" meant to refer to a general standard or is it supposed to mean each particular individual's potential?', 'what exactly *is* a "socially and economically fulfilling" life?'. These, of course, are extremely important questions and – as you will have seen in the main text – are not the sorts of questions that health promoters usually either raise or address – which is all the more reason for taking this opportunity to discuss them in detail with the students.

I suggest, that once these questions have arisen (as they inevitably will in experienced groups), or once you have highlighted them, a discussion of what these phrases might mean in *reality* is begun. Students are bound to raise theoretical issues simultaneously ('is it necessary for everyone to have an economically fulfilling life, whatever that means?', 'should resources be taken from better off individuals/European countries to supply basic opportunities for the worst off?') but your aim, at this stage, should be to focus on *what this target actually looks like*. For example, you might decide first to discuss the idea of *basic opportunity* and to ask students to say what this implies for them, materially. Responses may include: public hospitals, social support (state benefits of various kinds), schools, higher education, meaningful and well-paid employment, and so on. Quite different responses are possible, of course: privatised health services, no welfare safety net (to stop malingering etc.), parent-choice voucher-funded schooling, employment as provided by the free market with no state intervention and no minimum wage, and so on. If you have a variety of responses, so much the better for the purpose of lively discussion.

continues

continued

Step 2

Again it is important to focus mainly on the practicalities of achieving these goals: what will have to be done? how much will it cost? what sacrifices will have to be made? what other opportunities will have to be foregone? how much funding should go to hospitals? how much to schools? how much should be state-controlled? how many of these developments should be left to democratic choice?

Do not spend too long on this step. Your aim is merely to show the practical complexity of the second **Target**, and to make students fully aware of the hard (and often politically charged) choices that will have to be made to bring the WHO's idealism to fruition.

Step 3

At this stage in the group work you should switch students' attention from the practical to the theoretical. Ask them to *argue* for the specific goals and methods they have identified, even if they do not agree with them or the WHO's position. In other words, ask students to defend their practical understanding of *basic opportunity* with philosophical arguments – if only rudimentary ones. For example, if students have made out a mostly practical case for a free-market version of basic opportunity (i.e. if they have described a situation in which opportunities exist for those prepared to take them, and one in which opportunity to do fulfilling things is understood to stem primarily from freedom from restraints and barriers against the pursuit of desired goals) then ask them to justify it.

To this end you might permit them to discuss any *evidence* they have available that this sort of basic opportunity tends to increase social and economic fulfilment. But you should also try to prise out what they *mean* by these forms of fulfilment, and why they have seen fit to characterise basic opportunity not as, say, dependent on the state provision of welfare but as dependent on minimal state intervention. Ask: 'what, in your view, is a socially and economically fulfilled person?', 'what relationships does and should this person have with other people (aggressive, competitive, supportive, collaborative, etc.)?', 'why do you think such a person is living a good life and for what reasons is this life better than any alternative good life?' Such a conversation should lead naturally to Step 4.

Step 4

At this point you should either have the student expand, in general and without reference to the WHO's target, on her political philosophy – pointing out that if she agrees with the practical description of *basic philosophy* she has defended she must therefore hold a certain sort of position in political philosophy – or you should do the expansion, or get assistance from someone qualified to do so (perhaps a philosophy graduate looking for casual employment?). Whatever way you decide to approach the challenge, you must aim to demonstrate that it is not possible to talk meaningfully of 'basic opportunity' and 'socially and economically fulfilling lives' without attaching these notions to a political philosophy. (In

continues

continued

this example the student's political philosophy is individualistic and libertarian. If she is not aware of them, such a student might be told of books by such writers as Hayek, Nozick and Friedman – and also of critiques of these works.)

TARGET 5

5. **By the year 2000, there should be no indigenous measles, poliomyelitis, neonatal tetanus, congenital rubella, diphtheria, congenital syphilis or indigenous malaria in the Region.**

Unlike **Target 2** this **Target** is primarily ranged against disease and illness, and so is a little less broad and ambitious than the former. This basic distinction should certainly be pointed out, and you should also explain – and go on to demonstrate by means of the four steps – that **Target 5** is nevertheless most definitely debatable.

Step 1

This may seem obvious, but it is worth asking the students to identify briefly what these targets imply. Will these diseases disappear *because of* increased hygiene, nutrition and exercise; mandatory immunisation programmes; or mass education programmes, for instance?

Step 2

At this point matters get a little more interesting. There will, presumably, be unanimous agreement that measles, poliomyelitis and so on should be eradicated. However, it does not necessarily follow that there will be agreement on either:

i. the ways in which the diseases ought to be eliminated

or

ii. the cost of so doing.

In order to give full substance to the later Step 3 discussion, it is important to have the students at least spell out the options for a programme designed to achieve **Target 5**. These options may include the possibilities indicated in Step 1 above, perhaps with further suggestions or perhaps in some combination. Whatever the case, your aim should be to show that these methods are not necessarily either equally effective or equally ethical, and also – if possible – to foster disagreement between members of the group. (If your students are anything like those I've had the pleasure of teaching over the years you will not need to work too hard to foster disagreement. It would be surprising – in my experience especially in groups of women students – if immunisation were not itself a major issue. It is also highly likely that students will have different opinions about the worth of compulsory programmes of any kind in adult populations.)

continues

continued

You should aim to have students spell out, in as much detail as possible, first which means of preventing these diseases they favour, and then what strategy they would choose. For instance, if a student prefers to concentrate first on hygiene, nutrition and exercise, ask him to provide evidence that this will work, and then ask him to say *how* these aspects of life will be improved. Will this be left entirely to personal choice, perhaps on the assumption that these changes follow economic growth (assuming that this is occurring at the time)? Or will individuals and families be offered incentives of some kind by government? Or will there be punishments and sanctions for bad dietary habits and for not exercising? If immunisation is to be mandatory how will this be enforced? Will children not be allowed to enrol for school unless they can prove they have been immunised (as happens in some States in America)? Whatever practical option is selected, how much should be spent on it? And – crucially – what is the maximum percentage of a nation's GDP that ought to be invested to achieve **Target 5**?

Step 3
At this point turn directly to the Exercise instructions, and ask the questions listed at Step 3. This will lead to an interesting discussion where, again, you should try to foster dissent (this is most likely to arise with the questions 'who will benefit most?', 'who will be disadvantaged?' etc.). When this happens you should aim to draw out your students' *reasons* for their views and claims. You should attempt, in particular, to begin to draw attention to the fact that students' preferences are neither arbitrary nor random, but reflect their broader views (even if these are only aesthetic ones) about social relationships, responsibilities, structure, order and planning. You might, for example, point out that it is unlikely that a student will argue passionately for a carefully planned, state-funded programme of education and legislation, with sanctions for those who do not adopt disease-avoiding behaviours, and in all other matters be a strong supporter of individual choice and 'the battle to roll back the frontiers of socialism'. That is, *you should try to begin to show that there are connections – even at the apparently neutral level of disease prevention – between the chosen goals, the chosen methods, and one's vision of a good society* (is a good society regimented, well-ordered, liberal, anarchistic, one in which its people fear the power of the state, one in which its people feel safe and relaxed, one in which everyone has say and so on?).

As with **Target 2**, your discussion should lead naturally to Step 4.

Step 4
Since students may slide into Step 4 without noticing, it is a good idea to announce that the group is now to consider this step explicitly. You might then, for instance, at least begin to explain the *social differences* between (i) the state operating a wholly mandatory, automatic system of childhood immunisation and (ii) the state offering a comprehensive education programme to all parents on the pros *and* cons of immunisation, including such relevant facts as the financial

continues

continued

interests of providers of drugs, the economic benefits, the risks to some children, and so on.

You might choose to explain that option (i), roughly, is one form of socialist practice and has been known to be highly effective in so far as uptake and prevention of some of these diseases is concerned,[26] and that option (ii), while less effective in the above sense, has other benefits: it involves people in decision-making, it tends to respect their choices, it can enhance their knowledge and their levels of confidence – and that this might, roughly, be described as a form of social democracy.

TARGET 16

16. By 1995, in all member states, there should be significant increases in positive health behaviour, such as balanced nutrition, non-smoking, appropriate physical activity and good stress management.

Step 1

Like **Target 5**, **Target 16** looks fairly straightforward at first sight. Who could reasonably object to 'significant increases in positive health behaviour', after all? However, experienced students of the philosophy of health promotion, and certainly those who have satisfactorily completed and understood the exercises to this point in the book, will quickly recognise that there is more to discuss here than meets the naïve eye. For example, there are theoretical issues about the nature of positive health and its relationship to ill-health (see Chapter Six), about whether not smoking is obviously and always part of what it is to be positively healthy (see Chapter Three), and about what is meant by 'appropriate physical activity' and 'good stress management'.

Put like this, as theoretical issues, many pragmatically minded health promoters might be inclined towards a 'so what?' reaction. 'What does this pedantry matter – eating properly, not smoking, exercising sensibly and dealing with stress are so obviously a part of a healthy life that we really don't need to agonise over this any further.' Presumably out of frustration, it is common for even experienced students to come out with statements like this. If you do get this response then refer the students to key pages of this book. And, for a speedy demonstration that there really *is* a problem here, ask them to do Step 1 again: suggest that they list the practical goals of this **Target**. For instance, have objectors define what is meant by 'balanced nutrition' and have them defend *their* plan, with evidence, against the many alternative nutrition guides. Or have them define ideal stress levels for people, again with evidence, and again against the opinions of other, dissenting authorities.[46]

Further, to ensure realism, have dissenting students explain what 'appropriate physical activity' and 'good stress management' actually *are* for a deeply

continues

continued

committed computer scientist who hates exercise in any form, and who enjoys the alternative highs and lows of facing and achieving tight deadlines. Given this conundrum students can only decide to:

a. insist that he should exercise up to the recommended level for his age and fitness

b. accept that it is up to the individual to choose

or

c. aim for a compromise.

But in each case there are practical (and ethical) difficulties, which the student should be made aware of. If a then how can the health promoter ensure that the scientist exercises, and why is this worth doing at the expense of the scientist's unhappiness or even increased stress? If b then the WHO **Target 16** is not fundamental after all. And if this one is not fundamental why are the others fundamental? (In other words, you might use this example to challenge the ultimate authority of the **38 WHO Targets**.) And if c, what is the practical and moral force of aiming for less than normally appropriate physical activity and of causing a previously content person to change his behaviour in an unwanted way? Of course there may be reasons, but these would need to be spelt out by the student.

Step 2
You should take a similar approach to that recommended for **Targets 2** and **5**. Ask students to identify the most desirable practical means of achieving the goals they have specified, and to say why. And if they have compromised effectiveness or efficiency for some other reason (the person's wishes, or cultural sensitivities) then ask them to explain how and why they *rank* their practical goals.

The aim of this step is to show that there is a range of different methods, that there are reasons for choosing one or the other, and that these are inevitably at least partly theoretical reasons. Hence, Step 3.

Step 3
Again follow the model offered by the teaching instructions to **Targets 2** and **5**, and pick out those aspects which seem to you (and the students) most nearly to do with a vision of the good life. The idea of good stress management might be a good source of discussion, and will enable you to move to Step 4.

Step 4
The students' view of stress and their view of the role of individuals within society are related. A person who regards stress as a positive, driving force will be inclined to favour a demanding, competitive system in which people need to push themselves hard to succeed. It does not necessarily follow, but for someone who thinks of stress this way, a capitalist system would seem well-suited. It is overly

continues

continued

simplistic to say this but, just to illustrate the possibility, a person who sees stress as a negative thing is more likely to favour a state which provides numerous safety nets and guarantees, and enables her to relax when she feels the need, or even freely to withdraw from stressful situations (a challenging job, for instance) without social penalty (see the discussion of well-being in Chapter 6).

TARGET 24

24. By the year 2000, all people of the Region should have a better opportunity of living in houses and settlements which provide a healthy and safe environment.

Step 1

Like **Target 2**, it can be an overwhelming challenge to spell out this **Target** in practical detail, which is precisely why you should insist that students try to do so. What, for instance, is a 'better opportunity' – the choice of moving to a new house, or the impossibility – without choice – of living in poor housing following a national scheme of demolition? What is a healthy house? One which is free from disease-causing problems or one where a person can feel she belongs? (These are not necessarily compatible categories.) What is a safe settlement? Safe from what?

Don't overdo these questions, especially if students have already completed earlier exercises in the same session, but do insist on confronting the accusation (possibly the silent accusation) that this is more pedantry. By having students explain in practical terms what a healthy house looks like, where it should be located, and so on, students can grasp the magnitude of the challenge – and the more detail they spell out the more this will begin to look at least partly like personal preference – or prejudice – which is what you should constantly be seeking to bring to the surface.

Step 2

How are these developments to be brought about? Who will pay? Who will suffer? (There surely will be suffering since people do not, as a rule, like change.) From *what* or *whom* are the settlements to be protected? How is this protection to be carried out (fences, barbed wire, extra police, enforced and maintained standards of hygiene, a ban on private cars in each settlement?).

Steps 3 and 4

What sort of vision of society springs to mind when students think of and describe their ideas about healthy housing and safe settlements? Their practical choices are bound to be informed by implicit theories, health promotion as a 'movement' is very bad at acknowledging this, and you are insisting that your students, at least, confront the truth.

continues

continued

Does the settlement look like Milton Keynes? Does it look like Sydney? Is it a small commune where the traditional family has been eschewed in favour of shared responsibility for child-rearing? Is it a farm? Is it a mining community? Must it have a health centre? Must the health centre be medically based? How will the settlement be run? Who will make the decisions? If there are disagreements about what 'safe' *means* as far as a particular settlement is concerned, then how will these be resolved?

Force the students to think hard enough for long enough about **Target 24** and the *very task of doing this* actually becomes one of raising and thinking through questions of political philosophy (which is exactly what many of the questions in the paragraph above are). If this does not convince them that there is much more to promoting health than setting woolly targets and (mostly) trying to get people to avoid disease, then I am unsure what will.

EXERCISE SEVEN

WILLESVILLE POLITICS

1. Recall the health promoters who work at the Willesville District Health Promotion Unit. Take any *two* of them and attempt to draw their 'health promotion tower' and its base (as in Fig. 11). In other words, attempt to explain, as far as you believe you plausibly can, their respective political philosophies.

2. Now consider the practices of any health promoter known to you, and draw his or her 'health promotion tower' and its base.

3. Finally you may find it interesting to draw your own tower and base.

Note: it may be useful to have completed Step 5 of Exercise Six before attempting to draw your tower.

Teaching notes for: Willesville Politics

The aim of this exercise is to reinforce students' beliefs that health promotion and political philosophy are *necessarily* linked. Students should read the opening dialogues carefully (especially Dialogue One), and must try to *spell out* the links between at least two Willesville health promoters' statements about what they would like to do for Diane, and their probable political philosophies.

Dependent on the amount of detail students are prepared to consider, the exercise might be regarded as a fairly light task, run over an hour, or it might develop into a serious and extensive analysis of the relationship between health promotion and political philosophy. This is up to you and your students.

continues

continued

POLITICAL PHILOSOPHY

You should be aware that *political philosophy* is, essentially, sustained contemplation on the social world meant to produce reasoned answers to the questions: *what is the best way to arrange human activities and relationships in society?* Thus political philosophy clearly shares a common interest with health promotion. At the very least both enterprises must have a view on what is truly valuable in human life, and the practical consequences and recommended policies of both are bound to be shaped by this view. At the moment, the difference between political philosophy and health promotion is that political philosophers are explicit about what they think and why they think it, whereas health promotion theorists are not.

The importance of this connection cannot be overstated. *One's agreement or disagreement with both the methods and targets of health promotion depends ultimately upon the way in which one understands the social purpose of human lives.* Health promotion cannot *seriously* be undertaken without reference to the concerns of moral and political philosophy. You should try to ensure that students fully grasp this point.

AN EXAMPLE

Take two of the health promoters – Martin Miller and Carol Jones – whom we meet in the opening dialogue of the main text. They have different ideas about practice *and* they hold different political philosophies. Their 'towers', in descending order, would include the following considerations and points of view:

Martin assumes:

 i. that heavy drinking is a *fundamental* problem

while Carol assumes:

 i. that heavy drinking is a *symptom* of social malaise

Martin assumes:

 ii. that work with individuals can solve this problem

Carol assumes:

 ii. that work with individuals is at best tinkering and at worst irrelevant

Martin assumes:

iii. that individuals are largely (or even entirely) responsible for their behaviours

Carol disagrees. She believes:

iii. that individuals are only partly responsible for their behaviours

continues

continued

Martin assumes:

iv. that individuals are rational and self-interested

Carol thinks:

iv. that individuals have basic needs that must be met *before* they can truly express their self-interests

Martin assumes:

v. that individuals have certain duties as members of society

Carol assumes:

v. that the state has duties to its citizens which must be fulfilled *before* citizens can be said to have duties to the state

Martin assumes:

vi. that prevailing social arrangements are generally satisfactory

Carol assumes:

vi. that prevailing social arrangements are generally *un*satisfactory

It is obviously an over-simplification, but nevertheless fair to say that Martin has a conservative political philosophy while Carol holds a socialist one.

PRACTICALITIES

Physical aids can often be valuable, even when teaching philosophy. For example, the use of cards may be productive in running this exercise. You might have students write pertinent sentences – such as those which might have been written by Martin and Carol (see above) – on cards, and then have them rank these sentences (one on top of another) in order to construct their own towers. Or you might have some cards (perhaps 50–100) already prepared. If so you could ask students to put them in related groups – actually have the students physically do this – and then to go on to construct their own towers from these possibilities:

Whichever your approach to the exercise you will need to demonstrate:

i. that it is possible to detect political philosophies from the study of groupings of practical health promotion aims and methods

ii. that health promotion is *not* a random activity (randomly constructed towers just do not make theoretical sense)

and

iii. that the towers do not construct themselves, but are constructed according to people's political outlooks.

If possible you should emphasise the above points during discussion.

continues

continued

Further Possibilities for Discussion

You might, once you have discussed the students' 'towers', like to speculate on whether it makes sense to describe health promotion as a *movement* at all. You might, dependent on how the discussion goes, propose not only that health promotion is *not* a movement, but that health promotion *per se* does not exist. Perhaps you will decide to put it to the students that different political philosophical points of view exist, together with a wide range of intervention strategies and social policies ultimately based on them: all – misleadingly – called health promotion. You might then ask the students if they think this is a problem.

For my part I do not think it is necessarily a problem. Rather I believe that the exposure of pluralism is an inevitable, and beneficial, stage in the development of health promotion as a reflective discipline. Once health promotion is seen as value-*soaked* it becomes essential – indeed morally essential – that each variety of health promotion makes its prejudices explicit. It becomes vital that each form develops a respectable justification of its prejudice and practice: that each – in other words – develops a decent theory of health. And once this happens, openness and clarity ought to follow automatically. For instance, it should no longer be sufficient justification for a research project or a policy change that it is 'generally health promoting'. Where pluralism is a fact, any researcher or policy-maker should be obliged to explain what *kind* of health promotion she is advocating.

Furthermore, once pluralism is *thoroughly* exposed then the theoretical ground of health promotion can be seen not to be fixed and permanent, but to be territory to be argued for. For example, the more clearly it is shown that medicine and 'work for health' are *historically* rather than *necessarily* related, the better the chances of free and open debate about health promotion priorities.

In sum, as the prejudiced roots of health promotion are revealed, it is my belief that the 'movement's' advocates will become compelled to produce theoretical defences of their particular positions.

But do your students agree? Do you agree? Why? Why not?

The Outsider

SCENE ONE

It is three weeks later. For the last fortnight (mostly in the afternoons and evenings) Diane has been acting as a health promoter. Because James needed the help, and because she expressed an interest, Diane has mainly been working on a Young Person's Drug and Alcohol project. In addition to spending time reading the extensive literature on the subject she has been using her journalistic skills to interview young people in local pubs and clubs. Diane has also been producing her normal quota of words for the Willesville Chronicle, *and feels very tired.*

At the moment Diane is in a town centre bar in the early evening, waiting to meet James. She has arrived a few minutes too soon. Even though she is by now very well aware that 'the healthy choice' would be to have a soft drink Diane has ordered a double gin and tonic, and is chatting easily to the barman.

DIANE: You're not kidding. I'm full on at the moment. I write for the *Chronicle* and I've been working as a health promotion officer for the last couple of weeks.

BARMAN: Two jobs eh? You must be coining it.

DIANE: Not exactly. *(She takes a drink)* I've only got the one real job at the *Chronicle* but I wanted to find out what it is like to be a health promoter. I reckoned it must be a lot more interesting than it seems. And I thought I might be able to sell the story to a bigger paper – you know, a career move? *(She laughs ironically)*

BARMAN: It's not turning out so good then?

DIANE: Well it is interesting, I knew I'd have to make some compromises but I'm finding it hard to justify what I'm doing. I can see that I might be doing some good but I reckon I might be doing harm too – or maybe I'm just wasting my time and someone else's money. And I really don't know how to turn it all into something for the Sundays. It's too subtle. It's not sexy enough. I suppose I should've done something like AIDS work, but then that's not news so much these days. People are bored with AIDS.

BARMAN: So, what are you doing?

Health Promotion, Second Edition: David Seedhouse
© 2004 John Wiley & Sons, Ltd: ISBNs 0 470 84732 8 (HB); 0 470 84733 6 (PB)

DIANE: I'm part of a local initiative to help kids drink sensibly and not take drugs.

BARMAN: Yeah? I'm right behind you there. You should see the state some of them get into Fridays and Saturdays.

DIANE: I know, I know. But on the other hand they don't exactly do what they do unprompted. There's peer pressure, there's the ads, there's wanting to be grown up, there's the thrill, there's the risk, there's the social scene, there's a need – maybe – to overdo it, to rebel, to be young . . .

BARMAN: Sure. And then there's the drinking and driving, the fights, the vandalism, the distress to parents. There's injury, and even death. Last year a whole car full of teenagers were killed outright after they'd been drinking. One minute whooping it up here, the next nothing.

DIANE: I know that too. I wrote the story up. I guess I just don't know what angle to take on this whole thing. It is more complicated than I'd supposed. Or maybe I'm just making it more complicated than it actually is. *(She grins)* And then perhaps I should take the 'responsible host' angle. What do you say to that? Don't you think you and your bosses have got a responsibility here too? I mean, you sell the stuff. Don't you think you should stop serving when you think a kid has had enough? Don't you think . . .

MAN AT THE BAR: A pint of that lager when you're ready please mate.

BARMAN: Sorry sir, I was just having an interesting discussion with the reporter here.

MAN: A reporter? Who for?

DIANE: The *Chronicle*.

MAN: Oh, that useless rag.

DIANE: Thanks a lot. I might agree with you, but that wouldn't make me a bad reporter. I do what I can. I have to make a living, but that doesn't mean I don't have standards.

MAN: I didn't say you were a bad reporter.

DIANE: You implied it though didn't you? . . . Perhaps you didn't. Maybe I'm just too tired right now.

MAN: Yeah? Why? *(He begins to drink thirstily)*

DIANE: Well as I was saying to Justin here . . . oh he's gone . . . I'm doing a project – off my own bat – to live the life of a health promoter for a month. I thought it would help me write a good feature for the *Chronicle* and that it might be something I could write up for a quality national – but I can't get a good hook on it, I don't really know what to think about what I'm doing. There's a lot more politics than I thought.

MAN: You don't sound much like a journalist to me. *(To the Barman)* Another Export please.

DIANE: That's strong stuff isn't it?

MAN: *(A little irritated)* So what if it is?

DIANE: I'm sorry. That was really rude of me. My 'job' as a health promoter is mostly to work on an alcohol and drug abuse – I mean misuse – project, so I'm full of facts and figures about booze, and the damage it can do. Sorry . . . My name's Diane Grant by the way.

MAN: Forget it. I'm Andrew. Andrew Wilson.

DIANE: *(After a short silence)* What did you mean I'm not like a journalist? I suppose you reckon that a journalist will find a story even if there isn't one, and sod the truth? Is that it?

ANDREW: Not really. It was you saying you didn't know what to think. It's not good for you to think too much. What you're doing obviously bothers you. Journalists should be more detached than that.

DIANE: You're probably right. Maybe I'm not meant to be a journalist. But what about you? You sound like you know a bit about journalism. What do you do for a living?

ANDREW: I work at Adams' Meat Packers. On the beefburger belt as it happens.

DIANE: But you're well-educated. What happened?

ANDREW: What do you mean?

DIANE: *(Blushing slightly)* Well, obviously you could . . . should have a better job than making burgers.

ANDREW: Why? I don't like it much but then I don't much like the idea of working in an office, having a suburban house with a twee garden, watching the kids do what all the other kids are doing . . . I don't want to be part of a mindless cycle . . . I want my life to have a point to it.

DIANE: There's a point to Adams' meat factory?

ANDREW: It's a means to an end, that's all. Things are not ideal at the moment. I had to come back from an adventure a few months ago . . . My mother was dying and I had to do what I could. She's gone now and I'm doing what I have to to save up for the summer. Then I'm off on my travels again. I could never stay here but so long as I know I can escape to the train or the road across Europe and beyond, then I can bear the drudgery. It's not forever.

DIANE: I'm sorry about your mother.

ANDREW: *(Looking downwards)* That's OK. It's over with. That's all. Cigarette?

DIANE: I don't smoke.

ANDREW: A drink then?

DIANE: OK. Just one. A G and T.

ANDREW: Another Export and a G and T please.

DIANE: So Andrew, if you don't want convention what do you want?

ANDREW: I want the unexpected. I want fun. I want different experiences. I want travel. I want risk. I want to stay alive, properly alive.

DIANE: *(A little embarrassed by the poetry)* It must really hack you off working with mince-meat then.

ANDREW: It's a way out. As I said.

(They drink in difficult silence for a minute or two)

ANDREW: You think I drink too much don't you? *(He pushes his empty glass toward the barman)*

DIANE: If you do this every night and if you keep it up 'til closing time then yes I do. Fill it up for him please.

ANDREW: What if it makes me happy?

DIANE: You might think it makes you happy but it costs you a lot of money, you must get hangovers, perhaps you get into other sorts of trouble... scrapes with the law, I don't know and then there's your long-term health too.

ANDREW: What if I know all that and still choose to do it?

DIANE: Do you choose? Aren't you pressured into it? Couldn't you take off on your travels earlier if you cut down?

ANDREW: I guess. But you're not listening. I don't live my life like that. Most people seem to behave as if the point of life is to stay safe for tomorrow. It's like they permanently postpone *really* living. They'll get to it soon, you know, like John Lennon said: 'life is what happens to you while you're busy making other plans'? They just have to see to the family first, or the career, or the pension, or the mortgage. It's like they assume there'll be some idyllic time in their sixties or something. But I want immediate kicks, and then I want to move on some more. Six months is as far ahead as I ever want to think.

DIANE: I don't know. I think you think you are in control but I don't think you are really. I don't think you are any more in control than the average cog in the wheel, the average Joe in the street with a wife, two kids, three bedrooms, and commuting to do. And it isn't going to get any easier. You aren't so young...

ANDREW: I'm 42.

DIANE: As I say. Your options are getting less and... that's partly your fault. Look, I don't want to fall out with you, and my friend will be here soon, but wouldn't you just consider your health for a minute. I bet you don't exercise do you?

ANDREW: I cycle to work and I cycle when I'm travelling if you must know.

DIANE: That's good. So if you could just bring the drinking down and stop smoking then you'd be in better shape still. Look I'm the last one to condone some of this patronising health education stuff but it's a start – and I do have some leaflets here you might like to read *(she hands him some material on drinking limits and stop-smoking strategies she happens to have in her bag)*. I could put you in touch with some good support people if you want, and we could take it further eventually...

ANDREW: *(Looking at her uncomprehendingly)* You are a journalist after all. You haven't heard a word I've said. Those things don't matter to me.

DIANE: They'd matter if you get ill before you save enough money for the summer. Then you'd be sorry, surely. I mean, it is a very uncertain existence you have isn't it? Are you sure you really want to live like this? Don't you think there are alternatives you might enjoy more?

ANDREW: You don't understand a thing. If I get ill then I'd accept it. It is a price I am willing to pay – I don't want to pay it but I am willing if I have to. So long as I'm able to live now and to save for the next trip – the next unknown journey then that's OK. Stop smoking. Stop drinking. That's pathetic. So long as I have got the chance to move on then I'm happy. So long as I've got the choice then that's enough. That means accepting the consequences of my own choices, sure – but I must have the choice or there's no point.

DIANE: You're just not making sense. There's something illogical about what you're saying but I can't put my finger on it . . . Anyway I have to go now, my friend's just come in. It has been interesting talking to you though Andrew. Look after yourself. *(Getting down clumsily from her stool)* Excuse me. Bye.

ANDREW: *(With a kindly smile)* You too. Good luck.

SCENE TWO

Diane is speaking with the philosopher from her 'phone at the Chronicle. *It is the next morning.*

DIANE: It's not that I'm worried about Andrew Wilson – though I couldn't help feeling, well, maternal toward him. What bothers me is . . . is, I don't know *what's* bothering me!

I worked out early on that health promotion is ideological – though I didn't realise quite *how* ideological it is until you convinced me that prejudice must always come first – and I thought that this would help me to be an . . . intelligent . . . health promoter. Not for me, I thought, handing out stock advice and work sheets. I wasn't going to be an all-jogging, low-fat health fanatic. So what did I do? I told the bloke to cut down the booze and to quit smoking!

But then surely this is what *any* good health promoter would do, whatever the type. The fella obviously drinks too much, he smokes like there's no tomorrow, and I *know* he would feel better if he could cut down. So I tried to talk him round – just gently, you know – and I left him some of our literature that he could take or leave. I can't see what is wrong with that. So why did I feel such a fool?

Andrew Wilson wasn't a client, and didn't ask for my advice. An opportunity just arose – I wasn't even looking for an opportunity actually – and I took it, in a very small way, and offered him information and support if he wanted it. As it turned out he didn't want it – and he . . . well, I think he thought I was ridiculous – and said he didn't want it, so I stopped straightaway.

I can't put my finger on why I'm so bothered about it though. As a health promoter I have to do something, don't I? It *is* complicated, but I can't sit on the fence forever. Whether I'm a medical health promoter, a social health promoter or a good life promoter (and I'm not, by the way) I do have to make some sort of stand somewhere otherwise there'd be no point. I understand what you say about politics – and I accept your logic – but this just doesn't seem relevant 'on the shop floor' most of the time. In the real world the health promoter must do what she can, surely.

. . . You think I've got some misconceptions? I need to have a better theoretical base so that I can feel confident in doing the small things? You might be right. But what are these misconceptions? Where am I going wrong with all this? Why can't I get a proper grip on health promotion, even after all I've learnt? What am I missing? And why can't I just adopt a version of one of the types of health promotion, and stick to that? What is so wrong with them anyway? After all, any alternative you can come up with will also be politically prejudiced won't it? Please help me get to the bottom of this – and soon!

The Outsider Problem

Andrew Wilson poses a considerable problem for those who would promote his health. All current types of health promotion, conservative and radical, propose ways of life which Andrew does not want. He wishes to smoke. He wishes to drink. He is excited by risk-taking. He does not want to settle down and raise a family. Sooner or later health promoters of any type are bound to question the wisdom of Andrew's behaviour and each, in any case, is committed in general to a form of society which does not favour Andrew's goals.

What, then, are they saying about Andrew? He is not insane, he is not ill, and he is not ignorant. Nevertheless current forms of health promotion are bound to judge Andrew at best as misguided, and at worst as thoroughly irresponsible. This, of course, is a consequence of the fact that the political philosophies of each type are incompatible with Andrew's – and these clashes highlight the toughest of theoretical tests for health promotion. What do health promoters do about people who do not share their professional goals?

WHAT IS AN OUTSIDER?

There are many types of Outsider,[70,71] but if they have one thing in common it is that at least one (and often more) of those things that are most deeply meaningful for most of us – love, family, career, loyalty, honour, fitness – are trivial or even meaningless to the Outsider:

> If you are living a very ordinary dull life at low pressure, you can safely regard the Outsider as a crank who does not deserve serious consideration. But if you are interested in man in extreme states, or in man abnormally preoccupied with questions about the nature of life, then whatever answer the Outsider may propound should be worth your respectful attention. The Outsider is interested in high speeds and great pressures; he prefers to consider the man who sets out to be very good or very wicked rather than the good citizen who advocates moderation in all things.[70]

Outsiders discussed in philosophical works and depicted in literature tend to be obviously extreme – strikingly out of step with the rest of the world. People like this are so extraordinary that health promoters can safely ignore them – there are so few of them to worry about, and in any case they seem to be quite beyond the reach of health

Health Promotion, Second Edition: David Seedhouse
© 2004 John Wiley & Sons, Ltd: ISBNs 0 470 84732 8 (HB); 0 470 84733 6 (PB)

promotion. Imagine a health promoter trying to tell Nietzsche not to get overexcited, or a 'know your limit' expert advising Hemingway to drink only 20 units of alcohol a week. That would be ridiculous.

However, health promotion's Outsider problem is far more pervasive than the occasional encounter with an impossible maverick. The everyday problem is more subtle. The real Outsider problem for health promotion is that most of us are Outsiders some of the time. Health promotion's Outsider need merely be an unconventional person – one who does not always behave according to the values espoused by a particular form of health promotion. A health promotion Outsider may be the deep-sea diver, the mountaineer, the fitness fanatic, the heavy drinker, the carefree teenager, the 'fast-lane' nightlifer – indeed anyone who 'lives in the present'.[70] Or she might be happy to be habitually lazy (never exercising, not ideally hygienic), or she may be deliberately set against standard public health interventions (refusing immunisation for her children, sacrificing the best nutrition to avoid products made with fluoridated water), or she may just find satisfaction in regular smoking and alcohol consumption.

It is difficult to see how any health promoter who claims that certain behaviours are indisputably healthy can deal intelligently with such disobedience. He might claim that the Outsider is simply wrong, or possibly insane – or perhaps he might allow that the Outsider's values can sometimes supersede 'health values'. But these strategies each carry deep conceptual difficulties which can be tackled only by means of a developed theory.

THE CASE OF ANDREW WILSON

Consider just one Outsider, as an example. Let's take the case of Andrew Wilson. Although he is by no means the most extreme of Outsiders Andrew presents a daunting challenge to any form of health promotion. Here's what we know about him:

- he is middle-aged
- he is well-educated
- he is a rebel – he rejects the conventional life
- he has a temporary, low-paid factory job
- he is single
- he is probably an only child
- he is recently bereaved (his mother died)
- he smokes tobacco
- he seems to drink heavily
- he likes to travel independently – to be trapped in one place, especially England, is difficult for Andrew to bear
- Andrew seeks adventure, difference, risk – that is what makes him feel alive
- he does not want to think beyond the next six months
- he cycles, and enjoys it

EXERCISE EIGHT

EVERY QUESTION IS AN ETHICAL QUESTION

You are a health promoter. You have met Andrew Wilson as part of your 'Outreach' work. You wish to promote his health, and to do so thoughtfully. Therefore:

a. List, in order of importance, the aspects of Andrew's life you would most wish to work on.
b. Explain why you have ranked this list as you have.
c. Explain any practical steps you would take to promote Andrew's health.
d. Explain the points at which you would *cease* to try to promote Andrew's health.
e. Clarify any clashes of value there may be between Andrew and you.
f. Where there are clashes explain which values – Andrew's or yours – ought to take priority.

Teaching notes for: Every Question is an Ethical Question

This interesting exercise can develop in all manner of ways, and can be an important catalyst for deep controversy, drawing out of students their previously implicit moral and political positions.

———————◆———————

For the purposes of illustration, here is a brief and selective summary of one student's exercise answers. She was basically a **medical health promoter** who took her cue from the UK *Health of the Nation* document. No one else in the class agreed with her so, unsurprisingly, she began her report defensively:

> I know it's unfashionable, but I firmly believe that some behaviours are unhealthy because they are likely to cause damage to a person's body and mind. I also believe that people do not realise the consequences of what they are doing to themselves until these actually happen. Therefore I believe that health promoters, who do know what bad things can happen, have a duty to protect people from these harms to their health. Here are my answers to the exercise questions:

continues

continued

    a. his drinking
       his smoking
       his relationships
       his nutrition
       his exercise
    b. From what we have been told Andrew is a heavy drinker, and he drinks each night. He gets drunk in the pub every evening of the year, I believe, and that is simply not good for anyone. Deal with that and you could begin to work on the rest, but unless you tackle his alcoholism then you won't get anywhere...
    c. If I had targeted Andrew I would first try to educate him about the dangers of drinking, and I would also try to involve him in other group activities – and if these happened to be organised by Alcoholics Anonymous I would not object one little bit...
    d. I would not give up on Andrew. I do not believe he knows what he is doing, at least not so far as his drinking is concerned, nor his smoking for that matter. Maybe in the other areas I would back off if he told me to, but otherwise I believe I should carry out my duty to promote health...
    e. I would say that these are obvious. I believe in health and fitness, in a long and happy life, and Andrew is making some very serious mistakes
    f. Health values should take priority, though if they did there would still be room for other values.

It is important to point out that these answers are not problematic because they have been generated by a version of **medical health promotion**, rather *any answers* to this exercise will be ethically challenging just because this is the nature of health promotion. If your group happens to be of one mind, it will be harder for you to demonstrate this *essential controversy*, but it will always be possible (you might, for instance, suggest a plausible alternative set of answers, one which your students will at least see the sense of, and begin to debate the ethics of these).

In the example of the answers above, you might prompt the student as follows, without putting her under unnecessary pressure:

a. Why are Andrew's relationships of concern to health promoters? By what right can a health promoter intervene in Andrew's social life if Andrew does not request an intervention?

continues

continued

b. What is a heavy drinker? Is this category a matter of fact or a matter of opinion? You might like to discuss the raising of the officially recommended safe drinking levels in the UK mentioned in Dialogue One.

c. How can you be sure that the steps you propose to improve Andrew's health will not be counter-productive?

d. What is the source of your *duty* to promote health? Is the duty created by the fact of your employment as a health promotion officer? Is it a moral duty? Or is it both? Whatever the case, is it a *supreme* duty or are there potential reasons why you ought not continue to promote Andrew's health?

e. How can we tell whether one sort of value is better than another sort? What are the rules? What is the formula for finding this out?

f. What is the difference between health values and other sorts of values? When (if ever) can other sorts of value take precedence over health values?

No doubt countless other questions will suggest themselves to you, and you will enjoy a stimulating debate.

At the end of the session students should appreciate that they *each* have areas of their thinking about the *purpose* and *justification* of health promotion that require further development and support by argument.

THE OUTSIDER DILEMMA

As a health promoter – whether you favour **medical health promotion, social health promotion, good life promotion, go for it health promotion** or **mix 'n match** – the Outsider sets you a serious dilemma. Let's spell it out some more.

It is the nature of a dilemma that a person believes she *must* do two things but cannot because to do one will automatically make it impossible to do the other. In the case of Andrew Wilson (and with Outsiders in general) the two aims are:

1. *to ensure that Andrew is as healthy as possible* (which means the health promoter must somehow change some or all of Andrew's habits and/or life circumstances)

and

2. *to treat Andrew with respect, as a competent adult* who knowingly makes choices and is prepared to take the consequences (to treat him as a person who hopes and expects these consequences to be good, but who knows they may not turn out that way).

Of course, it is possible to overcome this dilemma instantly, by ignoring 2. However, it is unlikely that any credible form of health promotion would wish to do this.

THE DILEMMA FOR MEDICAL HEALTH PROMOTION

Recall the rationale of **medical health promotion**:

MEDICAL HEALTH PROMOTION

Health exists in the absence of disease, illness, injury, handicap, and the like
Disease, illness and injury are bad in themselves
Disease, illness and injury are also bad because they prevent people's normal functioning
Disease, illness and injury are disruptive (they cost people normal life opportunities, and they cost nations both working days lost and the price of treatment and prevention)
Bad health is experienced by individuals. Therefore the basic target of strategies to improve people's health should be behavioural change/lifestyle change, in order to minimise social disruption
Prevention of bad health should be undertaken where it is shown to work and where it poses no threat to the stability of a society

This gives the following specific dilemma:

The **medical health promoter** must seek both:

1. to ensure that Andrew is as healthy as possible – which in this case means that she should seek, by the quickest and most effective means, to change those aspects of Andrew's lifestyle which make him susceptible to disease and illness

and

2. to treat Andrew with respect, as a competent adult who knowingly makes choices and is prepared to take the consequences.

Remember that Andrew is not ignorant of the risks he is running and has chosen to take his chances in order to enjoy his present life to the full. Can the **medical health promoter** escape the dilemma? What are the options? The most obvious is to argue that it is not truly a dilemma, that a **medical health promoter** is obliged to seek only one of the two goals and that as a **medical health promoter** her obligation must lie in ensuring that Andrew is as healthy as possible *even if* this means overriding his wishes. But cast so starkly – as it must be in the absence of a decent theory of health promotion ethics – this solution offers a disquietingly impoverished picture of human life, one in which not being diseased matters more than anything else. And the reality *is* indeed this stark for **medical health promotion** as it currently is. The **medical health promoter** might like to express a wish to be reasonable and balanced and not to be 'healthist', but the Outsider problem does not allow her to sit on the fence. Either she is committed to **medical health promotion** or she is not. And if she is committed to it then she must be supremely committed to it: either that or she must come up with a more mature and flexible understanding of health and health promotion – an understanding of sufficient calibre to resolve the dilemma.

Nor is it an answer to ignore Andrew as an individual. It is not an answer for the **medical health promoter** to say that her work – as a campaigner say – is carried out at the 'population level', and that she need never confront individuals in this way. This is no answer because the public health work of medical health promotion has broad implications – it changes the social climate (and so may well indirectly pressurise Andrew), it influences government policy, and the money it consumes could be spent differently – it could even be spent helping people to live more unusual lives.

Nor can the **medical health promoter** argue that she ought to respect Andrew's choices in general, but not those that are bad for his health. For without the benefit of a coherent theory of health she will not be able to distinguish between Andrew's 'health choices' and his 'other choices'.[23]

THE DILEMMA FOR SOCIAL HEALTH PROMOTION

Recall the rationale of **social health promotion**:

SOCIAL HEALTH PROMOTION

Health exists in the absence of disease, illness, injury, handicap, and the like
Disease, illness, injury and handicap are bad in themselves
Disease, illness, injury and handicap are also bad because they prevent people maximising their life potentials
Disease, illness, injury and handicap (and therefore health) are unevenly distributed across differently privileged social groups
The causes of disease, illness, injury and handicap are manifold. Sometimes, however, it can be shown that they are the result of how people either choose to or have to live
Where disease, illness, injury and handicap are the result of broader social inequities health promotion ought to attempt to change these social conditions (be they bad housing, poor community amenities, inadequate education, debilitating employment or whatever). Behavioural change is not necessarily out of the question but it is inappropriate to attempt behavioural change without at the same time attempting to remedy socially caused health inequalities, and therefore without at the same time attempting to empower the most unfortunate members of society to live healthier lives

This gives the following specific dilemma. The **social health promoter** must seek both:

1. to ensure that Andrew is as healthy as possible – which in this case means that she should seek, by the most effective means, to change those aspects of Andrew's lifestyle *and* those features of society which make Andrew susceptible to disease and illness

and

2. to treat Andrew with respect, as a competent adult who knowingly makes choices and is prepared to take the consequences.

Can the **social health promoter** escape the Outsider dilemma? Like the **medical health promoter**, her only option seems to be to relegate one of the goals to something less than a duty. And, as a **social health promoter**, it seems she must, to be worthy of the name, decide that her duty lies with the first goal *even if* this means overriding Andrew's wishes. But in this case, what will she be implying about Andrew's life?

If the **social health promoter** takes this line she is surely committed to the position that because of inappropriate social conditioning and circumstances Andrew is somehow being forced to make unhealthy choices. But this is to assume that only some sorts of social circumstance produce competent decision-makers, and this assumption can only be based on values (the evidence is that Andrew is making consistent choices – the problem is that the **social health promoter** does not value them).

Alternatively, of course, the **social health promoter** might take the Stacey line and opt for the second solution to the dilemma, and allow – or even encourage – Andrew to make the choices he deems best for himself. But this is hardly an adequate way to deal with the dilemma, for in this case health promotion becomes nothing more than general and unconditional support for whatever choices any subject wishes to fulfil. Unless it is prepared to take a stand, health promotion vanishes.[6]

THE DILEMMA FOR GOOD LIFE PROMOTION

Recall the rationale of **good life health promotion**:

GOOD LIFE HEALTH PROMOTION

Health is partly to do with the absence of disease, illness, injury and handicap, but is more than just the opposite of these negative factors. Good health, in its fullest sense, means complete well-being
Disease, illness, injury and handicap are bad in themselves, and well-being is good in itself
Disease, illness, injury and handicap are bad because they prevent normal biological and social functioning. Lack of well-being is bad because this means that a person's life as a whole (including his thoughts, beliefs, attitudes, and values) is not as it should be
The prevention and treatment of bad health, and the promotion of well-being are beneficial for many reasons (cost-effectiveness, less pain, a happier world, and so on). Primarily, though, these things should be done simply because it is important that people live flourishing lives

This gives the starkest dilemma of all. That is, the **good life promoter** must seek both:

1. to ensure that Andrew is as healthy and fulfilled as possible – which in this case means she should seek, by the most effective means, to change all those aspects of Andrew's lifestyle which are not compatible with his having a good life

and

2. to treat Andrew with respect, as a competent adult who knowingly makes choices and is prepared to take the consequences. (Unless she believes that this is not part of a good life, but this is hardly likely, at least for a Western **good life promoter**.)

It seems the **good life promoter** must opt for the first choice, so things boil down to this: Andrew believes he has some well-being and is likely to gain more through his actions and plans, while the **good life promoter** does not and is committed to changing Andrew's life. Such a rudimentary conflict requires some further thought. What is going on, and how has this version of health promotion become so excessively forthright?

EXERCISE NINE

YOU ARE AN OUTSIDER

In this exercise you are required to play the part of an Outsider. To do so, take the following steps:

1. Decide on an 'Outsider behaviour' for yourself.

2. Outline a general health promotion policy that might be espoused by either **medical health promotion, social health promotion** or **good life promotion**.

3. Carefully note how this poses the Outsider dilemma, as stated on p. 137 above.

4 In your role as an Outsider, mount the most convincing argument you can that the health (or good life) promoter should leave you alone.

Teaching notes for: You Are An Outsider

It is not easy to predict how this exercise will go. Much depends on the type of student, on the extent to which they espouse conventional health promotion approaches, and on their willingness to have some fun. However, assuming a reasonable level of open-mindedness, this exercise can be very stimulating, and can provoke lively debate about both prejudice and evidence.

1. Your first task, as teacher or group leader, is to ensure that students select plausible 'Outsider' behaviours. If the choices are too outrageous the exercise will not work. It is the more subtle 'Outsider' behaviours which pose the greatest challenge for health promotion.

continues

continued

Appropriate choices might include Andrew Wilson's behaviours; excessive long-distance running (over 100km per week, for instance); a wealthy young man who enjoys the high life – especially eating the richest foods at the best restaurants without any thought about salt, fat and cholesterol content; a devout religious person who keeps unconventional hours and has no friends outside his religious circle; a middle-aged woman who secretly smokes marijuana each day to relax after work; a person who is unemployed, lives in a drab high-rise flat in an inner city, who has a nocturnal existence in various night-clubs, and who says he would not change this for anything; a person who has been unemployed for so long he no longer seeks work but has a satisfying life as a member of a rural motor-cycle gang. These cases will pose different degrees of challenge to the different forms of health promotion. As group leader you should aim to have students pair up a particular behaviour with that form of health promotion which is likely to have most trouble dealing with it.

2. You should next help students select a version of *one* form of health promotion, and encourage them briefly to outline the key contextual and behavioural changes this type of health promotion would be seeking in the name of health. **Good life promotion** is the easiest form to specify – all students need to do is to state a preference for a life of moderation, balance, employment, convention, and so on. Because this is easy to do it may be better to have most students concentrate on versions of **medical health promotion** and **social health promotion**, and have them state how these forms might specify healthy living.

   Whatever the case, it is important that all involved in the exercise are as *specific as possible* about the content of steps 1 and 2.

3. After this, spend a little time spelling out the Outsider dilemma again. Emphasise that a health promoter who believes in a particular account of health *and* who believes that people should be treated as adults, seems to face an impossible dilemma if her understanding of health conflicts with that of the person or persons whose health she would like to promote.

   Encourage discussion, for a few minutes at least, about possible ways around the dilemma. These include opting directly for one of the choices; questioning the competence or knowledge of the subject; and putting forward an account of health which is either *limited* theoretically and practically, or in which health is a 'secondary value' or of less importance than some other preferences. However the conversation goes, your task is to pull out the *further* implications of adopting any of these solutions to the dilemma: what would it *mean* for the health promoter to call a subject incompetent? Where should the health promoter draw the line? What values are more important than health? and so on.

continues

continued

4. Most of the exercise is now completed. The main point of steps 1–3 has been to clarify students' thinking about different types of health promotion, to bring them up against possible ethical limits, and to have them take seriously ways of living which run counter to mainstream thinking about healthy lives.

Now you can thoroughly enjoy the remainder of this exercise. One productive way to do this is to have students take sides and argue against each other – though be careful to select only those students who are capable of, and willing to, role-play consistently.

A BRIDGE TOO FAR – HEALTH PROMOTION'S ILLEGITIMATE SLIDE INTO WELL-BEING PROMOTION

As we have already noted (Fig. 7, point 3, Fig. 9, point 4, and during the discussion of *fundamentalist health promotion*) there is an increasingly popular view in some health promotion circles that the promotion of health in the traditional, medical sense can merge smoothly and inevitably into the promotion of well-being. This view has been given some (rather thoughtless) support by recent interest in measuring 'quality of life', and by the proliferation of measures[72] which purport to be able to do this. Nevertheless, the idea is profoundly mistaken, and needs to be thoroughly exposed as such.

Why is it so important to *show* that health promotion cannot be well-being promotion? Why go to so much trouble to demonstrate that **good life promotion** can never resolve the Outsider problem unless it promotes the life the Outsider chooses? There are three main reasons. Firstly, it *is* possible to resolve the Outsider dilemma. Indeed it is possible for **medical health promotion** and **social health promotion** to resolve it so long as these forms are willing to accept a theory of purpose which sets theoretical and practical limits on health promotion interventions. To appreciate this, and its importance for the future of health promotion, it is very useful to be able to point to an example which fails, as **good life** or **well-being promotion** does. Secondly, there are only two ways in which **good life promotion** can escape the dilemma. One is to prove that it has discovered an objective good life; the other is to show that the Outsider's choices are objectively wrong. It cannot do either of these, of course, but nevertheless versions of **good life promotion** seek to move from what they regard as *evidence* of unhealthy (or wrong) behaviours to *evidence* of bad lives. It should be obvious by now that this move is conceptually flawed, but it is worth the risk of a little repetition to emphasise it further.

This leads to the third reason for spelling out, as fully as possible, the ethical limitations of **good life** or **well-being promotion**. Because some influential groups of health promoters have so much invested in retaining a broad appeal, and in insisting they are in step with the WHO and its fashionable declarations, there is a lot at stake.

There is a health promotion industry, and it is a comfortable place to be if you don't think too hard and don't rock the boat. This cosy arrangement cannot last forever, because of its lack of theoretical grounding – sooner or later the edifice will crumble, but those who live in it are not going to allow that to happen without a fight. That is why their mistakes need to be laid totally bare. It is almost certain that most establishment health promotion authorities will ignore the arguments you are reading now – this is the stock tactic of all vested interests, after all. However, the more plain the errors are to see the less chance there will be of the industry continuing to get away with them for too long.

LACK OF ANALYSIS

Despite the current interest in measuring well-being, it must be said that it is not possible to do it. Not one existing 'measure' of well-being and quality of life offers even a half-plausible explanation of what these terms might mean. Instead, labouring under the *illusion of shared meaning*, they tend merely to ask such vague questions as:

> To what extent are you experiencing difficulty in the area of:
>
> 1. managing day-to-day life
> 2. household responsibilities . . . [73]

or

> During the last four weeks, how much of the time has your *physical health* or *emotional problems* interfered with your social activities (like visiting with friends, relatives etc.)?[74]

or they ask people to report *both* their levels of capability (how well they can walk, run, handle relationships and so on) *and* their levels of life satisfaction (whether the subject has felt 'full of life', 'down in the dumps', 'calm and peaceful', and so on),[75] simply assuming that these are obviously commensurable aspects of life.

The conceptual difficulties of well-being and quality of life measures and surveys mirror those of health promotion itself. Without proper theoretical underpinning, well-being and quality of life surveyors will either not notice, or will not see why they should worry, that:

i. the multitude of different questionnaires do not ask the same questions, and so cannot give the same results
ii. the questionnaires are bound to make value-laden assumptions about the nature of well-being and so are bound to guide respondents' answers in significant ways
iii. the surveys seek to give technical content to a notion which is irreducibly subjective in part (and therefore not translatable into such technical forms)[76,77] and
iv. crucially, even if an agreed gold standard measure of well-being could be negotiated this would inevitably be only one – albeit official – account of well-being among a range of alternatives (each ultimately differently politically inspired). What is well-being for one group of people (or for one culture) is not necessarily well-being for another. (For instance, most of the current crop of questionnaires focus first on the individual whereas many non-Western cultures focus first on the family.)

Despite these points, the measurement of 'quality of life' and 'health status' has become a growth industry in recent years. And as it has grown its exponents have tended to use increasingly technical words and notions to describe their activities: for instance, the various measures are commonly judged according to how 'valid' and 'reliable' they are. Unfortunately, however, scant attention has been paid to the 'validity and reliability' of these terms themselves: in what sense, for instance, can a questionnaire meant to establish levels of well-being be 'valid' in the absence of any explicit understanding of the nature of the key term?

It is beyond the scope of this book to discuss these matters properly. But if you are interested you might like to read *Health Care Analysis* **4**[5] (available from any local university library), which is devoted to this very theme.

EXISTING WORK WHICH SHOWS THE IMPOSSIBILITY OF OBJECTIVELY ASSESSING WELL-BEING

It is not that the surveys are not yet precise enough and will come right over time. The problem is ultimately conceptual, as previous theoretical work (done over centuries) has shown.

Psychological Interpretations of 'Well-being'

Psychologists have been thinking about the nature of well-being for over 30 years:

> ...there would seem to be no small merit in being able to measure and consequently monitor [well-being]. For example, if medical personnel were able to measure subjective well-being, an indication of a patient's quality of life preceding, during and following a treatment would be available: this not only making rational discussion of quality versus quantity of life possible, but also providing additional information for use in decision-making when alternative treatments are possible.[78]

If an instrument capable of measuring well-being accurately could be designed, then it might come to be as useful as: '...the clinician's thermometer: with a sensitivity to changes of a not necessarily long duration, and...[be able to]...measure a state...'.[78] But it is one thing to find a term useful for the purposes of communication between professionals and for general taxonomy – yet quite another to say that the term stands for something definite, and represents the ultimate practical goal of health promotion. In fact, while there is some consensus amongst psychologists that well-being is 'constructed' out of three components – life satisfaction (which is said to be cognitive), positive affect and negative affect (which are said to be experiences) – beyond this the nature of well-being remains mysterious:

> Proposals for a distinction between inner and outer dimensions of well-being are considered promising but speculative at present...Although considerable research into subjective well-being exists, the structure of well-being is not yet well established or researched...[79]

WELL-BEING IS NOT OUT THERE

But of course it is a matter of logic that psychologists who hold different life values will continue to advance different accounts of well-being. Psychologists interested in finding out more about well-being are not searching for an independently existing thing; rather they are attempting to *manufacture* a helpful notion or concept. The notion of well-being (just like the notion of health) does not exist separately from human beings' theories about it, and so cannot be discovered in the way that the relationship between heat, volume and pressure can.

There are several other theories of well-being in existence. These are not meant necessarily to have practical implications, but again they differ, and it is surely impossible finally to resolve these differences. Aristotle had an explicit theory of well-being, a state he described as eudaemonia,[80] and there are at least three modern philosophical accounts of well-being on offer. The three are traditionally divided into: 'hedonist', 'desire fulfilment' and 'objectivist' theories,[81] and are worth a brief review.

The Hedonist Theory of Well-being

The hedonist theory holds that an individual's well-being is determined by the extent of the 'felt satisfaction' we experience during our lives. Hedonists believe that the only factors that contribute directly to individual human well-being are our experiences of pleasure, enjoyment, or satisfaction. All other good things are of instrumental value only.

According to one version of the hedonist theory, the level of an individual's well-being can be 'totted up' by giving a positive value to the pleasurable episodes experienced by a person during her life, and a negative one for unpleasant episodes.[82] More general varieties of the hedonist position assess well-being not by calculating the value of fragmented experiences, but by trying to assess a person's life satisfaction as a whole.

Although the hedonistic idea is appealingly simple at first sight, the assessment of human well-being by calculating the difference between pleasurable and unpleasurable episodes is far from straightforward. For example, to derive a realistic assessment of a person's 'pleasure level', at the very least the duration and intensity of her pleasures and pains must be taken into account. Furthermore, not all pleasures and pains are of the same quality – the same sources of pleasure and pain can be experienced differently according to the sensitivity of the person experiencing them. For example, although two people of normal hearing listening to an excellently performed piece of music will receive the same auditory stimulus, and may both have a pleasurable experience, if one is a music teacher and the other understands nothing of music other than knowing what he likes, they may well each enjoy the same piece but will almost certainly do so in significantly different ways.

If an advocate of the hedonist understanding of well-being tries to sidestep the details – and says instead that well-being simply means 'general life satisfaction' – he then faces the difficulty of developing a conception of life satisfaction clear and determinate enough to be useful to those who would like to promote it in practice. He must, for example, explain the relationship (if there is one) between life satisfaction and the more short-lived pleasures. Is life satisfaction only partly to do with pleasures? If so, what proportion of pleasures has to be taken into the reckoning? Do all pleasures carry the same weight? Is it possible for pains to add to life satisfaction? And so on. But once the advocate of the hedonist theory begins to take these questions seriously he ceases to be a pure hedonist (since he begins to admit that it is possible to understand well-being without necessarily referring to directly pleasurable experiences).

The Desire Fulfilment Position

According to this position human well-being is brought about by the fulfilment of desires, wants or preferences. The central idea is that life goes well for us to the extent that we get or achieve what we desire.[82] Desire theories of well-being are broader than hedonistic theories since we do not always desire those things that are directly pleasurable to us. Indeed we can desire some stressful, trying states because we think that it is important to experience such things.

Like hedonism, the desire theory is a subjective theory of well-being in that it insists that only the subjective mental states (the desires or preferences) of an individual can determine what constitutes her well-being.

Objectivist Theories

According to objectivist theories (such as the *fundamentalist* good life view described earlier) well-being depends upon conditions and circumstances which have a positive value for *any* life which includes them. Within these theories well-being is typically said to be generated by success in one's work, or in giving one's children a good start in life; to involve states of character, such as courage, humour, integrity, or self-understanding; and to be at least partly based on good relationships with other people.

The problem with objectivist theories is that sooner or later they become paternalistic, and if they are applied to the lives of those who do not agree with their content they are nothing other than the imposition of *blinkered* prejudice on unwilling recipients.

THE KEY CONCEPTUAL ERROR

Ultimately of much deeper significance than the ubiquitous *illusions*, the reason why it has become fashionable to think that health promotion ought to be **well-being promotion** is that some health promotion theorists are unknowingly perpetuating a conceptual error. As we saw in Chapter Five, these theorists seem seriously to believe that conventional health promotion can slide sweetly into well-being promotion: that 'negative health promotion' can become 'positive health promotion' without even so much as a blip. This mistake is in danger of becoming the latest trend in health promotion, and so it is essential to show precisely what is wrong with it.

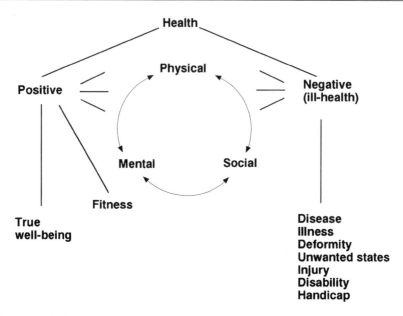

Figure 14   A model of health (reproduced with permission from R. S. Downie, C. Fyfe and A. Tannahill, *Health Promotion: Models and Values*, Oxford, 1990, Fig. 2.3)

POSITIVE AND NEGATIVE HEALTH: THE ERROR EXPOSED

Once again, Downie, Fyfe and Tannahill offer a prime example of the error. They are by no means the only culprits – indeed it is hard to find theoretical work in health promotion which does not commit this error in one way or another. Downie et al. have been singled out merely because their work is an attempt to synthesise so much that is conceptually ill-founded in contemporary health promotion – and so provides a perfect foil for constructive criticism. At one place in *Health Promotion: Models and Values* they explain that positive health is made up of 'true well-being' and 'fitness' and that negative health consists of 'ill-health' (see Fig. 14).

As far as it is possible to make sense of this figure (and the authors' explanation of it) the idea seems to be:

1. that preventing negative health can cause positive health
2. that health promotion has the twin goals of preventing negative health and promoting positive health
3. that positive health can *also* be caused in ways other than preventing negative health.

The authors are rather careless in their use of terminology in this discussion. It is permissible – they say (p. 24) – to *substitute* positive health for well-being in their Fig. 2.2 (Fig. 17 in this text) but in their Fig. 2.3 well-being is depicted as an *offshoot* of positive health. But it cannot be both and, as far as I can see, this immediately renders their account incoherent: either positive health is the same as well-being or it is not. But let this pass.

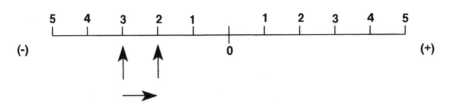

Figure 15 Health as a continuum (reproduced with permission from R. S. Downie, C. Fyfe and A. Tannahill, *Health Promotion: Models and Values*, Oxford, 1990, Fig. 2.1)

Figure 16 This is not the case

As we have seen the authors are aware that the relationship between positive and negative health is not a simple one since positive health is not wholly of the same family as negative health. Indeed, they rightly point out that the picture is not as drawn in Fig. 15.

To put it slightly differently, it is not the case that positive and negative health are related as integers on a continuum (Fig. 16), where the addition of a positive number will *automatically* move the pointer from –3 to –2. Rather it is as shown in Fig. 17.

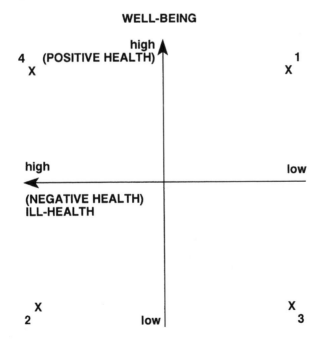

Figure 17 The relationship between (positive health) well-being and (negative health) ill-health (reproduced with permission from R. S. Downie, C. Fyfe and A. Tannahill, *Health Promotion: Models and Values*, Oxford, 1990, Fig. 2.2)

(Note that positive health can be substituted for well-being and negative health can be substituted for ill-health – as is allowed by the authors, at their p. 24.)

This (amended) figure claims that people who have negative health do not automatically lack positive health (or well-being) since these are different – though related – sorts of thing. Thus Downie et al. argue that it is possible to have high levels of both positive and negative health simultaneously:

> This person [number 4 on the diagram] is experiencing a high level of well-being despite a high level of ill-health. Such people may feel in peak physical condition, unaware of an advanced malignancy, or may be terminally ill but well-adjusted to their fate, at peace with themselves and the world.[6]

It is also possible to have other combinations, as shown by the Xs in their figure (Fig. 17). However, these details are of little importance overall. What does matter, however, is the authors' claim that positive health (which I am interpreting as interchangeable with well-being) and negative health are not on a single continuum. They are correct in this assertion *but* they have not developed this insight to its logical conclusion because they want to synthesise **medical health promotion** and **good life promotion** (along with all the other elements listed in Chapter Five). This mixing of negative and positive health *cannot be done*, and the full logic would have made this clear. It only looks as if it can be done if matters are left at **Type One** level (see p. 33 above) – i.e. if the various meanings are left reassuringly fuzzy. But to leave things like this is to miss *everything* of ethical import in health promotion – and a more devastating oversight is impossible to imagine. The full reasoning is as follows.

THE STEPS

In order to show that well-being and negative health are not necessarily related, and so are not necessarily poles on a continuum, assume for the moment that well-being means *contentment* (undoubtedly one plausible interpretation – and perhaps easier to comprehend). This gives a continuum which looks like Fig. 18. Now, if a person contracts a disease it is *likely* that she will also become less content (see Fig. 19).

However, as Downie et al. point out, it is not *certain* that this will be the case. It may be that a person contracts a heavy winter cold, but that life is generally going very well, she feels she needs a good rest away from work, and the chance to be with her young

Contentment ——————————————————— **Negative health:**

Disease
Illness
Deformity
Unwanted states
Injury
Disability
Handicap

Figure 18   The contentment–negative health continuum

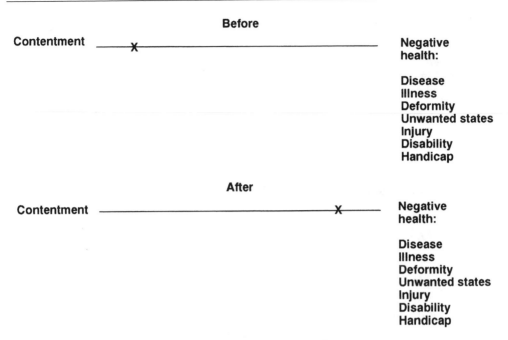

Figure 19 Level of contentment before and after contracting a disease

daughter who is away from school and who otherwise would be in the charge of a nanny. In this case a simple continuum will not represent the situation – it cannot cope with a person being just as content with life *and* having an increase of negative health. There must be two crosses, not one, and they split as in Fig. 20.

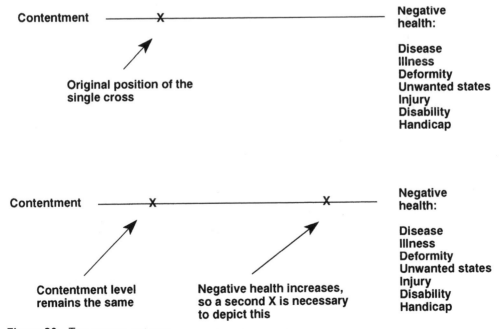

Figure 20 Two crosses, not one

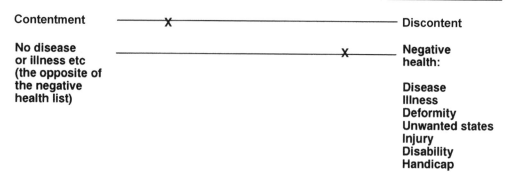

Figure 21   A realistic depiction of the person with the winter cold

The only way to deal with the reality of the situation is to use at least two continua (Fig. 21).

It then becomes possible to describe other situations where contentment and negative health are not tied together. For example, a person with a stable chronic condition (diabetes, low back pain, or angina) can obviously have fluctuating levels of contentment as depicted in Fig. 22. Furthermore, it is quite possible that a person's negative health could increase at the same time as his contentment increases. For example, a person may learn pain and life-management skills – and come to accept his status – and so become more content even as his pain worsens (Fig. 23).[83]

It should be quite plain that although the two continua may be related, they are by no means always related. Contentment *can* fluctuate *quite independently* of disease status – and disease status can fluctuate quite independently of contentment (in the case of a symptomless disease, for instance).

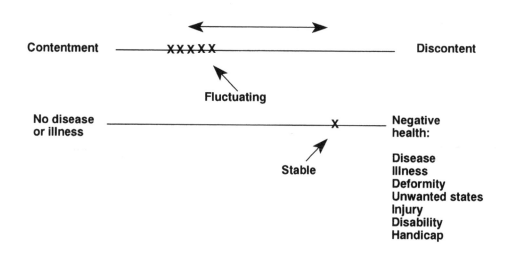

Figure 22   Fluctuating contentment–stable clinical condition

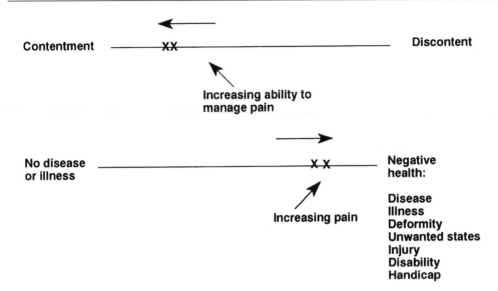

Figure 23   No necessary relationship

THERE IS NO NECESSARY RELATIONSHIP BETWEEN NEGATIVE HEALTH AND WELL-BEING

The basic mistake is that, even in their Fig. 2.2 (Fig. 17 in this text), Downie et al. insist on *some* necessary relationship between ill-health (negative health) and well-being (positive health). On their account, and in their figure, it is *impossible* to refer to the one without also referring to the other. But herein lies the error – the relationship is actually coincidental – and this is crucially important ethically, as we shall see in Part Three. Well-being and negative health are separate ideas – indeed they are qualitatively different (well-being has a necessarily subjective element – negative health does not). *Well-being and negative health are no more necessarily related than happiness and a person's height, or misery and the weather, or arrogance and a person's employment.* These pairs *can* (and often do) have a bearing on each other but they need not have and – like health and well-being – there is no good reason to put them together on a chart as in Downie et al.'s Fig. 2.2. It just *looks* like a necessary connection (a) because it is becoming the accepted convention and (b) because no one has seriously considered that it might be mistaken. So a norm has been established – health and well-being have become associated by intellectual default, and the health promotion edifice has grown ever more ethically suffocating.

To repeat: the relationship between health and well-being – or health and the good life – is contingent. The health continuum and the well-being continuum are separate. If you want a quick demonstration of this then all you need to know is that almost *any* other sort of continuum could replace the 'ill-health' continuum in Downie, Fyfe and Tannahill's original figure. Just for example, consider Fig. 24.

Assuming that well-being means contentment, it is obviously possible to have a low level of education and high well-being (X1), a low level of well-being and a high level of education (X2), and so on. It happens all the time.

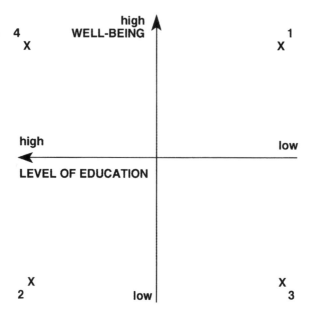

Figure 24   The relationship between well-being and level of education

Any other continuum will do, for example Fig. 25.

Again, I assume my contemporary dance skills are minimal but nevertheless I do (I believe) sometimes experience high well-being (X1). Equally, I once witnessed an excellent contemporary dance troupe whom I have good reason to believe (from the message they wished to convey) had worryingly depleted well-being levels (X2).

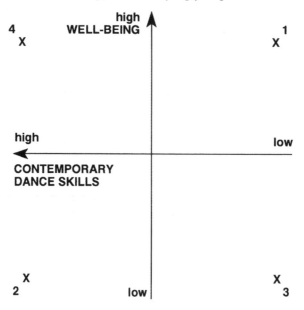

Figure 25   The relationship between well-being and contemporary dance skills

If virtually *any* other continuum can be linked with well-being then there is no special connection in the case of health. There just seems to be because a group of people at the WHO, for some reason, once came up with an intellectually barren 'definition of health', it became dogma, and this supremely unsound idea has been propagated ever since – so much so that in some quarters it is almost heresy to challenge it:

> The central concept of health promotion, and the launching pad of many of its most exciting ideas, is health itself. Accordingly, we begin with an examination of the concept of health, taking as our initial text the much quoted and universally criticized World Health Organization (WHO) definition of health:
>
>> Health is a state of complete physical, mental and social well-being, and not merely the absence of disease or infirmity.
>
> *This definition makes several important points for our purposes.*
>
> First of all, it involves a distinction between health negatively defined – as the absence of ill-health – and health as a positive state – seen as the presence of well-being. Developing this distinction, we assign a substantial amount of our next chapter to the delineation of the negative and positive dimensions of health, and their complex interrelationships. We broaden out from the WHO conception of positive health to include fitness in addition to well-being. (p. 2)[6] (My italics)

It is *worse* than the Emperor's New Clothes. It is surely impossible to 'broaden out from' the state of completeness the WHO describes, but the myth has become so deep-seated, and the various theorists are so keen to build further on the WHO's hallowed foundations, that additional nonsenses are continually clipped onto them.

The problem, of course, lies in the italicised sentence in the quote above: *this definition makes several important points for our purposes* – we can fit it with our prejudices and use it to our advantage, in other words. But not every idea can legitimately be made into the shape you want it to be. If it could there would be no intellectual standards and no role for careful deliberation. But there are philosophical standards, they can be applied to practical effect, and there is really no excuse for failing to heed their logic.

WELL-BEING PROMOTION SLIDES INTO ARROGANCE

For the **good life promoter** it is not enough only to focus on negative health. Rather it is Andrew's well-being as a whole which needs to be improved. But unless the good life promoter shares Andrew's outlook (which is unlikely and is certainly not the case with the form of good life espoused by Downie, Fyfe and Tannahill) the situation is that however much Andrew may think he has well-being the good life promoter will be convinced he does not.

Good life promoters *must* claim privileged knowledge of well-being, and are *bound* to declare that it is possible to achieve objective or true well-being, or they will have no case:

> 'Well-being' sometimes means no more than people's subjective estimations of mood or level of happiness on a given occasion. In this sense, they themselves are the only authority on their well-being, and there is no implication as to how they have come to be in that state or how long it will last. If they are 'feeling great' then they have a high degree

of subjective well-being whether that state will last minutes or a life-time, whether it is brought about by being in love, going for a swim, good weather, or alcohol.

> Subjective well-being, however, may be spurious...[and]...may arise from influences which are overall detrimental to an individual's functioning or flourishing, and/or to society...we must look to a more objective assessment of well-being. In doing so it is important to pay attention to the <u>origins</u> of feelings of well-being. (p. 18)[6]

That is:

> Subjective well-being...must stand up to some sort of outside scrutiny if we are to consider it to be a true state of well being'...(p. 18)[6]

And:

> A great deal of wisdom has been accumulated over the centuries about the kinds of activities which make for a flourishing human life. (p. 18)[6]

However, while it cannot be denied that *Homo sapiens* has thought long and hard about what makes a good life (and that it is often possible, generally speaking, to distinguish wise words from foolish ones) it is equally indisputable that the resultant wisdom, taken as a whole, is not only made up of an astonishing diversity of ideas but that these ideas often conflict with each other. There is not one consistent body of wisdom about the flourishing life and in pluralistic societies – never mind between societies – any claim to know objectively the constituents of a worthwhile existence must be treated with the utmost caution.

For the **good life promoter** the continua are represented by Fig. 26.

Yet if **Andrew** were to think in the same terms the picture would be that of Fig. 27.

Note that while the lower continuum (disease–absence of disease) would be pictured identically by the health promoter and Andrew (because there are various

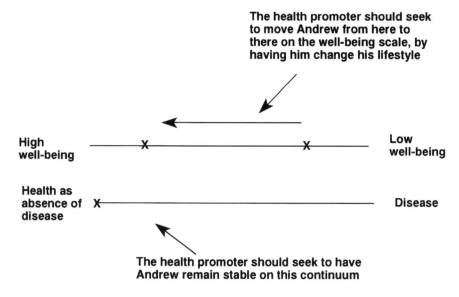

Figure 26   The point of view of the good life promoter

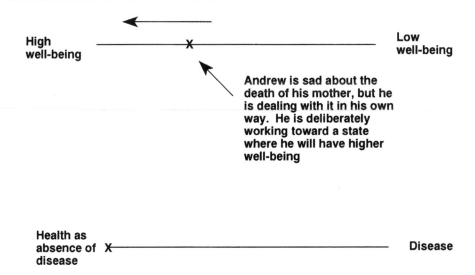

Figure 27   Andrew's point of view

measurables and facts involved)[84] the higher continuum – the well-being scale – appears quite different because this is entirely the realm of value and prejudice.

A False Link

Andrew disagrees with the **good life promoter**. The **good life promoter** disagrees with Andrew. This is a matter of prejudice. Perhaps recognising this, the health promoter who seeks to promote well-being *and* health seeks to give the impression that he can link what is not linkable – that is, the health promoter seeks to justify a prejudice by appeal to evidence that has nothing necessarily to do with that prejudice. The health promoter justifies his bias by pointing to disease, which has objective elements. And since disease is more objective, and the health promoter has linked well-being to it in his scheme of things and in his diagrams, it can *look as if* advice on well-being springs automatically from the same source as advice about disease and disease prevention (and that the expert on negative health promotion is therefore also and equally an expert on well-being promotion) – but this is an illegitimate conclusion. It can be that disease prevention increases well-being but it does not have to do so. If Andrew judges that it will not in his case then it will not.

It is a fact that different people understand well-being in different ways. Straightforward life experience shows this. Most people will be able to think of people who consider well-being to mean 'happiness', others who think of well-being as 'positive stress', others who conceive of well-being as 'frequent intellectual stimulation', and yet others who feel that to have well-being means 'to be tranquil'. Life just shows that not everyone considers the same feelings to be indicative of well-being. To take a more specific example, feelings of frustration during a difficult course of education will be interpreted by some people as representative of well-being, but not by others. Some people will see the struggle as worthwhile, as doing them good, as making them happier, as offering needed stimulation – others will judge it negatively,

Well-being = happiness	Well-being = positive stress	Well-being = frequent intellectual stimulation	Well-being = tranquility
↑	↑	↑	↑
Means or Origins = (often) a wide social network, an outgoing personality, an ability to do desired projects, satisfaction with oneself and one's position . . .	Means or Origins = (often) a demanding job, constant vigilance, constant self-motivation, finding fresh challenges and trying to meet them . . .	Means or Origins = (usually) a good standard of education, an environment where new learning is possible, intellectual hobbies, no mind-numbing TV . . .	Means or Origins = (perhaps) financial support, a relaxed attitude, ability to deal with stress, quiet surroundings, a job with no responsibilities, a rural home . . .

Figure 28   Four commonplace accounts of well-being, with a selection of possible 'means' or 'origins'

as making them miserable, as upsetting their peace of mind, as causing them stress. Different interpretations abound (see Fig. 28). The nature of well-being is forever disputable.

THE OUTSIDER PROBLEM IS A TOUGH NUT TO CRACK

The Outsider problem is the acid test for any form of health promotion. To solve it a health promoter needs:

a. to offer a theory of health promotion which can accommodate different outlooks and behaviours (without having to countenance *all and any* outlooks and behaviours)
b. to find a way both to promote health and not always to override the competent Outsider's choices
c. to have concrete practical health promoting tasks to do which can be of value to insiders and outsiders alike.

This is not an easy challenge. Currently no health promotion type can adequately meet it. The only way to deal properly with the Outsider problem is to apply a careful theory of health promotion, based on a proper understanding of prejudice, as Part Three will show.

SUMMARY

THE TASK OF THE PREJUDICED HEALTH PROMOTER

I am aware that some of what I have tried to explain in Part Two may not have been easy to follow. However, I submit that the reason for this is that health promotion has got itself into such a terrible conceptual mess – into such a muddle – that it is impossible to sort it out tidily. Many of the mistakes are related, often subtly, and several of the theorists' ideas are inconsistent. The best that can be done is to clarify the central difficulties so that they may be avoided in future, and to set out key points on which to base a developed and practical theory.

To sum up the progress made in Part Two:

1. All health promotion begins with values (it is prejudiced).
2. Health promotion values drive the evidence.
3. Any form of health promotion which claims otherwise (and so claims not to be prejudiced) is labouring under the most profound illusion – it must at least be *necessarily prejudiced*, and any which claims *not* to be prejudiced will therefore exhibit *blinkered prejudice*, and this does not have a place in health promotion.
4. The philosophical task of any health promoter (who is after all working in a field vastly more ethically complicated than most other professions) is:

    i. to understand that he must be prejudiced
    ii. to explore his prejudices (and constantly to try to act on *reasoned prejudice*)
    iii. to develop the most consistent account of his prejudices
    iv. to attempt to justify his prejudices to others, and so to explain his activities and the reasons for his activities *openly* to others (note: this does not, of course, mean that he must prove that his prejudices are *right* – though it is possible to prove that some *methods* work better than others. Rather he must show how they *make theoretical sense*, and hope that others will agree.)
    v. to be open to the possibility that his prejudices might change – that there may be better reasons for holding other prejudices
    vi. to work out the sources of his prejudices.

5. The health promoter must:

    i. Try to understand the political basis of his prejudices.
    ii. Try to understand the political bases of other people's prejudices.

6. The health promoter must seek a form of practical health promotion that is theoretically grounded. That is, he must seek a form of health promotion beyond **medical health promotion, social health promotion**, and the rest. Either that or he must work to develop a proper philosophical account of his favoured form.

Naturally, the theory offered in the final Part of this book is prejudiced too. But this is not a difficulty since its prejudice and political philosophical basis are freely acknowledged (so that others can judge whether or not they share its values). What is most important is that the theory is constructed in such a way as to avoid, as far as possible, the imposition of a blinkered prejudice about ways of living on other people. I know I am prejudiced, and I know other people have different prejudices. I want to pursue mine. I assume other people want to pursue theirs. The form of health promotion I advocate seeks to allow this – it wants to allow the pursuit of prejudice, within certain limits that the theory implies. As such it is the complete opposite of well-being promotion, as I shall try to explain.

The Foundations Theory of Health Promotion

An Introduction to the Foundations Theory of Health Promotion

FOUR REASONS TO BE THEORETICAL

Health promotion is a political enterprise rooted in human values, choices and prejudices – and these add greatly to its capacity to mislead. Their presence can create a powerful illusion, that even when health promotion is saturated with values, it is a neutral endeavour. The problem is that to those who share its values, any form of health promotion will tend to look perfectly acceptable. And this is the **first reason** why health promotion must develop decent theories about itself: since the goals and methods of health promotion are always prejudiced they are always contestable and therefore always require justification – however obviously right they might appear to be.

The **second reason** why health promotion must – as a matter of urgency – develop a philosophical tradition is that, unlike most other health work, it is often done without the permission (and often without even the knowledge) of the recipients. Doctors, nurses and other practitioners tend to work mainly with individuals and families and – where their patients are competent – will (normally) inform them of what they intend to do and why, and seek their approval. The main reason for this (other than common courtesy and contractual obligation) is that it can never be taken for granted that the health worker's interpretation of what is best will be shared by the potential recipient of care. Health worker and client may have different goals, may have contrasting beliefs about the value of what is being proposed, and may interpret success and failure differently. Because of this, in most forms of health work it is thought to be essential to place *limits* on interventions.

And in order to draw limits – for instance, in order to say I will *not* intervene if a competent and knowledgeable patient tells me to stop, or to say I *shall* continue where I have good reasons to believe that the patient misunderstands the evidence and will ultimately benefit – a theory is required. These matters are far too important ever to be decided by anything less.

Health Promotion, Second Edition: David Seedhouse
© 2004 John Wiley & Sons, Ltd: ISBNs 0 470 84732 8 (HB); 0 470 84733 6 (PB)

The **third reason** why health promotion must develop mature theories of purpose is to make itself *explicit* – to make itself a properly public enterprise and to expose itself to wide and informed debate. If health promotion is actually promoting the practical implications of various political philosophies then – at least in those societies where openness and accountability are considered to be central social values – the public is entitled to know what is going on.

Fourthly, health promotion should substantially improve its theoretical basis for internal reasons. In the absence of thoughtful theories of purpose health promoters can reach only superficial agreement about policy. Without underlying theory to allow thoughtful comparison of the effectiveness, efficiency, politics and ethics of the various alternative forms, health promotion advocacy cannot possibly be anything more than a matter of 'who shouts loudest wins'. It cannot, in other words, be anything more than *Willesville health promotion* until its philosophies are developed and expressed.

ONE THEORETICAL BASIS FOR HEALTH PROMOTION

In the final Part of *Health Promotion: Philosophy, Prejudice and Practice* I offer to you, and to all other health promoters and their official bodies (including the WHO), a theoretical basis for health promotion work. To begin with I outline, in summary form, a theory that **health is the foundations for achievement** (more detailed accounts of this theory can be found in companion texts).[23,84,85] And after this I add further detail to the theory with specific reference to health promotion.

GENESIS

The **foundations theory of health promotion** is derived from conceptual analysis of the meaning of health, from study of some other theories of health, from empirical observation of work actually done in the name of health, and from certain untestable beliefs (certain types of prejudice) about the morality of social arrangements. My analysis of these matters has led me to conclude that any plausible account of health must understand the purpose of health work to be the identification and – wherever possible – removal of obstacles to worthwhile (or *enhancing*)[23] human potentials. That is:

> Work for health is essentially *enabling*. It is a question of providing the appropriate foundations to enable the achievement of personal and group potentials. Health in its different degrees is created by removing obstacles and by providing the basic means by which biological and chosen goals can be achieved.

> *A person's (optimum) state of health is equivalent to the state of the set of conditions which fulfil or enable a person to work to fulfil his or her realistic chosen and biological potentials. Some of these conditions are of the highest importance for all people. Others are variable dependent upon individual abilities and circumstances.*

> The actual degree of health that a person has at a particular time depends upon the degree to which these conditions are realised in practice.[23] (Quotation slightly changed from original.)

This idea can be depicted in the abstract (see Fig. 29).

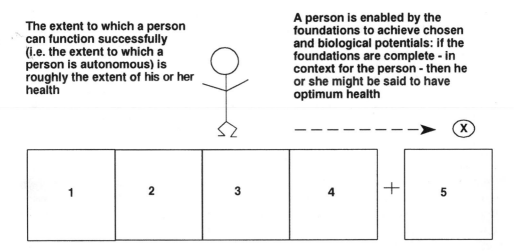

The extent to which a person can function successfully (i.e. the extent to which a person is autonomous) is roughly the extent of his or her health

A person is enabled by the foundations to achieve chosen and biological potentials: if the foundations are complete - in context for the person - then he or she might be said to have optimum health

If the person begins to move towards, arrives at, or is driven towards Ⓧ, then additional provision or maintenance of the stage might be necessary

Figure 29   An abstract depiction of health

The boxes in this figure may be described either as *conditions for* health or *constituents of* health (though ultimately only the latter understanding can be sustained).[84] Their importance, whichever way you look at them, is that they provide a platform for action – a stage for autonomy. According to the **foundations theory** if a person can stand upon the four central blocks in good order then she will have a high level of health. If her boxes are missing or in bad shape she will have a low level of health.

How many different sorts of boxes there are, their exact content, and how important each is compared to the others is arguable, varies according to circumstance, and is at least partly a matter of judgement. On the **foundations theory** the numbered blocks shown in Fig. 28 have the following general substance:

> Some of the foundations which make up health are of the highest importance for all people.
>
> These are:
>
> 1. The basic needs of food, drink, shelter, warmth and purpose in life.
> 2. Access to the widest possible information about all factors which have an influence on a person's life.
> 3. The skill and confidence to assimilate this information. In most societies literacy and numeracy are needed in older children and adults. People need to be able to understand how the information applies to them, and to be able to make reasoned decisions about what action to take in the light of that information.
> 4. The recognition that an individual is never totally isolated from other people and the external world. People are complex wholes who cannot be fully understood separated from the influence of their environment, which is itself a whole of which they are a part. People are not like marbles packed in boxes, where they are a community only because of their forced proximity. People are part of their surroundings, like cells in a single body. This fact compels the recognition that a person should not strive to fulfil personal

potentials which will undermine the basic foundations for achievement of other people. In short, an essential condition for health in human beings who are aware of the implications of their actions is that they have an awareness of a basic duty which follows from their living in a community.

Other foundations for achievement 5 are bound to vary between individuals dependent upon which potentials can realistically be achieved. For instance, a diseased person, a person in a damp and dilapidated house, a person in prison, a fit young athlete, a terminal patient, and an expectant mother all need the central conditions which constitute part of their healths, but in addition they require other specific foundations in order to enable them to make the most of their present lives.[23] (Quotation slightly changed from the original.)

Boxes 1–4 are intended to be analogous to central supporting conditions (points 1–4 in the quote above) without which a meaningful life is impossible. Box 5 is meant to represent various forms of additional support which may be needed in difficult circumstances (possibly, though not necessarily, in life crises). When faced with unexpected or unusual difficulties people sometimes find that the four central boxes, even if they remain in excellent condition, are of much less use than usual. If people are 'falling over the edge' of their platform (for example, on suddenly learning that they have a serious medical condition) they will need the support of a fifth box. That is, they will require: '... other specific foundations (necessary) to enable them to make the most of their present lives... '.[23] The content of Box 5 depends entirely upon the nature of the problem at hand. Thus the fifth box may represent medical services and support; improved facilities for a disabled person; hospice care for a terminally ill man; special protection and counselling for a battered woman, and so on. The fifth box is needed when a particular life problem becomes bad enough to impede significantly a person's movement on the platform formed by the other four boxes. Box 5 then either permanently extends the platform, substitutes for an irreparably damaged central box, or is the means by which a person is enabled to climb back onto her normal platform.

HEALTH, NOT MEDICINE, IS THE FOCUS

It will be immediately obvious that this notion of health does not have traditional medical provision as its focus. This is not a problem or an error, rather it is a logical consequence of the fact that work for health seeks to remove impediment to human achievement, and that those problems that can be tackled by medicine do not automatically constitute a *special category* of impediment.[84] Just as a person will become substantially immobilised in his life in general if he becomes seriously diseased or injured, so he is equally likely to be severely impeded in life if he does not have a home, or possesses no useful information, or has not been educated, or does not realise the extent to which he is formed by and depends on the existence of a community of others.

TARGETING

Because of this logic, it may appear that the **foundations theory of health** implies that *any* effort to help people live better lives is work for health. However, while the theory certainly does extend the idea of health beyond medical endeavour, it nevertheless sets practical and ethical *limits* on the role of health workers (including health promoters). The task for any genuine health worker who is working with either an *individual* or a *small group* is to recognise the importance of the foundations for that individual or group in context – to identify with or for each individual or group those foundational components which are lacking, or those which are most in need of renovation – and then to work on those aspects of the problem so defined, in a way most appropriate to the skills of that health worker. Thus the **foundations theory** begins to offer guidance to individual health workers, and helps to establish practical priorities.

LIMITING

There is a very important limit to work to promote the health of individuals and small groups:

> ...work for health cannot be fully comprehensive – not all work should be thought to be health work. Such a state of affairs is not possible, nor is it desirable to have professional interference in the name of health covering all aspects of individuals' lives. *Once suitable background conditions have been created, the achievement of the particular potentials that have been chosen is up to the individual and not the concern of health workers, although permanent maintenance work will often need to be carried out on the foundations.*

> The analogy of work for health is very close to the work needed to lay the foundations of a building. *Obstacles such as poor drainage, subsidence, awkward outcrops of rock (analogy: disease, illness, poor housing, unjustified discrimination, unemployment) have to be eliminated or overcome in some other way. Then firm foundations and reinforcements have to be added (analogy: good general education, confidence in thinking things through personally rather than relying on what one has been told, good opportunities for self-development). But, unlike the case of building construction, work for health should stop here.* What a person makes of the foundations he has is up to that person, as long as he possesses at least the essentials of the central conditions. Given this then an individual must be allowed to become the architect of his own destiny.[23] (Quotation slightly changed from the original.)

DIFFICULTIES

There are naturally very many theoretical and practical problems with the **foundations theory of health**, some of which I have dealt with in detail elsewhere,[23,84] some of which I have yet to confront, and some of which I shall discuss later.

It is worth briefly mentioning two possible difficulties, to help introduce the theory. They are these:

1. The content of the boxes is wholly prejudiced.
2. No measures of health are indicated, and therefore the foundations theory is ultimately as vague as – or vaguer than – every other interpretation of health.

The first apparent difficulty is actually not a problem at all. As I have argued at length already, values are necessarily implicit in any suggestion about how to bring about better health. The real problem is that these values are often disguised so that it *seems* that what is at issue is largely a technical matter. The **foundations theory** directly challenges this misperception by making its own prejudices explicit.

As for the second concern, it is quite possible to set comprehensive practical standards. However, for a variety of reasons I have so far resisted using the theoretical framework as a basis for detailed assessment of the success or failure of work for health. Rather my main aim has been to establish a justified *backcloth* for measurement – not to specify precisely how this measurement should be made. However, in order to make the theory comprehensively useful to health promotion practitioners, further general specifications, and more detailed practical targets, are necessary.

Some further detail is given in the remainder of this chapter. The idea of rational fields presented in Chapter Ten and illustrated in Dialogue Seven of this edition of *Health Promotion: Philosophy, Prejudice and Practice* adds significantly to the practicality of the foundations theory. In addition, at the time of writing, a computerised decision-making toolkit based on the foundations theory is in development (see www.vide.co.nz). The conceptual basis of this toolkit will be fully explained in a future publication, provisionally entitled *Values-Based Health Care*.

The Trouble with Assessing Success Without a Specific Theory of Health

Consider the enormous difficulty of assessing success in health promotion *without* the benefit of a theory of health.

At the moment the expressions 'health gain' and 'health outcome' are used, extremely vaguely, to stand for 'success' in health services and health promotion.[86] Most commonly the phrases are used to describe:

> A. the *simple* results of health service or health promotion processes
>
> For instance, the number of heart by-pass operations performed per year, or the number of Diagnosis Related Groups (DRGs) treated at hospital X at cost Y, or the number of people discharged within a given time, or the number of smokers who have not smoked for X months following health promotion programme Y, are totted up and said to represent the health outcome or to indicate the level of health gain.

Or,

> B. the *converse* of measurable health problems.
>
> For example, by curing infection, or by reducing population morbidity, or by eliminating immobility by hip-replacement operations, health is said to be gained *in inverse proportion* to the type and degree of the original problem.

It is vastly easier to include health gain in quantifiable calculations if it is limited to the above 'end-points' than if it is not. The increase in a person's *physical* mobility before and at a specified time after a hip-replacement operation can be reasonably well quantified, whereas an increase in happiness, fulfilment and life opportunity is, as we have seen, notoriously difficult to measure. However, while the limits set by A and B above may make some measurement possible, there is no reason other than convenience why these and not more general indicators of the success of health service and health promotion activities should be used. Indeed, since the point of health services is generally thought to be the restoration of people to normal lives (where possible) it seems to make more sense to think of health gain as the move towards or gain in 'normal living' brought about by a health intervention. Yet once *this* is conceded (as it is by several health economists)[87] then the notion of health gain becomes so open-ended that it cannot realistically be measured.[88] The open-ended health gained as the result of a successful coronary by-pass operation then becomes not just the discharge statistic or the antithesis of the original clinical problem, but the extent of fulfilling life the recipient can enjoy that he would not have enjoyed without the operation. In other words, once you move beyond *convenient* measures, and if you do not possess a sustained theory of health, then your criteria for success become *unlimited*, and you slip insidiously into **good life promotion**, with its many and serious attendant problems.

A further implication of opening-up the notion of success in health work is that health is not gained only as a result of explicitly intended health promoting interventions.[89] If health gain is held to be somehow equivalent to a more fulfilled life then very many activities can create it. For instance, health might be gained as an unemployed person gets a job, or as a person finds new direction in life through a course of education, and so on. But if health promoters were to take this idea seriously then it would become enormously difficult actually to do health promotion in the face of so many complexities.

ASSESSING SUCCESS WITH A THEORY OF HEALTH: DEFINING THE NUTS AND BOLTS OF HEALTH PROMOTION

Because many contemporary 'measures of health' are conceptually weak, and since the **foundations theory** can solve some of the practical problems of those methods which assume health promotion to be evidence-driven (and therefore not to need a theory), it is worth briefly illustrating how the **foundations theory** begins to generate useful measures of success beyond the individual level.

CLOSED, SUBSTANTIAL HEALTH GAIN

In order to talk more meaningfully about success in health promotion it is necessary to add more specific content to the boxes which make up the health stage (see Fig. 30).

To enable precise quantification each sub-section of each box would obviously need a great deal more elucidation: what level of nutrition is adequate? what sorts of employment are fulfilling and which are not? what are good levels of literacy? and so on. Equally obviously, these matters are in fact so complex, context dependent, contestable and flavoured by prejudice that *unequivocal* practical measures are surely out of the question. However, this is not to say that clear general standards (as well as guidelines for unusual circumstances) cannot be established. The point of *beginning*

1	2	3	4	5 — ADDITIONAL OR CRISIS SUPPORT
A home to call her own for everyone in a particular society	Open access to the widest possible information	Education to good levels of literacy and numeracy	The constant awareness of one's belonging to a community—the awareness of the interests of others and of one's dependence upon others' thoughts, on their physical and cultural support, and on their productivity	Access to life saving and sustaining medical services
Protection from death, assault, and undue coercion	Assistance with the interpretation of information (e.g. legal, medical, technical, bureaucratic)	Education to enable a good level of unsupported interpretation of information		Access to medical services that enable the restoration of normal function for the individual (ideally to restore the person to the full platform, left)
Adequate daily nutrition	Encouragement to find, to explore, retain and act on information	Open, continuing education without bar of age	A constant awareness of one's duty to develop oneself and to support others—and so to develop the community	
Assistance, whenever required, with defining and (in some circumstances) pursuing purposes/life plans	Encouragement of open discussion of information (public seminars, sponsored 'open info' sessions, public service talkback radio and television)	Encouragement of self-education throughout life		Access to special context dependent support in medical crises
Meaningful, fulfilling employment			The constant understanding that citizenship involves not only individual fulfilment but a commitment to the larger civic (global) body	The continuing fulfilment of special needs—the absence of which would constitute crisis

Figure 30   The foundations with more specific content

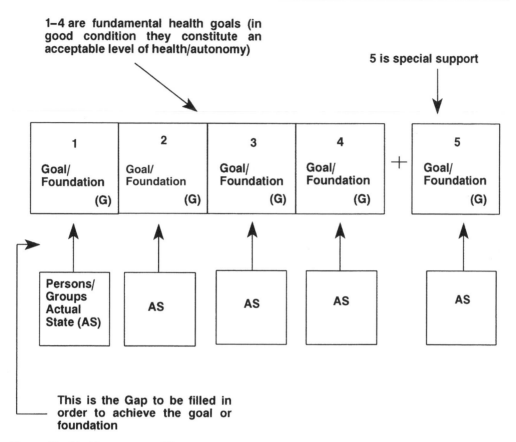

1–4 are fundamental health goals (in good condition they constitute an acceptable level of health/autonomy)

5 is special support

Figure 31 Health gain as gap filling

with theory is to make plain (and so open to debate) the various reasons why these standards are considered appropriate.

On the **foundations theory** the point of having practical standards would, in the first place, be to set egalitarian targets that should be achieved for all people in a given society (see the 'foundations tower', Fig. 36 on p. 186). For this reason the theory explains 'health gain' as follows. If it is correct to conceive of 'health need' as a *gap* or a *difference* between an actual state (AS) and a goal (G)[90] then working for health is essentially a question of 'filling the gap' between a person's or group's (or even a whole society's) actual situation and the desired or desirable goal (or improved state of health). This can be depicted as in Fig. 31.

Of course this remains a very crude idea. But note four interesting points. First, the need is not the goal itself but is for those things which 'fill the gap' and so bring the person or group up to the 'goal state'. Second, the extent to which the 'gap is filled' is the extent of the health gain. So, if a person is suffering a bacterial infection (if she is in that particular AS) and is cured by antibiotics without side-effects, she will have been restored to her full platform and the health gained could be said to be the difference between her previous AS and G (Box 5). To give another example, if a person is homeless (and has been in and out of mental institutions partly as a consequence of his homelessness) then he plainly needs a home – he requires this to fill the gap between his AS and his Box 1. That part of his stage is missing and he needs it back to enable him to move freely on the rest of his stage. To find a home for such a person would be to promote his health.

Thirdly, while being cured of infection, or obtaining a decent place to live, may well have innumerable open-ended benefits, the way in which the **foundations theory of health** is structured means that the health gain is finally achieved when the goal state is achieved. As I have mentioned here, and explained in greater detail elsewhere,[91] one of the most important ethical limits set by the foundations theory is that the attention of health workers ought to be limited to the provision and maintenance of fundamental foundations – beyond that it is up to the individual to make of her life what she can. And this crucial limit should be paralleled at the level of general health promotion provision and responsibility. The primary aim of **foundational health promotion** work ought to be restricted to closing the gaps between people's actual states and their possession of a sound platform for achievement. Once this platform is established people's performance on it (and the nature and level of the well-being they achieve) must be up to them. And so the further benefits which may accrue following foundational support should *not* be described as health gains. On the **foundations theory** the idea of health gain becomes both rich in meaning *and* finite. (Note also that on the **foundations theory** there is no sense whatsoever in talking of positive and negative health.)

Fourthly, according to the **foundations theory** it is possible (and I think necessary) to begin to distinguish *different sorts of health gain.* Those means necessary to close the gaps between ASs and the foundation goals or boxes might be called **primary health gains**, once in place (and these could be quantified given a clear enough – and flexible enough – definition of standards). On the **foundations theory** primary health gains are the most important sorts of health gain and should be a fundamental social priority. Where fundamental gaps exist which could be filled (in other words, where primary health gains are possible but not yet achieved in a society) resources should be switched in order to achieve them. In reality it is inconceivable that this would happen overnight, particularly quickly, or perhaps even at all. However, any serious health policy based on this theory would seek as soon as possible to have the primary health gains met (Fig. 32).

TECHNICAL ISSUES

There are countless technical and philosophical difficulties with this basic scheme. Some are soluble (see the rewritten or updated sections of Ref.[23] for some suggestions of how an holistic understanding of health can nevertheless be perfectly practically focused), and some are perennially disputable (as is the case with any theory or method which proposes ways of distributing social goods).

How, for example:

(i) does one compare the value of the gaps between ASs and different sorts of G?

Figure 32 Giving real and limited content to the term health gain

And what if,

(ii) under the same box, person (A) can go from:

[AS] ――――――→ [boxes][G]

and person (B), starting in the same place, can go only from:

[AS] ―→ [boxes] [G]

and will never manage to achieve G fully? What if one person can be fully and inexpensively cured of a life-threatening illness and another, even when cured, requires lifelong, financially costly support even to allow a bearable existence?

The foundations theory in general cannot be precise about these difficult problems. However, since the theory is that the point of health work is to create and increase autonomy it can be said – in response to the first question – that the relative value of the different boxes should be decided, in practical context, by reference to the various amounts of autonomy (movement in life) that will be created by providing each one. In other words the challenge is to discover which box, if it is missing or deficient, poses the greatest obstacle to a person's fulfilling progress in life. Furthermore – in answer to (ii) above – since the theory is essentially egalitarian in that it is meant first to support the weakest members of society, each person should be brought as near as possible to the foundation level. That is, person B should be supported as fully as possible either until it is unrealistic to press for further improvements, or until that support becomes so costly of resources that it begins to diminish the strength of the foundations of other people.

SECONDARY HEALTH GAIN

If benefits are possible beyond the provision of fundamental foundations for everyone then a plethora of rationing dilemmas emerges. Who should receive what treatment or extra life benefit before who else and why? According to my theory the only way in which health gain makes sense is as an addition to the foundations. So where policy-makers have the luxury of deciding between extra benefits they should act so as to maximise the foundations of all. Thus, my theory urges that *as a matter of policy all new technology, research and investment in medicine and health promotion should be bought or undertaken with the explicit and demonstrable intent of improving the lot of everyone* – that is, the first thought of any policy-maker or legislator should be – to what extent will this innovation bolster the foundations (at least potentially) of *all* citizens? Again, this idea does not give precise practical guidance in all cases, but by stating the purpose of collective health policy in principle, it at least makes coherent planning a possibility.

And some cases will be fairly easy to decide. For example, if a purchasing health authority has to choose between investing in a life-extending measure for patients suffering from Alzheimer's disease which does not significantly improve their quality of life, and an equally financially costly health promotion measure to significantly improve road safety – then according to the foundations theory they ought to opt for the road safety measure. Or if a government department has to decide whether to screen for very rare conditions that may affect only very few people, and their budget to help the poorest members of society is already inadequate, then they should not screen. Of course not everyone will concur with these decisions, but this is inevitable in a pluralist society and at least the decisions I favour could be made with overt justification, with the advantage of an underpinning theory.

The precise calculation does not matter that much so long as the basic intent is clear and understood. Where there are hard choices, and where the notion of 'foundation expansion' does not help the decision, then at this point, but not at the initial stage, other explicitly stated and argued criteria must be brought in. These could include such considerations as degree of benefit, future benefit to others, relative costs – and might even include versions of the QALY[87] (as a secondary decision-making measure) so long as the application of these methods did not undermine the basic foundations policy (Fig. 33).

BENEFITS

Naturally I do not claim that the **foundations theory** can provide all the answers. Sometimes it can offer clear practical guidance, sometimes it can suggest a general direction for policy-making in health promotion, and sometimes it is of no use. But what is most important is that the theory openly acknowledges that setting health priorities is indisputably a political matter, argues that policy should be first decided at that level, suggests a theoretical basis for doing so, and insists that any technical measures should be consistent with that primary base.

First principle - make policy so as to bolster the foundations of all. So, aim to move thus:

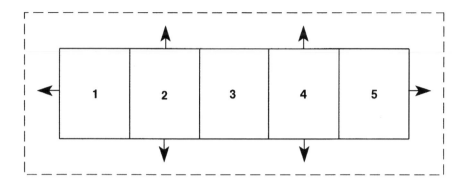

— = old foundations

- - - = improved foundations

Second principle - ration according to a clear, overt and theoretically sustained method in those cases beyond 'foundation expansion'.

Figure 33 Fundamental principles of rationing for health

Thus the theory:

i. offers clarity of general purpose to health promoters
ii. explicitly drives techniques, methods and models and is not driven by them (for instance, any policy-maker who endorses my theory must simply reject the non-egalitarian QALY approach to health promotion, at least until the basic foundations are in place for everyone)
iii. is clear about what is *not* to be rationed (whereas under most other approaches all support services are potentially open to rationing)
iv. explains how *closed* health gains can be understood and potentially measured
v. is explicit that what matters at bottom is human autonomy/functioning/ movement/doing/capability
vi. offers a general guide to health and health promotion policy-making
vii. is clear that it is not possible to be absolutely precise over the tough 'micro' decisions, but offers various decision-making methods that enable deep and systematic reflection about them.

And what all this means is that health promotion must be seen both as an endeavour to help individuals and also (and ultimately) as a task for governments. They, and only they, are able to ensure that everyone has the foundations for achievement.

Tough Questions

Over the years the foundations theory has become rather large and complex. There are, however, some frequently asked (tough) questions whose answers may help explain a lot (and see also Ref. 23).

QUESTION ONE

The foundations theory of health is meant to apply to all people – perhaps to all human beings – and yet its foundational blocks seem to apply only to competent adults; to people capable of assimilating information, of learning, of feeling part of a community, of making informed choices. Not all health work is done to help such privileged people – much of it is directed toward improving the lot of people with mental illnesses, people who are for one reason or another incompetent (severely intellectually disabled people, unconscious people, senile people and very young children). Isn't the foundations theory biased toward the interests of competent adults? How could the foundations theory be applied to help, or to help decide what best to do for, a severely damaged neonate?

ANSWER ONE

That is an interesting question. The short answer to it is:

a. the theory is meant to apply equally to all those beings judged to be persons or potential persons
b. because of the way the world is (i.e. because people live in grossly unequal circumstances) the theory is biased *in favour* of the disadvantaged – not against them
c. of course the theory can help decide what best to do for the severely damaged neonate.

In order to give a justified long answer to the question it is necessary first to recognise the limitations of the foundations diagram (Fig. 30). The blocks in the illustration are analogous with only some aspects of the theory. Essentially they illustrate:

Health Promotion, Second Edition: David Seedhouse
© 2004 John Wiley & Sons, Ltd: ISBNs 0 470 84732 8 (HB); 0 470 84733 6 (PB)

a. The idea that in order to discover to what extent a person is healthy you not only have to look at her as a body and mind, you also have to examine the state of certain 'enabling conditions'. These may be either internal or external to her. If they are in good order they will allow her to move or perform well in her life in general. In principle this consideration applies equally to all people (we all have internal and external conditions), though in reality the content of our 'enabling conditions' is obviously often very different.

b. That although some people do not have a full set of foundations, we all (including the neonate) need at least *some* to survive, and still more to thrive.

c. That the purpose of health work is to offer the firmest possible opportunities for movement for particular people in particular contexts. That is, the health promotion task is to build and maintain a stage most appropriate to the achievement of a particular person's most fulfilling and/or desired (biological, intellectual and/or emotional) potentials. The task is to create autonomy, thoughtfully, for everyone.

d. The way in which health workers can (i) conceive of the general nature of their task and (ii) identify practical priorities when working with individuals and groups. For instance, where a health worker seeks to promote the health of an intelligent, well-off business woman who wants to quit smoking the focus will be on realising a *chosen* potential, where the worker seeks to promote the health of an unborn child by encouraging a mother not to drink alcohol (and so avoid foetal alcohol syndrome) the focus will be on realising a *biological* potential – by having the child born within a normal range.

e. That there are theoretical, ethical and practical limits to the interventions that can be made in the name of health. If the point of health work is to liberate fulfilling human potentials then *all* human potentials – not just the physiological ones – are possible targets for the work. And if you take this idea seriously then work for health must be *self-limiting*: if you have deliberately established a good set of foundations for a person or a group then you have effectively excluded yourself from future involvement unless you are specifically asked. If, for instance, you have offered information on safe sex to a teenager; if you have given him skills to avoid being coerced, if you have educated him about social conditioning – if, in other words, you have raised him to a position where he can make informed choices without undue pressure, you will – in these respects – have created a good degree of health (or autonomy) for him and will therefore be obliged to cease intervening if he requests it. In other words, your job will have been done.

It also follows that given a reasonable set of foundations different people's biases should be treated with equal respect (for instance, a health worker should not glibly override a Jehovah's witness' request not to receive blood). And there is an obvious implication that while it is acceptable for individuals knowingly to damage their own foundations it is not acceptable for them knowingly to damage other people's.

The foundations *diagram* is meant to offer guidance in the above general ways. It is *not* meant primarily to help answer the question: is this person healthy? For this it is better to turn to my written account of health, which is more explicit. In particular, note that:

> How many different sorts of boxes there are, their exact content, and how important each is compared to the others is contestable, varies according to circumstance, and is at least partly a matter of human social judgement.

If you just take the diagrammatic version it *looks* as if, to be healthy, a person should be informed, educated, have a sense of community and so on, and that she may then become unhealthy as she encounters a crisis – as she begins to fall off her stage. But this is one of the points where the image fails to capture the theory. It looks as if these crises happen only to already healthy people, or perhaps that the movement towards the edge may be voluntary, and/or that medicine/special health services are somehow always supplementary to the four central conditions. But I do not mean any of this – it is a distortion generated, I confess, by my inability to find a more exact illustration.

To try to clarify a little: first, the stage is not *actually* separated into discrete blocks. Figure 30 is merely a crude representation of complex, interacting reality. Really to assess the state of a person's health it is necessary to take a general view of a person's potentials and the obstacles in the way of the achievement of these potentials, and the nature of the potentials obviously varies considerably between different people. So, in this sense, a more accurate representation of the foundations would be to have the four boxes plus Boxes 5, 6, 7 and so on to indicate the number of additional foundations required to create autonomy for different people in different circumstances. That is why I say:

> Other foundations for achievement are bound to vary between individuals dependent upon which potentials can realistically be achieved. For instance, a diseased person, a person in a damp and dilapidated house, a person in prison, a fit young athlete, a terminal patient, and an expectant mother all need the central conditions which constitute part of their healths, but in addition they require other specific foundations in order to enable them to make the most of their present lives.[23]

(Note, though, that the content of these boxes cannot just be anything – it must be genuinely foundational.)

Second, it is also a little misleading to call Box 5 (which in fact stands for a lot of alternative boxes) 'crisis support'. It is probably better to say 'additional support', though if it were not present its absence would usually constitute a crisis. (For example, this box can represent continuing home care for a quadriplegic car accident victim, bereavement counselling for a gravely troubled spouse, antibiotics for a deep gash in the hand, etc.)

Thirdly, it is possible, on the foundations theory, at least to begin to assess a person's health even if that person does not, or even cannot, possess most of the central foundations:

> *A person's (optimum) state of health is equivalent to the state of the set of conditions which fulfil or enable a person to work to fulfil his or her realistic chosen and biological potentials.*[23]

Take careful note that this says that a person's state of health should be assessed by looking at *the conditions which fulfil or enable a person to work to fulfil her realistic chosen and biological potentials*. With this in mind, consider a severely mentally disabled person who is said to have a 'mental age' of three years. Information and education are not *realistically* much use to her, and therefore the lack of these things does *not* damage her health. However, even given these considerable constraints on her autonomy it is still possible to work on those areas of her life that can be improved in order to give her as much freedom as possible (even if this is only freedom from discomfort, boredom, ridicule – whatever may be a liability to her).

Turning to the damaged neonate, once again information and education are not (yet) relevant (though they will be if the health worker is trying to increase the health of the baby and her parents, and the health worker has decided to regard them as a single group). Nevertheless, the state of the infant's health can be assessed – and practical steps taken – in accordance with the foundations theory, in the following way. First it will be necessary to ask two questions:

1. what is the present state of those conditions (*including* the [potential] person's physical and mental capabilities) which fulfil or enable the person to work to fulfil her chosen and biological potentials?
2. can the state of these conditions be improved?

Now, say the child is impeded by *spina bifida*, there may be a question about whether to perform an operation or not, and so the basic question might be recast – will the operation enhance the baby's health? Well, if it looks like an operation will change a foundational condition and enable the infant to *work to fulfil* (in this case the work will at first be solely biological) worthwhile potentials then it will be *work for health* and, other things being equal, should proceed. However, if the operation will not improve the foundational condition – and will not even potentially improve other foundations either – then it should not be done. That is, if it will not create autonomy (if it will not reduce pain, if it will not contribute to future movement, and certainly if the child is expected to die soon in any case) then there is no justification for it on the foundations theory, though there could be on other theories, dependent on how they have been constructed.

So, in the neonate case I accept that the metaphor is less than perfect, but I think the *theory* is still viable. At a push you could see the health work task for the neonate (as illustrated in Fig. 30) as being first only within Boxes 1 (food, warmth etc.) and 5 (special obstacle removing medical care), but with the long-term view of establishing a solid and full set of foundations. However, I think it is better to understand this non-graphically, as initial work to establish vitally liberating physical potentials (assuming the neonate stands a fair chance of good development if operated on).

One further point, in the italicised quote above you may have noticed that 'optimum' is in parentheses. I admit I have had difficulty with this issue over the years, and this is the clearest statement I can manage to date. The problem is that if 'the set of conditions' 'fulfil' a person's 'realistic chosen and biological potentials', or even merely 'enable a young person to work to fulfil' her potentials, then it seems to follow that the person may therefore already have an *optimum* state of health (and this *is* what I want to say). However, I also want to explain that the foundations may not be in optimum condition, but that this does not mean that the person is unhealthy – just that he has a lower degree of health than he might have. Thus, disregarding 'optimum', I also want to be able to say that *any* state of health is equivalent to 'the state of the set of conditions that enable a person to work to fulfil etc.' A person in bad health (the cancer sufferer, the starving child, the man with MS) may not be enabled, by his or her foundations, to work very well at all but so long as *some* work is possible the person should still be described as having some degree of health. The general rule still applies – the health worker should assess a person's health by looking at the state of the foundations. If a person is not able to work *at all* – biologically and intellectually – to fulfil her realistic chosen and biological potentials then she will be dead.

In sum, the foundations *diagram* is inadequate because:

i. The boxes are not necessarily of equal value. That is, in the case of the neonate only Boxes 1 and 5 are of any relevance, whereas in the case of the person who asks for help to quit smoking only Boxes 2 and 3 or perhaps only 1 and 4, depending on the policy the health promoter adopts, are important.

ii. Sometimes one box can/has to substitute for another, or parts of others. For example, as depicted in Fig. 34. That is, a person's entire life may be collapsing due

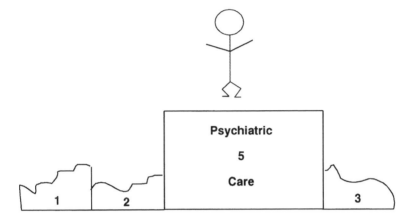

Figure 34   One box can substitute for another or others

to a psychosis, in which case it may be that Box 5 (which in Fig. 30 is represented only as 'special support' and which may therefore appear extra or additional) becomes the central or possibly the only foundation, at least for a time.

iii. Sometimes the 'extra' box can be dominant, and can be permanent. For example, as in the case of Fig. 35.

Figure 35   Special needs support for Ann,[23] a paraplegic following a road accident

iv. The boxes do not necessarily display the *internal* parts of a person's health in proper proportion. The boxes as depicted emphasise the external conditions or aspects of people's health in order to redress an existing imbalance (at the moment we tend mistakenly to think of a person's health as mainly or entirely an internal matter: 'how are you feeling today? how is your cough? I hope the sickness is receding'). However, both the internal and external conditions are to be regarded as of potentially equal importance. Which of them actually happens to be of most importance is decided by the particular context. For the person requiring intensive care following a boat explosion the focus must be on internal aspects of his platform. For the unhappy person who needs motivating – who needs to be inspired in order to flourish – the external aspects of his stage (information, education, a sense of purpose) will be the most important (see the Introduction to Ref. 23 for an expanded explanation of this holistic philosophy).

QUESTION TWO

How does the foundations theory of health promotion solve the Outsider problem?

ANSWER TWO

The foundations theory can solve the problem because it sets a theoretical limit on its prejudices. The general choice of the foundational boxes, and of course the foundations image itself, is inevitably the product of my broad political prejudices. I *believe* that these general boxes are actually central to the creation of autonomy in life, but I cannot definitively prove this, and their value is at least partly dependent on the form of society in which people have to live. It is also part of my broad political philosophy that people's choices should be respected, unless there is good reason not to, and people should be as free as possible (consistent with similar freedom for others) to create the shape of their own lives. For this reason, *prejudiced work for health is limited by the extent to which the targets of the work are capable of forming and acting on their own broad prejudices.* Elsewhere,[84,85] I have referred to an *Autonomy Flip*. This is a point at which work to *create autonomy* in a subject must by and large cease; a point at which the health worker must first bow to or *respect the autonomy* of the individual or group she has been trying to support – even if she disagrees with him, her or them.

The foundations theory allows health promoters to promote foundational health in Outsiders – it allows them to work on Boxes 1–4, and to do more *on request* – but it also compels them to respect the choices of the competent Outsider, even those who smoke and who drink heavily, and all the other things people such as Andrew Wilson wish to do.

To spell this out further, no theory of health can be entirely neutral about life goals, but some theories are more neutral (at least in their effects) than others. The foundations theory is prescriptive up to a point (any practically useful theory has to be) but it is designed to leave it up to the individual to decide what to do, as far as possible. All the foundations are asserted in order to encourage this.

The theory says that certain prerequisites (Boxes 1–4) – safety, shelter, information, education, confidence, a feeling of purpose – are necessary to any reasonably autonomous human existence. If these prerequisites are in place then a person may be described as having at least a reasonable level of health – indeed he may be described as having a fair degree of health even if he does not have any of the sorts of well-being described in Fig. 28.

The provision of further supporting conditions (Box 5), appropriate to the individual in question, may make the individual healthier. He should, for instance, have disabling problems of disease and injury attended to – but this is to be done to ensure that he has the best possible level of personal mobility, and so that he is able to determine and pursue his own best interests (in other words, to move freely on the strongest attainable platform). The fact that the subject might choose to pursue goals he thinks are in his best interests and the health promoter does not, and the fact that he might change his mind about his best interests from time to time, is generally speaking no reason to interfere and insist that he should be consistent. We are all of us inconsistent in our 'global' thinking on occasions.

I believe that health work ought to be based on this theory of health rather than theories of well-being (which fail to solve the Outsider problem) because the foundations theory does *not* prescribe desirable goals universally, whereas theories of well-being are all inclusive – they are universal in their condemnation or approval of ways of living. It might, of course, be objected that the foundations theory of health contains a notion of well-being – and so is paternalistic too. It might for instance be argued that I suggest shelter and education as central conditions because I believe these things to be good for people, and that therefore I do have a theory of well-being after all. However, while it is true that I suggest general, practical means I do not suggest any specific ways of living. Nor do I say that these means are objectively the 'origins' of well-being. They may not be for some people, and if these people so decide then I argue that they should be allowed to destroy their foundations. I do not think they should be allowed to destroy the foundations of others without permission but even this is not to claim that these are 'objective means'. As the WHO rightly recognises (but does not yet adequately explain), these things tend to be the *prerequisites* for a fulfilling life – even though they are not necessarily so.

In sum I am concerned first that people are able to *do* – not with what they do do. I am not, when I use this theory, ultimately concerned if people are self-destructive or unhappy (though personally I'd rather they were not). On my theory it is up to them to choose and to survive how they will – work for health is not work to make people happy, rather it is work to set people's creative potentials free. Once creative potentials have been liberated, people's actions are up to them.

QUESTION THREE

Is there *anything* objective about the foundations theory of health – or is every part of it generated by prejudice?

That, too, is a very interesting question. The short answer is that several aspects of the theory are, in some sense, objective – though it is also true to say, because the theory necessarily has its roots in political philosophy, that every part of it is coloured by prejudice to an extent. Let me try to explain how this might make sense.

Essentially the foundations theory has at least four objective aspects:

i. *Problems/obstacles/impediments that are matters of fact*
   The most general feature of work for health according to the foundations theory is that all work for health must, in some way, be directed against obstacles to the achievement of those human potentials which lead to various kinds of flourishing. These obstacles, whether physical, mental, social or environmental, are real in a way beyond subjective bias. A broken leg following a ski accident is, for instance, a brute fact (whether you like it or not you have a broken leg); as is a damp, cold house; as is unemployment; and as is a myocardial infarction. To the extent that such obstacles as these can be said to be objective problems, because it is cast against them, the foundations theory is objective too.

ii. *Whether or not the work for health is effective*
   The foundations theory is meant to enable the health worker to identify health problems, to rank them according to severity, and to decide which of the problems she is most equipped to deal with (taking the severity and urgency into account). In other words the foundations theory encourages the health worker to be practically specific, to identify clear targets for intervention, to spell out what will count as success and what will be considered failure, and to try to do those things which will have the greatest impact. Given this, the foundations approach can be assessed according to whether, or to what extent, it achieves what it sets out to do – and almost always this judgement will require much more than subjective opinion. The acceptance that one is prejudiced most definitely does not imply a disregard for evidence.

iii. *At least some enabling conditions will be needed*
   The central conditions of work for health (Boxes 1–4 in the figures) have been selected, according to certain preferences, from alternatives. This selection is undeniably prejudiced, and it is also true to say (I think) that there is no such thing as a universally objective need[91] since all needs depend on some purpose or other – even those needs for warmth, shelter, food and so on that make up Box 1 are not always necessary (the ascetic does not need warmth, the dying man does not need food, the person who wishes to commit suicide does not need oxygen, and so on). On the other hand, it is true to say that for the great majority of people the constituents of Boxes 1–4 are, or will be, necessary as a matter of fact if they are to have meaningful and productive lives – whatever society and whatever culture they live in. To this extent the theory is objective: some of the prejudices are necessary for any sort of creative movement in life.

iv. *Choice*
   In similar fashion, people's choices depend in part on what is, on what happens to us, on how we are programmed biologically and socially to react to events; and in

part upon how we prefer to react. However, as far as the foundations theory is concerned, the source of the choice does not matter. What *is* important, however, is that if a choice has been made by a person with a reasonable level of health (by a person with a platform in reasonably solid repair) then – for the health worker – that too is a matter of fact. The choice *is* – whether the health worker agrees with it or not – and the fact of that choice limits practically what the health worker who holds the foundations theory is able to do to or with the person she would like to help.

QUESTION FOUR

So any theory of health, including the foundations theory, must inevitably be prejudiced – even though not everything about the theory will be equally prejudiced. But to go a stage further, how are the foundations prejudices based on a political philosophy?

ANSWER FOUR

You will know from an earlier discussion (see Chapter Five) that it is not possible to identify exactly, and without dispute, the connections between types of health promotion, their implicit theories, and political philosophy. It is, however, possible to indicate broad connections between work for health and political philosophy, and sometimes possible to say that some aspects of some thinking about health promotion are clearly related to political philosophies of one kind or another.

As a general rule, the more detailed the theory of health, the easier it is to pin-point the political philosophy on which it is based. The foundations theory is detailed, and so it is easy enough to see a number of connections. For example:

i. The foundations theory of health does *not* accept that the prevailing social situation in almost all the so-called developed world is desirable. Great wealth exists in the hands of a relative few while very many do not have a full set of foundations, even though it is practically possible that they might have good foundations. People are homeless, jobless, friendless, apathetic, without hope, manipulated, deceived, and diseased, when a civilised redistribution of social goods would make it likely that at least some of these foundational lackings could be remedied. There are privileged people whose health could not be further improved (except perhaps for Box 4), who have excess resources which if offered to underprivileged people could create less troubled, less impeded lives. This is not only a matter of disease and illness – it is a matter of social justice, and so a matter of health promotion.

ii. The theory is egalitarian to the extent that it argues that the central conditions for health should – where this is not unrealistic[23] – be promoted for all persons as an absolute social priority, for if this is not done then avoidable *dwarfing* will continue to occur.[85] This egalitarianism is based on the belief – on the prejudice – that all persons are of equal worth even though they may be of unequal ability, talent,

Figure 36   An elementary illustration of the political base of foundational health promotion intelligence, productivity, and so on. It is also based on the prejudice that societies should be constructed so as both to reflect and to maintain this equal worth.

iii. The **theory** is liberal to the extent that it argues:

    a. that these central conditions should not be indefinitely large – that society should not impose equality beyond the provision of those things which the great majority of us require to give us the chance of a worthwhile life, and

    b. that the point of ensuring foundational equality is not equality for equality's sake but equal opportunity to be in a position to achieve. The theory assumes that it is a fact of life that, because of genetic and other biological differences, some people will be able to achieve more than others. Since the point of the foundations is to enable achievement, this achievement should not be fettered (at least in the name of health) by any other considerations than that the foundations for achievement of others should not be damaged – deliberately or otherwise – by the achievements of the most successful, and

    c. that a freely formed decision made by an informed and competent person should be respected unless there are compelling overriding reasons for not doing so.[92]

iv. The **theory** is utilitarian to the extent that, beyond the provision of the central functions and additional enabling support (Box 5), the planned further distribution of resources (for instance, medical services) may favour those citizens most likely to maximise the situations of all others (see Fig. 33). Note that the theory therefore holds that the maximising of social goods is a secondary goal. The primary goal is the equal treatment of persons even if this does not maximise other social goods.

QUESTION FIVE

In this case isn't the foundations theory of health merely a rather simplistic account of social justice, not health?

ANSWER FIVE

That is a very understandable comment. The short answer is yes, it is a simplistic account of social justice in that it contains no arguments explicitly about social justice (though there are countless books of philosophy that do this, and yet can prove their prejudices no more than I can). But primarily it is a theory of health. Confusion is bound to arise because it is not possible entirely to separate issues of health from social issues in general. The foundations theory of health has merely developed this truth to its logical conclusion.

Again, the full story can be seen by reading the books the theory was first developed in. But briefly – and at the risk of repetition – here are the bones of it that are most relevant to your question. Firstly, it is important to know that the foundations theory of health began solely as an investigation into the meaning of the word 'health' – solely as conceptual analysis. I was interested in these questions: what sort of word is health? To which other concepts is it most closely related? Logically, is the meaning of health the exact opposite of the meaning of disease? What, if anything, is the difference between a *theory* of health and a *concept* of health? These are purely philosophical questions, and in the beginning I had, as far as I am aware, no intention of extending the results of this abstract inquiry into a political argument. Of course, I brought to this conceptual analysis a multitude of semi-formed, part-articulated, but mostly hidden, beliefs and opinions about justice, about the good society, about the extent to which people are free and the extent to which we are socially determined, about duty, about personal responsibility, about welfare, about the obligations of the state, about medicine, about nursing, about the power imbalances between the different health professions, about poverty and deprivation (which was and still is inescapably obvious in many parts of the North-West of England), about the class system, about what I saw (and still see) as the criminal waste of human talent as the best life chances almost invariably went to those who were already the most privileged...all these prejudices were believed by the brain doing the analysis.

The extent to which these thoughts coloured the philosophical investigation of health is unclear to me, but there must have been some influence (perhaps the choice of examples to analyse, the selection of the ideas of other philosophers, the often unstated assumption that health matters equally to everyone). Whatever the case, as soon as the investigation moved beyond the conceptual it was *bound* to become political and my prejudices were then also bound to affect the analysis (I assume this applies to all social philosophy – to all academic commentators and commentaries on social issues).

The next stage in the investigation of the meaning of health was, of necessity, not only conceptual. There are other theories of health in existence, developed not only by philosophers,[93] but by theologians,[94] biologists,[95] medics,[96] political scientists,[97] nurses[98] and others.[99] It was necessary to study these theories, to see where they disagreed with each other and also to try to work out what they each (and actual health care practice too) had in common. It turned out that they are all directed, in one way or another, toward the detection and if possible prevention or removal of obstacles of various kinds to human potential of various kinds – and thus, conceptual analysis and observation of other thinking and practice began to be combined.

And from this point the philosophical and practical questions became increasingly entwined. In fact they just *are* entwined, only I had not realised it before. I know now that it is impossible to answer practical questions properly without also answering (or at least asking) philosophical ones, and *vice versa* too – for very many philosophical questions. What's the point of work for health? What is a successful health intervention? What ought to be the doctor's role? At what point should a nurse begin to care for a patient and at what point should she stop? In scarcity, what is the fairest distribution of medical resources? Philosophy and practice are inseparable in these conundrums (for instance, success needs both to be defined and observed, the extent of a doctor's role is an ethical as well as a technical matter, the question 'when should a nurse begin to care?' can be properly answered only by defining practical triggers for caring *and* by working out what it means to care).

To illustrate further: take the first of the questions in the paragraph above: 'what's the point of work for health?' How can this be answered? There seem, at first, to be two possibilities: it can be answered theoretically *or* it can be answered practically. Theoretically, for example, the point of work for health might be said to be 'to enable' or 'to empower'. Practically, the point may be said to cure this sickness, to repair this injury, to overcome this excessive anxiety. But are these different sorts of answer? Clearly they are not. The theoretical answer has been derived partly from experience – enabling or empowering is often the result, and is always intended to be the result, of practical health work: the very meaning of health comes about through social endeavour – health does not have a wholly asocial, ahistorical meaning. Equally, however, the practical answer is not exclusively derived from atheoretical behaviours and practices – there are *reasons* why sickness and injuries are dealt with: they tend to be painful, unwanted, debilitating and *disempowering*. We do not merely respond unthinkingly to such problems but attach different sorts of value to our efforts to solve them: we can give relief, we do not wish to see others suffer, we can foster renewed independence, we can ultimately increase our economic wealth by restoring people to health – and, sometimes, we can decide *not* to treat (the therapy will do no good, the person wishes to die, the therapy will in some way cost too much). Even if we do not know it, what we do reveals these values.

And once this irrevocable connection between theory and practice is recognised any attempt to separate health from broader social controversies becomes unsustainable. Aside from the fact that at least some illnesses are caused by social conditions and injustices, as a matter of logic, if the point of medicine is to enable people – to restore their function or to create improved function – then there is no theoretical difference between this sort of technical intervention and other sorts of intervention we do not conventionally think of as health work. For example, an employment agency can sometimes alleviate a person's depression by finding her a job – and so restore or improve her social functioning – just as well if not better than a solely clinical intervention. Obviously there is no ultimate barrier between official and technical/ medical work for health and other interventions done to enable people.

And once *this* is accepted I think it becomes easy enough to see how matters of health provision and matters of social justice are necessarily related. It should also be clear that it is *not possible* to put forward a serious theory of health *without* at the same time offering at least a rudimentary account of social justice – it just cannot be done. Even if you argue that all there is to health work is medicine, and that the only reason for medicine is to prevent or cure disease, you are necessarily committed to the view that the reason diseases are bad is what they prevent people doing (otherwise why are they a problem?), and so you are therefore also committed to the view that autonomy (or, people being able to do things they want to) is a good thing. And given this you must – you cannot avoid it – at least decide whether every person's autonomy is *equally* important. If you say it is, and if society beyond medicine is not geared up to ensure that this prejudice is realised in practice, then you are bound to be critical of the existing current set-up, which you *must* say is unjust. And if you say that the autonomy of *some* people is more important than that of others (for instance, if you think that the most talented and successful people ought to be treated before other people in society, or ought to be allowed to pay for better and speedier treatment if they wish to) then here too you are committed to a position on social justice. Namely, that it is just to treat people unequally even in the medical realm. If you have a view about the importance of health, health services and health promotion you also have a theory of social justice. Perhaps your theory is not spelt out, perhaps it is almost entirely implicit or almost entirely a matter of extrapolation from your position on health – but you hold it nonetheless.

The End of Illusion

Diane is sitting at her desk in the Chronicle's *open-plan office. She has just about finished her stint as a health promoter, and has written a challenging article about her experience. She has included the sort of stuff the* Chronicle's *readers will expect – pictures taken in a gym, pictures of smiling people with 'Stub out Smoking' T-shirts on, a picture of a local dignitary opening an Alcohol Free Youth to 21 club, and so on – but she has set all this within an article she's called '**What's the Point of Health Promotion?**' In her piece she has raised – gently but firmly – some 'big question marks' as she puts it. How much does all this cost? Does it work? Has health promotion got its priorities right? What are the priorities? Who are health promoters to tell you that you should stop smoking? Whose life is it anyway? She's also half-way through a piece for the* Sunday Examiner *(the health editor has made some encouraging noises) in collaboration with the philosopher, and she's feeling pretty pleased with herself.*

Just then the delivery girl arrives with a bundle of the latest issue of the Chronicle, *the one with her article in it. She picks up a copy and eagerly opens it.*

Diane's face is turning red as her anger grows. How could he do this to me? *she thinks. Aggressively, but for no particular reason, she opens the paper at other pages, and then stops cold. Her face drains of colour.*

Diane throws the paper aside. She storms into the Editor's Office.

EDITOR: Diane. You might have knocked.

DIANE: And you might have told me you weren't going to run my article.

EDITOR: I did run your article.

DIANE: You cut out everything that was worth printing.

EDITOR: That's a matter of opinion.

DIANE: I've spent four weeks researching that article and I gave you something that is actually stimulating – something that might get people thinking for once.

EDITOR: That isn't your job and it isn't the *Chronicle's* job. We're a local paper, not a vehicle for your pseudo-intellectual ramblings.

DIANE: (*Genuinely hurt*) They're not. I tried really hard with this. I got a balance. If only you'd given it a try you would've been surprised.

Health Promotion, Second Edition: David Seedhouse
© 2004 John Wiley & Sons, Ltd: ISBNs 0 470 84732 8 (HB); 0 470 84733 6 (PB)

8

Willesville Chronicle, Friday 6 December, 2002

HEALTHY WILLESVILLE

by Diane Grant

Willesville's Health is on the way up—it's official. According to our Health Promotion Unit, as a town, we are:
- smoking less
- exercising more
- losing weight (in all the right places).

However, not all is rosy. Drinking is on the increase, and the healthy trend does not cover those on lower incomes.

What can be done? Staff at the Unit offer a range of advice. Best suggestions are:
- drink low alcohol beers
- don't go it alone if you find it hard to exercise
- join an exercise club
- spurn smoking and drinking ads—lung and liver disease is not glamorous
- look after yourself—mind and body. You only get one chance.

Your Health — Your Responsibility

That's the message from the Unit. It is all too easy to take the unhealthy option—we are even encouraged to do so by some non-health industries—but the buck stops with you. You decide what you eat, what you drink, and whether you exercise. No-one does it for you.

But the Good News is that the Unit is there to help. To get started, or to keep going—when it gets tough, give the experts a call.

For details on Healthy Lifestyle call the Willesville HP Unit on 528-7952.

Diane Grant's Tips for Healthy Living
I was a health promoter for a month. If you want to be healthy, and want my advice, then:
- QUIT SMOKING
- CUT DOWN ON THE BOOZE (but not too much if you are over 40—a little tipple each day *can* keep the doctor away)
- EXERCISE 3 TIMES A WEEK, 20 minutes or more (but ask your doctor first)
- EAT LESS FOOD (WHY NOT GO VEGGIE FOR A WEEK?)
- RELAX
- ENJOY YOUR FRIENDS

Willesville FC on the Up

After three dark years in the lower reaches of Division One, Willesville FC look set to mount a challenge for the Premiership promotion play-off places. Since manager Paul Newstart took over from David 'Big-Time' Splatt there has been a new mood at the City reserve.

In an exclusive interview with the *Chronicle* Newstart said: 'As Mr Rough always used to say – you've got to control the centre of the Park. It only takes a second to score a goal. Clean sheets are what we pay the goalie for.' Club owner Nigel Umbro commented: 'Paul has no money to spend, which is just as well given our recent history.'

Willesville Chronicle, Friday 6 December, 2002   9

Closure cloud over Adams'

by Bill Lading

Cost cutting measures are to close Adams' Greenlane meat packers.

CEO Norman Stanhope says management will shut the Willesville factory next Friday, and can offer no guarantees about units in Glenfield and Albany.

He has been holding talks this week with local Union representatives. There may be some redeployment of staff to the main Campbell Town works, but up to 200 Greenlane workers will be permanently laid off.

Other cost cutting measures include a reduction in the car and van pool and a ban on the use of cellphones.

Mr Stanhope is confident that these measures will ensure the long-term health of Adams Co.

Experts Predict Property Slump

The residential property market in Willesville is forecast to deteriorate over the next six months.

Professor of Property Studies at Willesborough University Garry Howse says 58% of the panel predicted a decline in the market conditions, while 34% anticipate the market will remain steady. Only 5% expect any improvement.

The majority say market confidence and sales will decrease markedly over the next three months for all residential property categories in Willesville and outlying suburbs.

"Their opinions suggest that prices for lower priced houses should stay relatively stable", says Professor Howse. "However the middle and upper markets are expected to show considerable downward movement. Comments noted the impact of economic and political uncertainty and rising interest rates."

MISSING PET MYSTERY

The Willesville vanishing cats and dogs saga continues. This week 7 local owners have reported the disappearance of much-loved family pets.

"We can't understand it", said Constable Dibble. "The animals are here one minute and gone the next. It's as if they have disappeared into a black hole, however people can rest assured that we are looking into it. At first we though it must be a kids' prank or that unscrupulous thieves were selling them on. But the pets are disappearing in broad daylight, and they are not even pedigree animals."

Animal Protection Leagues, at a loss to explain the mystery, are on the look out for strays. "Perhaps they are being abducted by aliens" said Mr F. Mulder, a well-known local veterinarian. "My assistant tells me not to be silly, but how else do you account for it? 100 missing pets in less than a month has got to be more than coincidence."

Police are advising local pet-owners to keep their animals indoors and to watch out for strange lights.

Mrs Slocum, a Willesville resident, bewails the loss of her pussy

Another Rock Suicide

Andrew Wilson, 42, of 14 Cedar Drive, Willesville was found dead at the foot of Castle Rock on Wednesday.

He had recently returned from India to care for his mother Sarah. Mrs Wilson died six weeks ago from a long illness.

Sometime Wednesday evening it is thought Mr Wilson climbed 'the rock'—a notorious suicide spot—whereupon he took his life. A note was found in a coat pocket.

Inquest to be held Friday week.

EDITOR: If you want to write for the nationals I suggest you go freelance. I'm not having the *Chronicle* turned into a laboratory for Ms Diane Grant. If you don't want to work for us then just say so.

DIANE: You had no right to destroy my piece without telling me.

EDITOR: I have every right. I thought you knew I wouldn't run it actually. Look, calm down, won't you. Why don't you sit down?

DIANE: I won't. I am very angry with you.

EDITOR: I have edited your stuff before and you've been OK with it.

DIANE: It's a bit more than editing! And this is different.

EDITOR: Why?

DIANE: Because it's to do with justice.

EDITOR: What? I reserve the right to decide what goes in the *Chronicle* – you know that. Everyone here knows that.

DIANE: I don't mean that – though there are limits to what you are entitled to do. There are courtesies...but that's not it. What I mean is I think that we – people in Willesville, people most places – are being duped.

EDITOR: What a revelation! Come on Diane. We're all duped one way or another all the time – everyone knows it. You don't need to tell anyone that.

DIANE: Don't I? It's one thing knowing in general that politicians don't tell the truth but quite another thing finding out clear evidence that we are being conned.

EDITOR: What are you talking about?

DIANE: I'm talking about health. We're supposed to believe that the government is promoting health because it has Health Promotion Departments like Willesville's all around the country – that the government is concerned for the people, that it wants us to live healthy lives – yet it is all basically either a front, or a way to make people feel guilty, or a way to cut costs to hospitals by keeping people out of them.

EDITOR: But what's wrong with that? It seems OK to me. I couldn't work out what you were writing about in your article if you really must know. Telling people to quit smoking, eat better and so on – that's what health promotion is. Simple as that. Don't you think you're making things just a teensy bit over-complicated Diane?

DIANE: Don't patronise me. I'm not complicating things. It just is complicated. But if you want it down to basics those health promotion units aren't promoting health. Perhaps just occasionally they improve a few people's health but mostly they are wasting their time.

EDITOR: I see. Health promotion units *don't* promote health. Very penetrating I'm sure.

DIANE: (*Fiercely*) You really are a very stupid person aren't you Derek? You are simple so life is simple and that's all there is to it.

EDITOR: You be careful what you say.

DIANE: It doesn't matter what I say because you censor it – remember? I'm wasting my breath but I'll tell you what health is. Then perhaps you'll see what damage you're causing.

EDITOR: I don't want to know. OK?

DIANE: (*Ignoring this*) You know this chap? (*Pointing to the report of Andrew Wilson's suicide*) I met him. He drank too much and he smoked and obviously he was not as happy as he could have been, but I've come to believe he was healthy enough at the time I met him. He knew what he wanted. At the time he was able to choose what path to follow. He smoked, yes, but he didn't care if smoking is risky because he liked taking risks.

EDITOR: Come off it Diane. He's just killed himself and you say he was healthy? What is it with you?

DIANE: He was healthy until they shut Adams'. That's where he worked.

EDITOR: (*Sarcastically*) Oh I see. Shutting a meat factory is a health issue. Of course it is.

DIANE: Yes it is because that closure meant that Andrew Wilson was trapped. It meant that he couldn't get out of Willesville as he thought he could. It meant, as far as he could see, a sort of living death.

EDITOR: (*Mockingly*) You don't like Willesville much do you Diane?

DIANE: Just because closing Adams' hasn't got anything to do with medicine doesn't mean that it isn't a health issue.

EDITOR: Diane, shutting Adams' doesn't cause disease.

DIANE: It might do, it probably will in the end, and it probably caused Andrew's suicide, but that's not the point. Something – some event, some change – does not have to cause disease to cause less health. It all depends what you mean by health. And what you mean by health guides . . . (*stammering*) I mean it ought to guide – what health promoters do.

EDITOR: OK, suicide is a health issue. I accept that. So why don't you go and do an article on suicide in Willesville. I'd allow that.

DIANE: I'm sure. I might very well not do any more articles in Willesville. But just tell me why you think suicide's a health issue and closing Adams' isn't.

EDITOR: Someone who commits suicide is mentally ill. They should have received medical treatment to stop them killing themselves. And if someone tries and fails then he usually needs one doctor or another to help pick up the pieces. Obviously suicide is a health issue.

DIANE: So what you're saying is that someone who is depressed has a health problem because their depression is making them behave abnormally and might even make them kill themselves – it's cutting down their options and they need help. Right?

EDITOR: Right.

DIANE: How is that different from Adams' workers who can't get another job? Their options are cut and they need help.

EDITOR: They're OK unless they have to go to the doctor.

DIANE: You can't justify that, I know you can't. You just think what many health promoters are forced to think, you associate health with medicine and so your hands are tied. Even if you say that health is something well beyond disease – as most health promoters seem to – you still have to behave as if it isn't.

I think it's all wrong. Say if Andrew had failed to commit suicide and had been badly injured. Say he needed life-long medical care, disability support, welfare benefits and all the rest. He'd get them because he'd been injured. He would be perceived to have a health problem. But the fact that his life is devastated through Adams' closing means that he gets nothing – just the dole. Don't you think that's crazy?

(And to think I gave him those leaflets. What an idiot.)

I've come to the conclusion that we should think of health as first to do with the basic necessities for people to live reasonable lives – homes, a feeling of purpose, good information – which they hardly ever get from the *Chronicle* by the way – education, a sense of belonging: the basic resources for everyday living. And then – if there is a crisis – they should get appropriate support. That can be medical support if necessary but I can't see any reason why it has to be medical. Nor can I see why that is always seen as the focus. It's all back to front. A life crisis is a life crisis and people need whatever support is necessary. If Andrew Wilson had been directed to a State Redundancy Centre, if he had been given a whole range of social and financial supports, if he had been given the chance to reassess his life, which is what I think he needed, then he wouldn't have committed suicide.

EDITOR: You don't know that.

DIANE: No I don't. But I do know that there would have been more chance of saving him. Why do we have so many hospitals and no Redundancy Centres?

EDITOR: We do have other forms of social support. He could've got help if he'd wanted it.

DIANE: The balance is all wrong.

EDITOR: (*Angry at being drawn into this*) Maybe it is but that's hardly suitable for the *Chronicle* is it? What do you think we are? The *Morning Star*? Political subversives?

DIANE: No. Of course not. But you are just as political as if you were. Being establishment is just as radical as any other political position. There is no such thing as a moderate.

EDITOR: This is the *Willesville Chronicle* we're talking about! The local rag for God's sake.

DIANE: Precisely. And it is all the more effective because it doesn't raise political questions.

EDITOR: I've had enough of this. You're obviously upset. You've been overdoing it. I want you to take a week off. Shake off these student fantasies. Come back. Do the job you are paid for. If you can't – or won't – then there's no place for you here. Understand?

DIANE: Too much and too late. Why doesn't any of this bother you?

EDITOR: Because I like things the way they are. And if people don't look after themselves that's their look out. So long as they don't bother me. Now I'm busy – and you've got a decision to make. Goodbye Diane.

Ethics and Health Promotion

MORE TOUGH QUESTIONS

QUESTION SIX

How can the foundations theory help health promoters in their practical work?

ANSWER SIX

This is the big question. In short, it has these answers. If a health promoter decides to adopt the foundations theory it will help her in the following ways:

i. It will give her a sense of *direction* – a clear picture of her professional purpose.
ii. It will help her to understand the *relationship* between her chosen theory of health and the vision of the good society from whence it sprang. And so long as she is comfortable with this interpretation of the good society she will feel confident that she is justified in doing what she does. Her work as a health promoter will no longer seem arbitrary but will be a theoretically explicit acknowledgement of her prejudices.
iii. It will allow her to establish a *theoretical framework within which to practise*. She will know which interventions fall within the bounds of the framework, and are therefore acceptable, and which are outside and so unacceptable. More of this below.
iv. It will allow her to set *clear targets for her interventions, to justify* this selection, and may possibly help her *assess* the extent to which she has succeeded.

CENTRAL ETHICAL DISTINCTIONS

Health promotion is obviously a moral endeavour, yet so much health promotion practice proceeds as if in an ethical vacuum. The foundations theory, however, openly

Health Promotion, Second Edition: David Seedhouse
© 2004 John Wiley & Sons, Ltd: ISBNs 0 470 84732 8 (HB); 0 470 84733 6 (PB)

acknowledges that ethics is all-pervading in health promotion and makes two crucial distinctions. The first between:

1. health promotion done specifically to assist a defined individual or group, and health promotion done more generally, to improve the health of populations

and the second

2. health promotion done on request, and health promotion done without a recipient or recipients asking for it.

Examples which fall into each category are offered below and – in conjunction with Exercise Ten and its accompanying guidance to teachers – are also used to show more fully how a health promoter can achieve i–iv above. These examples, and their discussion, are not intended as a comprehensive guide to the ethics of health promotion. However, if studied along with the rest of this book, and with reference to other competent works on applied ethics and moral philosophy,[100,101] then you will be well placed to develop a considered perspective on health promotion ethics.

FOUR ALTERNATIVES

The two distinctions mentioned above give rise to four alternative categories of intervention, as follows:

A. Health promotion done to improve the general public health *in accordance with* the clear wishes of all or most of the general public.
B. Health promotion done *on request* of a specifically defined individual or group.
C. Health promotion done to improve the health of a specifically defined individual or group *without* that individual or group *requesting it.*
D. Health promotion done to improve the general public health *without the expressed consent* of the general public, and/or done at the *request of a minority interest group.*

Before briefly examining the ethics of each of these possibilities it is worth recalling the foundations with a reasonable level of content, by looking back to Fig. 30, on p. 170. It is extremely important to bear in mind that a health promoter's work may be practically and ethically very different dependent on whether the figure ♀ stands for a single person, or a group with harmony of purpose or – as it may – stands for a group with different or conflicting interests, or stands for society at large.

ALTERNATIVE A

Practically speaking, the foundational health promoter who wishes to work on projects that affect the whole of society, and has a clear public mandate so to do, must:

a. review the content of Boxes 1–5
b. decide which boxes *in general* need most urgent attention and which she is best equipped to provide or maintain – and then decide on her most effective role

c. proceed to work on that box or those boxes with a view to improving the
foundations of as many *unidentified* people as possible.

For example, a foundational health promoter might reasonably decide that she is best
equipped to provide much-needed information about, say, breast cancer or how to
cope with unexpected unemployment – and set about writing brochures and books for
wide distribution. Or she might campaign for the provision of freely available adult
education, or she might decide to persuade supermarket chains to sell only pesticide-
free produce. There are countless foundational public health projects on which she
might embark.

Ethically speaking, given that the health promoter is honest about her *reasoned
prejudices*, then it is unlikely that there will be many ethical objections raised. These
tend to occur only where there is controversy about either the evidence or the
desirability of certain general policies (such controversy exists over immunisation
for children, for example, though this is often played down by those who are in
favour of it).[102] Unless resources are extraordinarily scarce, major ethical controversy
should not occur in *generally mandated* work according to the foundations theory
since the boxes will be seen to be basic requirements for a reasonably flourishing
life for almost everyone. However, because the idea of 'foundations for
achievement' is politically based, the likelihood of ethical dispute increases in
proportion to the difference between 'foundations politics' and any existing political
climate.

ALTERNATIVE B

Similarly, in normal circumstances alternative B poses few ethical difficulties. But this
is not to say that it never poses difficulties. In *principle* one might want to say that if
health promotion is a good thing, and if it is good that health promoters respond to
the informed requests of citizens for health promotion services, then there will be an
ethically trouble-free situation. However, in practice there is an obvious difference
between the case of the individual who has decided, after much thought, to quit
smoking tobacco and has chosen to consult his local health promotion team for
advice and help, and the case of ten passionately committed members of a
neighbourhood approaching the health promotion team for their professional and
financial support to help create a car-free neighbourhood, when several others in the
neighbourhood are opposed to the idea (this latter possibility might also be included
under alternative C).

In order to decide what best to do in these circumstances, it is obviously not enough
merely to say that in principle health promoters should respond to informed
requests for help. Rather, careful reflection about the merits of each request, and
about the health promoters' ability to respond to it, is required. This is not the place
to explain how such careful reflection might be done – for this, health promoters
should look elsewhere,[85,103] and should begin work on Exercises Eight, Nine and Ten
in this book, which help explain how the foundations theory can assist moral
deliberation.

ALTERNATIVE C

Unless the proposed project is clearly foundational, alternative C will require at least as much ethical deliberation as alternative B, and usually more, before the health promoter decides to proceed or not. Again, much hinges upon the circumstances.

For instance, there is a difference between a health promoter deciding, *without being asked*, to work each evening in the streets of Manhattan to improve the health of the homeless (by offering food, advice, a friendly ear, and perhaps some better possibilities) and desisting if his help is rejected, and a health promoter seeking to promote the health of lunchtime drinkers, without being asked, by campaigning vigorously outside and inside local bars to get the message across – and not desisting even when some of the drinkers ask him to. The health promoter trying to do something for the health of the homeless is trying to achieve basic – foundational – goals and the other health promoter is not, or at least is not in those cases where the drinking is light, chosen and pleasurable – in other words, where it is not a problem.

There will also be differences of method. The health promoter working with the homeless will, of necessity, be sensitive in his approach (in order to have any effect) whereas the health promoter working with the lunchtime drinkers will, of necessity, not be sensitive in his approach – he will inevitably have to be critical of the drinkers' drinking, at the least. Moreover, an important aspect of any ethical deliberation is to try to predict its likely practical results. For the health promoter on the streets it is likely that he can anticipate some success, perhaps considerable success if he can find a way to engender more fulfilment for his chosen subjects.[104] There may be considerable failures too, but most probably these will be experienced personally, by the health promoter (if his well-meaning attempts are turned away, if he is physically attacked, if he is robbed). For the health promoter campaigning against lunchtime drinking, he may be successful – he may find that he prompts action by drinkers already worried by their drinking, but he can also expect some ridicule, or even to reinforce drinking patterns amongst drinkers who become irritated by his attention, and who wish to make a pointed stand against him. All these things need to be taken into account in order to decide whether unsolicited health promotion is ethically defensible or not.

ALTERNATIVE D

So too with alternative D. Large-scale interventions to improve the public health are, in complex societies, almost inevitably paternalistic. It is impractical to consult everyone about such matters as anti-pollution measures, acceptable levels of food additive, seat-belt and crash helmet legislation, national childhood immunisation programmes, and so on. And nor is it possible to suit everyone when there is disagreement. In these cases, more than in the other three – what really matters is having, demonstrating, explaining and *abiding by* a defensible, explicit theory of intervention for health.

EXERCISE TEN

APPLYING THE FOUNDATIONS THEORY OF HEALTH PROMOTION

This exercise offers the opportunity to apply the foundations theory to two practical cases. Because there are important ethical differences between *working for the health of individuals* and *working for the health of populations*, two examples are given. The task is to work out, using the foundations idea, the most ethical and most effective way of promoting health in each case.

EXAMPLE I: THE PERSON WHO *MIGHT* LIKE TO REDUCE HER ALCOHOL CONSUMPTION

You are acquainted with a 30-year-old woman called Wendy. You happen to sit together on the morning train into town, and the topic of drinking and health arises in casual conversation. Wendy knows you are a health promoter and says 'Oh, I'm sure I drink too much. I certainly did last night. Perhaps I should cut down. What do you think?'

Using the foundations theory, what do you do?

EXAMPLE 2: RESEARCHING THE PUBLIC HEALTH

You are a middle-aged senior researcher in public health. For the last five years you have received, from your Health Research Council, a sizeable grant to ascertain the causes of cot-death. You believe you have discovered multiple factors, but would like to do further work to confirm these, as well as continue to provide education programmes to the most 'at risk' groups. You are quite sure that your work is firmly in the public interest.

You are under no contractual obligation to continue your research programme. You could choose other projects which may or may not receive funding.

Using the foundations theory, do you apply for a continuation of funding for cot-death research (which you are likely to receive) or do you embark on an alternative project (and so run a greater risk of not receiving funding)?

continues

continued

Teaching notes for: Applying the Foundations Theory of Health Promotion

EXAMPLE I

This is the easiest of the two cases. It should be attempted by students with access to Fig. 30 – the foundations with specific content.

As a first step, students should be encouraged to discuss the content of the image, decide if they are happy with it, and add further practical content as they wish. Ask them, for example: 'what level of information is adequate?', 'what specific content should appear in Boxes 1 and 4 in this case?', 'will Box 5 be necessary, and what is its content likely to be?' and so on. Remember that the content must always be of a foundational nature.

Once the scene has been set:

a. you must ask students which box they are focusing on and what its content is

and

b. you must constantly remind students of the *point* of the foundations theory.

To give one possible example:

Suppose a student offers the view that the key foundations are first *information* and second *education*. She might then choose to draw a set of foundations as in Fig. 37.

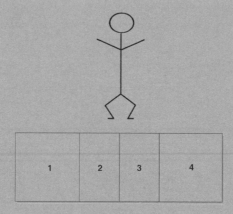

Figure 37   A suggested representation of Wendy's platform in the case of her drinking

continues

continued

Figure 38   A way of working with the Foundations in mind

You might respond to the student like this:

Okay, you've checked out what Wendy knows, found her knowledge lacking in Boxes 2 and 3 (Fig. 37), and will be working to *extend* Boxes 2 and 3 as in (Fig. 38).

You might then say:

Look what this will do to the foundations as a whole. It will expand the stage from the position in Fig. 37

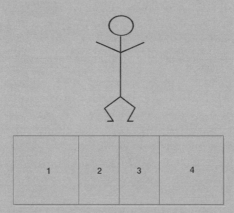

Figure 37   A suggested representation of Wendy's platform in the case of her drinking

to that of Fig. 39:

And this means – or should mean – that you will have succeeded in increasing Wendy's autonomy (and so her level of health) by your intervention.

As you spell this out, you will be achieving the second of your tasks – reminding students of the point of foundational work for health. Having done so you will be well placed to consider further issues. For instance:

 i. What if Wendy says, 'I don't want to hear this'?
 ii. What if Wendy becomes unhappy and begins to lose friends over the weeks, and you think your advice might partly be the cause of this?
 iii. What if the expansion of foundations 2 and 3 leads to a *contraction* of other foundations?

continues

continued

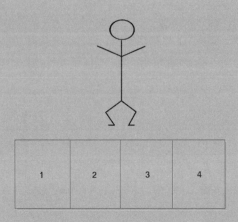

Figure 39

iv. What if you discover an additional problem in Wendy's life – a Box 5 problem – which her drinking is helping her cope with? What should you do in this case?

v. What if you discover that Wendy is an alcoholic, and her drinking is ruining her life?

The foundations theory can help form policy on each of these further questions, though it rarely if ever indicates a single policy. What the theory definitely does do, however, is to prompt thinking and reflection about theory and practice, which is what you are aiming to achieve.

Possible foundations responses to the above additional questions might include:

A. Stop
B. Carry on giving information until you are sure Wendy can make a competent judgement about her drinking. Then stop.
C. Examine the strength of Wendy's other foundations for achievement. Then stop.
D. Decide, with her autonomy in mind, if it is acceptable for the expansion of Boxes 2 and 3 to *shrink* others. Examine the size of the Box 5 problem. See what further support you could provide, or Wendy wants from you. Decide whether this is appropriate support. Reassess.

EXAMPLE 2

You should make two points in this case: first, where resources are limited, health promotion (and even whether to do any health promotion at all) is always a question of choosing priorities according to both values and evidence. Second, it is extremely difficult to establish what is in the 'public interest'.

continues

continued

This said, your educational task is as follows. First, explore some of the research (knowledge, disputes and controversies) about cot-death or whatever other public health area you have chosen to examine. If possible, provide a selection of background papers and extracts so that students can know something of the subject. Be prepared, also, to answer whatever questions you can about this background material.

After this, ask the students to imagine that they are the public health researcher, and are genuinely anxious about the best way to proceed to work for health. Again, display the foundations diagram (Fig. 30) with specific content, and have the students discuss and add to it as they will, within its theoretical limits.

Then encourage students to discuss:

i. The box or boxes on which the researcher can (or should) best work.
ii. The foundations benefits that may emerge from the research.
iii. The foundations benefits that may emerge if the researcher pursues alternatives, *or* if he is unable to do any further research (if his grant application is unsuccessful, for instance).

Figure 40

continues

continued

iv. Possible disadvantages and damage to the foundations.
v. The ethical issues which arise from seeking to study and intervene in a social situation where either no one has asked for your help, or where a *minority* special interest group has asked for your help. What are you trying to achieve? In what senses are your goals 'work for health'? How can you tell if there are better goals to pursue?

Be careful to spell out the context of the research. Does cot-death affect all social groups? The richest? The poorest? Is the society in question affluent as a whole (there are important differences between researching cot-death in Sweden and in India, for example)? How much is already known about cot-death? Is further education necessary? Are there more urgent social priorities?

As you have students reflect on these matters, as if they were the senior researcher, it would be very helpful to introduce the Ethical Grid[85] if you can. This device has been designed as an aid to decision-making in health care and – especially in its central (blue) boxes – is itself a version of the foundations theory. Roughly, the relationship is as indicated in Fig. 40.

If you are unable to use the Grid, then have students, in the guise of the researcher, ask the specific question – do I apply for a continuation of my research grant for research and education into cot-death? – and then analyse it with reference to the various categories of the Grid. In this way students will be able to ask practical questions (black), decide on general priorities (green), consider their personal and professional obligations (red) (if they believe they have any), and be able to say what they consider the basic rationale (or purpose) of their work to be in this case.[85]

A BRIEF DISCUSSION OF THE ETHICS OF ALTERNATIVE D: THE CASE OF FLUORIDATION

It is the practice of some nations with a temperate climate, in some if not all of their regions, to raise by artificial means the fluoride concentration in drinking water to one part per million (p.p.m.) (proponents of fluoride recommend a slightly higher level in cold climates, slightly lower in hot ones). These countries do this to improve the dental health of their populations without these populations having to do anything more than drink tap water or any beverage made with it (tea, coffee, beer, soft drinks, reconstituted fruit juices) sufficient to ensure an intake of around one mg of fluoride per day (about one litre of tap water in fluoridated areas). The hope is that since drinking tap water is, for most of us, an activity we take for granted, the dental health of the public can be improved with or without our knowledge. As far as our teeth are concerned it is quite immaterial whether we know what fluoride is, whether we know we are ingesting it, whether we approve of it, or whether we are worried about its presence.

There are many who find fluoridation to be, without question, a good thing. Some argue that if one finds ethical fault with fluoridation then one could find similar fault with *any* measure designed to protect the public (including road speed limits, pollution controls, regulations to prevent people swimming in dangerous waters, the prohibition of pesticides damaging to the environment, legislation to ensure safe drinking water and so on). Some advocates of fluoridation maintain that if all interventions done with the public interest in mind were to be subjected to close and constant scrutiny, public health measures would be unworkable. And what is more – they say – it is well known that fluoridation is effective and carries few if any risks, therefore it should be done and there should be no argument about it.

However, careful study of most of the practices we take for granted in the modern world tends to reveal that those things we assume to be safe, proven and ethically trouble-free, are very often deeply controversial, both as a matter of science and as a matter of value (the space programme,[105] AIDS,[106,107] immunisation,[102] fertilisers in farming,[108] medicine,[99] health promotion,[46,109] factory egg production,[110] and democracy[111] are all examples). And fluoridation is no exception. While there are those who claim that fluoridation can cause a reduction in tooth decay of between 50 to 70% higher than if it were not administered[112,113], others argue that the fluoridation of tap water offers no benefit and carries risks. For example:

> Tooth decay has been declining substantially over the past 20–30 years in both unfluoridated and fluoridated regions of the developed world.[114–117] In several developed countries, the decline commenced before the use of fluoride in any form became widespread.

> A result of these declines is that now there is little or no difference in average levels of tooth decay between comparable unfluoridated and fluoridated regions of at least four countries: Australia,[113] Canada,[118] New Zealand,[119] and the USA.[120,121]

and

> Scientists and health professionals who are questioning fluoridation draw attention to a body of evidence, published in reputable medical and scientific journals, that some people suffer from dental fluorosis, skeletal fluorosis, bone fractures and intolerance/hypersensitivity reactions from naturally and/or artificially fluoridated water. All these diseases have been confirmed by several independent studies and so could be regarded as well-established.[122]

Such authors conclude that, because of these doubts, mass fluoridation should cease and health promotion efforts should switch to practices that are better supported by the evidence:

> The comparisons of tooth decay in unfluoridated and fluoridated cities within Australia, New Zealand and the USA, together with the large declines in tooth decay observed in many unfluoridated cities, show that children can have good teeth without fluoridation. The problem is that nobody knows for certain what are the most important factors causing the reductions in tooth decay in

unfluoridated cities, such as Brisbane, Australia, and Christchurch, New Zealand. For instance, how important is the program of daily toothbrushing with fluoride toothpaste in some of Brisbane's primary schools? This program is not expensive, because it is carried out by schoolteachers rather than dental therapists. How important are changes in diet, and how important is better education of parents and children about oral health?

Despite these uncertainties, there is no doubt that improved diet reduces tooth decay. In particular, reducing sugar consumption and increasing the consumption of cheese and possibly wholemeal bread reduces tooth decay considerably.[123–125]

...In fluoridated areas, it is still the poor who tend to have unhealthy diets and have the worst teeth.[126–128,122]

(Any internet search under 'fluoride controversy' will uncover seemingly endless arguments and data, pro and con.)

That fluoridation is controversial is amply reflected by the fact that nations have different policies. Currently, in most English-speaking countries, over half the population has little choice but to drink fluoridated water (it is possible to buy filters to remove fluoride, but this is not cheap and in any case requires knowledge and the commitment to go to the trouble) yet the practice has been abandoned in Sweden, Holland and Germany.[122] Most of the people who are virtually obliged to consume at least five times the typically naturally occurring amount of fluoride are unaware that, were we to live elsewhere, we would not have to consume it. And this, if one is committed to the notion of an informed public (as most health promoters apparently are, and as is taken as read in *medical* ethics circles), must be of ethical concern.

And this is by no means the end to the ethics of fluoridation. For example, Diesendorf is of the view that the evidence in favour of fluoridation has been obtained selectively, and that many of the studies which purportedly show fluoridation in a good light were not based on controlled or randomised trials. He also points out, noticing a tactic reminiscent of that used by the UK HEA in its Smoking Guide (see pp. 66–67 above), that evaluative statements are regularly used by fluoridation's scientific proponents as if they are entirely factual. Diesendorf cites the use of the terms 'controlled fluoridation' and 'deficiency of fluoride' to describe *naturally occurring* levels of fluoride, and the repeated use of the statement 'fluoride is a natural substance' to suggest that it is therefore automatically harmless, come what may. In fact, he points out, only a small fraction of the world's population (mostly in India) ingests naturally fluoridated water with fluoride concentrates equal to or greater than 1 p.p.m.[122]

Such deceptions cannot obscure the ethical questions for Diesendorf. For instance, he asks:

Is mass medication, which is compulsory or expensive to avoid (ethically) wrong?

Is (the) medication (of people) with an uncontrolled dose (ethically) wrong?[122]

Diesendorf asks why – when it would clearly not be acceptable for doctors to prescribe drugs without recommending an appropriate daily dosage – is it acceptable for people's intake of fluoride to depend not on their following instructions, but according to how much tap water they consume, their age, or how much fluoride their kidneys are able to excrete?

Diesendorf notes (correctly) that since the risks and benefits are not objectively comparable (i.e. they are not of a nature that enables a simple comparison, as if they could each be placed on the same scale) then any assessment of them must also involve human values of some kind:

> There is no way of comparing risks and benefits without making value-judgements. For instance, how many cavities saved in a child's teeth are equivalent to a hypersensitivity reaction induced in a young adult or a hip fracture in an old person? How can we compare risks and benefits in the case of people who have lost their natural teeth as the result of factors not connected with tooth decay? These people receive no benefits from fluoridation, yet they suffer the risk of skeletal fluorosis arising from the accumulation of fluoridate in their bones over their lifetimes.[122]

FLUORIDATION AND HEALTH PROMOTION

Once again it is easy to see that the selection of a health promotion strategy does not depend only on evidence, and in the end must be decided according to certain convictions based ultimately on political philosophy. If you are of the view that health promotion is a:

> ...descendant of the great old regulatory public health measures which have had such an impact on the population's health over the last century[6]

and if you believe that it is fundamental to the functioning of a stable society that well-established institutions should be supported and maintained (even if these are plainly unjust when seen from alternative points of view), then it is highly unlikely you will even think to challenge conventional, established wisdom. Indeed, you will simply take for granted that:

> ...[f]luoridation of water supplies [can] prevent dental caries (and possibly also osteoporosis)[6]

and mention this casually, without reporting any counter-evidence or difference of opinion. Equally, if you are of the view that capitalist systems encourage the exploitation of citizens by other citizens in the interests of private profit, then you are likely to be suspicious of fluoridation – at the very least because someone will certainly be profiting from the process, and because most people will have no say in the matter. If you are of this persuasion then you may even arrive at the conclusion that:

> ...the fertilizer and aluminium industries promoted fluoridation initially because they were finding it very difficult to dispose of this toxic by-product. Research money from them and the sugar industry ensured the answers they wanted.[129]

But, to favour or oppose health promotion strategies primarily on implicit ideological assumptions is no basis for a mature discipline, especially one which obviously seeks to help other people. Rather, where complex matters of evidence and ethics co-exist, and where you need to decide whether to advocate a particular policy or not, it is best that you do so according to a considered theoretical basis open to public scrutiny. As things stand only the foundations theory of health promotion offers this help to practising health promoters.

QUESTION SEVEN

So what does the foundations theory of health promotion recommend in the case of the fluoridation of tap water?

ANSWER SEVEN

The theory does not, of course, mechanically direct the health promoter to the answer. However, the foundational health promoter considering whether or not to advocate, say, the continued fluoridation of the public water supply in her locality should be aware that she is, at least in the first place, contemplating the merits of alternative D. And she should certainly begin by asking two key questions. Namely:

i. Should fluoridation be continued here?
ii. If so, what *other* health promoting strategies should be put in place? If not, how should the change be managed in the most health promoting manner?

To answer these questions the health promoter not only has to get as much as possible clear about the evidence and ethics of fluoridation, she also has to make several specific decisions. She should start with the image of the stage or platform in mind. She might, then, begin her deliberations by asking: should fluoridation be continued in Willesville County? and next consider the four plus boxes which illustrate part of the foundations theory. She should ask: which of these boxes is of most relevance in answering the questions? Is each equally relevant, or does one dominate in this case? She should reflect on the issues raised by the content of the boxes at will, seeking to explore both whatever facts she can establish and aiming to clarify questions of value, and their relationship to the evidence. She might, for instance begin at Box 1 and ask – is fluoridation a basic biological or human need? Is fluoride essential in the way that food, shelter and protection from injury are essential?

If she were to take this line she would almost certainly have to decide that fluoridation is not necessary in the foundational sense: the evidence is disputed and even if fluoridation does produce the maximum benefits claimed there are alternative means of achieving them, means which do not rely on virtual compulsion. However, the foundational health promoter should be constantly aware that she could have chosen to begin her reflection at a different place, say at Box 4. If so, she might have taken a different line.

Whatever the case it is vital that the health promoter gets hold of as much evidence as possible, and that she understands that the way she interprets it will in part depend on her values. If she particularly values the status quo, if she particularly values interventions by the state in the interests of the people rather than leaving *everything* to individual choice, if she sees something important in the knowledge that in this respect at least all the citizens of Willesville are in the same boat, and if she also decides that fluoridation produces benefits at little or no risk, then it is likely that – at the beginning of her deliberation at least, she will favour retaining the policy.

Of course, whether she starts with Box 1 or Box 4, the foundational health promoter will also have to consider the importance of Boxes 2 and 3 (information) (education), and so must decide *what else* she will need to do, whatever her basic preference about fluoridation. She could, for instance, decide that since the pros and cons are so open to debate, her *key task* is to inform the public about the fluoridation controversy, to enable them to think about the evidence, its implications, and their options, carefully and calmly, and then either to follow a majority view (if she can obtain this) or try to enable those who want more, less (or even no) fluoride to find ways of fulfilling their choices. Alternatively, she might decide to offer the pros and cons to the public, to enable them to think carefully, *and* put forward her own point of view – whether for or against, in her capacity as someone who has had the time to research and to think seriously about the matter.

The Foundations Theory of Health Promotion Does Not Always Compel One Sort of Answer

Precisely because it allows for the introduction of personal and political values the foundations way of approaching health promotion does not spontaneously produce right answers. As we have seen, people with different political persuasions may look on the evidence in different lights, and so reach policy conclusions different from health promoters who see the issue from another political perspective, even if each has exactly the same evidence. However, necessary flexibility is not – at least on the **foundations theory** – a *carte blanche* for any conclusion. For example, on the **foundations theory** the health promoter is *obliged*:

  i. to consider as much of the evidence as she can reasonably muster (she should not merely take the verdict offered to her by one authority – she should look around and check out what she is being asked to believe)
 ii. to consider at least Boxes 1–4, and to include aspects of each in her decisions about both means and ends
iii. to offer as explicit a justification as she can whenever she decides to put a particular consideration above all other considerations. For example, if she regards fluoridation to be a basic need of more importance than the need to inform the public that fluoridation is controversial, then she must clearly explain why
 iv. constantly to bear in mind the ethical limits of her work (the platform analogy and cut-off points will help her in this).

QUESTION EIGHT

Is this a model? Are you suggesting that the foundations theory of health is yet another health promotion model?

ANSWER EIGHT

Obviously not. This is philosophy of and for health promotion. It is a rich and complicated tapestry of ideas which cannot be simply copied, and which cannot be followed as one would follow a flow chart. My hope is that health promotion practitioners, teachers and academics – but particularly practitioners – will take the time to study it, to understand it, and perhaps reject and amend parts of it, so that they can be theoretically in command of what they are doing, as befits any professional.

QUESTION NINE

What is the role of the state in health promotion?

ANSWER NINE

That depends on the political outlook of the government in power. An *entirely* non-interventionist government (surely a contradiction in terms) will not consider itself to have *any* health promoting role. More realistically, however, the health promoting role of the state – at least on the **foundations theory** – will be extensive. It is the state, primarily, which must lay foundations for achievement. It may wish to employ health promoters to *enforce* these foundations, to maintain them, or only to patch them up – but it is the state that is ultimately responsible for health promotion in most societies. Individual health promoters must do what they can where they can.

QUESTION TEN

What can health promoters forced into untheoretical practices do at the moment?

ANSWER TEN

Intellectually:

1. work out where they stand and why
2. work out how to defend this stance
3. thoroughly work out what this stance must imply in practice

Practically:

4. protest
5. do what they are asked to do but always in a way which is as promotive of **foundational health** as possible
6. argue the case for **foundational health promotion**
7. become active in health promotion movements at large

In general, health promoters who wish to work according to an intelligent theory of purpose must fight to be recognised as *thoughtful* professionals. If they choose to be foundational health promoters then they will acknowledge their preferences openly and will work according to a theoretical structure designed to limit any damage to others which their preferences might cause, and will be explicitly seeking to promote situations in which the preferences of their subjects can flourish. Because of this, in everything they do foundational health promoters will challenge untheoretical practice. The foundational health promoter can defend her decisions by appeal to both evidence and (ultimately) to political philosophy. If she does so consistently, and for long enough, she shall become part of a maturing discipline – one which can proudly and meaningfully say, 'our job is to promote health'.

QUESTION ELEVEN

How does foundational health promotion deal with the case of smoking we discussed earlier (see Chapter Three)? How does the foundational health promoter decide whether to proceed with Plan A or B?

ANSWER ELEVEN

By using the foundations theory it is possible to say that people *should* be helped to quit smoking, and to offer a full justification for this assertion. And because the foundations ideas are based on substantial theory, it is also possible to say when people *should not* be asked to give up smoking (even though much health promotion work currently proceeds as if there are absolutes in human life, such situations are actually very rare). Furthermore, the foundations theory enables those who use it to consider what else their position commits them to, and to reflect carefully on which means are appropriate and which are not.

Most importantly, the foundations theory of health promotion serves to put smoking into perspective since it inevitably places 'the smoking problem' amongst a broader set of health concerns. As Sonja Hunt has said:

> There is something seriously wrong with a society in which homelessness, poverty and racism are tolerated, even seen as normal, while smoking is regarded with horror. Smoking may well be an obnoxious habit but it is not nearly as harmful as sleeping in the street or a crowded bed and breakfast, living in constant debt in a cold damp house, going daily in fear of insult or assault, or facing a future devoid of dignity and respect.[130]

The foundations theory of health explains that such foundational factors are not just a *cause* of illness but they are *part of* a person's state of health because they profoundly affect that person's life. Where these foundations are lacking – and where their lack is an obstacle to a person's fulfilling development – then there is a health problem (whether or not the person is ill in a medical sense). Certainly these are social and educational problems, but they are also – logically – health problems too.

Smoking is a health problem for an individual if it is undermining her platform for living, and if she sees it as a problem. Smoking is not a health problem if it is what she wants and it is not undermining her platform. Whether or not smoking is a health problem depends upon your point of view. If you think that smoking is *always* a problem and is therefore necessarily a central concern for health promotion, then you are letting your prejudice run away with you.

Rational Field Health Promotion

It is not sufficient to know that prejudice pervades health promotion. In order to be a comprehensively honest health promoter you need:

  i. to make your prejudices explicit

and

  ii. openly to design practical strategies based on these prejudices, the evidence and your preferred theory of health (ideally, the foundations theory of health).

RATIONAL FIELDS

The foundations theory was explained in Chapters Seven and Eight, and its use in policy-making briefly explored in Chapter Nine. However, despite this theoretical detail and worked application, practising health promoters sometimes experience a distance between theory and practice. This new chapter, and the dialogue which follows it, show how rational field health promotion can bridge this gap.

Although much work needs to be done to refine it, rational field theory points the way ahead for reflective, mature health promotion. Once conventional health promoters accept the obvious truth that their form of health promotion is as prejudiced as any other, they can use rational field theory (and the rational field template) to make their planning fully explicit both to themselves and the intended targets of their work.

WHAT IS A RATIONAL FIELD?

(Note: the following explanation of rational fields is an edited extract from *Total Health Promotion: Mental Health, Rational Fields and the Quest for Autonomy.*[131])

All rational fields have the same basic structure.[132–135] They are formed by any kind of problem-solving behaviour, and can therefore be any size from minuscule to

Health Promotion, Second Edition: David Seedhouse
© 2004 John Wiley & Sons, Ltd: ISBNs 0 470 84732 8 (HB); 0 470 84733 6 (PB)

enormous. A rational field is initially created either by an instinct or a value-judgement or both. These instincts or judgements generate goals and sub-goals, strategies and sub-strategies, each of which maintain the rational field.

NATURAL AND MANUFACTURED RATIONAL FIELDS

NATURAL RATIONAL FIELDS

As a matter of fact the living world is composed of innumerable rational fields. A plant is a rational field, striving to grow and to propagate. A bacterium is a rational field, a cell in a body is a rational field, a gene is a rational field, organs in the human body are rational fields, a developing person is a rational field: anything that is instinctively purposive is a natural rational field. All the above examples have goals and sub-goals, strategies and sub-strategies, each of which maintain the rational field. If new problems emerge, each rational field may expand or adapt in order to try to deal with them. For example, in ideal circumstances a plant will grow and produce many seeds. If there is a drought, or if the plant is attacked by insects, or if there is excessive wind, then if it can it will adapt its goals and strategies accordingly (perhaps it will make only one fruit instead of many, or perhaps it will produce special chemicals to repel further insect attack, or perhaps it will grow extra roots as an anchor). The same is true of any natural, goal-directed system.[136]

This just is the way the world is.

A similar observation was made by Arthur Koestler, who believed that:

> A living organism is not an aggregation of elementary parts, and its activities cannot be reduced to elementary 'atoms of behaviour' forming a chain of conditioned responses. In its bodily aspects, the organism is a whole consisting of 'sub-wholes', such as the circulatory system, digestive system, etc., which in turn branch into sub-wholes of a lower order, such as organs and tissues...each member of this hierarchy, on whatever level, is a sub-whole or '*holon*' in its own right – a stable, integrated structure, equipped with self-regulatory devices and enjoying a considerable degree of *autonomy* or self-government. Cells, muscles, nerves, organs, all have their intrinsic rhythms and patterns of activity, often manifested spontaneously without external stimulation; they are subordinated as *parts* to the higher centres of the hierarchy, but at the same time function as quasi-autonomous *wholes*...[137]

Koestler gave examples of the autonomy of the *holons*: the human heart has several independent pacemakers, a strip of tissue taken from the heart of a chicken embryo and put in nutrient solution will go on pulsating for years, and transplant surgery clearly shows that individual organs can be 'quasi-independent'. Koestler also speculated that:

> Science is only just beginning to rid itself of the mechanistic preconceptions of the nineteenth century – the world as a billiard table of colliding atoms – and to realise that hierarchical organisation is a fundamental principle of living nature...[137]

Natural rational fields are in keeping with Koestler's idea. None are wholly independent – because of the world's interconnectedness – but any rational field must have at least one distinct purpose and strategy by which to pursue it. A rational field does not have to be seen as part of a hierarchy, and rational fields are often disharmonious, both within themselves and with other rational fields. Nonetheless, rational fields and *holons* appear to have much in common.

The Rational Field Template

CLASSIFICATIONS

VALUES

Goal X

Goal Y

Goal Z

STRATEGIES

MEANS

INSTINCTS

Figure 41   The Basic Rational Field Template

MANUFACTURED RATIONAL FIELDS

Manufactured rational fields are different from natural ones. They are also goal-directed (they must be to be rational fields), but they tend to be more erratic and unstable than natural rational fields, since they are formed by human assumptions and decisions made beyond-the-evidence. Manufactured rational fields are formed and sustained by *our* classifications of reality, *our* values, and *our* instincts (see Fig. 41 above). And it is these that are of greatest relevance to health promotion.

Manufactured rational fields can be as small as a plan to read a book with a glass of wine this evening, and as big as it is possible for any human institution to be. Conventional health services are manufactured rational fields, Microsoft is a manufactured rational field, Microsoft's marketing department is a manufactured rational field, and so is psychiatry, nursing, a badminton club, the law – every system designed by humans to achieve a purpose is a manufactured rational field.

Once we can properly recognise manufactured rational fields for what they are we can take control over them. Once we know what we are dealing with we do not have to fall into rational fields that suit other people more than they suit us, and we do not have to follow particular goal-directed paths in the false belief that these paths are all there is.

AN EXAMPLE OF A SIMPLE MANUFACTURED RATIONAL FIELD

A traveller unexpectedly lost in a foreign city, unable to speak or read the native language, must define a goal and devise ways to achieve it if she wants to regain her bearings. She might think: I don't want to be lost (a combination of value judgement and instinct which defines the field's perimeter), if I find the central railway station I will probably find a map (two related goals), if I draw a picture of a train with a question mark and show it around I may get directions to the station (two related strategies), first I need to find some paper (sub-goal)... and so on. By doing these things she creates a small rational field. As she formulates and tries strategies to achieve her goal the field expands. As soon as she is successful, the rational field dissipates.

Fig. 42 is obvious and elementary, but it nonetheless describes the components and structures common to all rational fields, however simple or complex.

AN EXAMPLE OF A MORE COMPLEX MANUFACTURED RATIONAL FIELD

Large organisations such as hospitals and commercial companies create and perpetuate vast and complex rational fields. Just like the traveller's field, these larger fields are initially created by classifications and value-judgements or instincts (we must treat disease, we must improve our brand recognition) which generate further goals and sub-goals, strategies and sub-strategies, each of which contributes to the rational field's evolution.

To describe the relationships between the goals, strategies and means of an organisation the size of BP, for example, would be a virtually impossible task – even

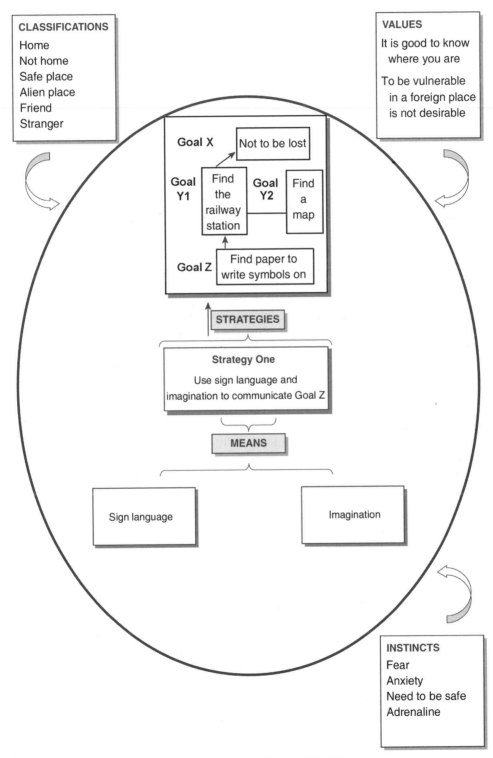

Figure 42 Simple illustration of the use of the basic Rational Field Template

the most determinedly extensive depiction of BP's rational field would be an oversimplification. Fortunately, however, the exact details do not matter for present purposes. They can be calculated as necessary for any particular total health promotion project – rather it is the basic structure and formation of rational fields that needs to be understood. If you know this then you can assess any manufactured rational field for coherence and value, and you can knowingly manufacture a rational field according to your own classifications and values.

Microsoft's **manufactured** rational field response to the surprise emergence of revolutionary software from a rival company might (again very crudely) be illustrated as in Fig. 43.

THE MAIN POINTS

At this stage, the main points to note about rational field theory are:

1. That even so simply expressed, the rational field template is useful because it enables decision-makers to state their most important goals, to check crudely whether these goals are compatible with each other, to define and lay out different strategies, to see how these impact on the goals (some may fit with one goal but not another, for example), to state the primary means for achieving any goals, and to assess whether the means, strategies and goals are coherent and efficient.
2. Even more important, the use of the rational field template makes it plain that a rational field is formed from beyond-the-evidence.[131] In addition to a simple internal field made up of means, strategies and goals, the rational field template shows three boxes – one for *instincts*, one for *classifications* and one for *values*. Instincts, classifications and values shape rational fields – they form their walls. Usually, in our social affairs, we tend not to notice or we play down these elements. But they are crucial for the rational field template. Only by stating and understanding them can we properly understand and judge between our rational fields.

Filling in the instinct, value and classification boxes can be an uncomfortable process; particularly for people who have never before conceived that their world is an option rather than a necessary reality. To have these very basic human judgements forced into the open can feel like a home invasion (which it is, in a way). But it is necessary if we are to be able to explore our thinking and policies open-mindedly.

Considerable personal judgement is required to complete the rational field template, and it may therefore be that some people fill in the values, classification and instincts boxes only sparsely, if at all. This, however, is a form of denial which must be overcome if total health promotion[131] is to succeed. There very obviously must be some values, instincts and choices in play, or else there could be no manufactured rational fields. In order to use the rational field template correctly health promoters must be honest about their biases (it can help to get other people – preferably people with different values and a different way of seeing the world – to assist in filling in the template. This way the health promoter can begin to decide whether she has been as fulsome as she might have been in listing the formative elements of her rational field).

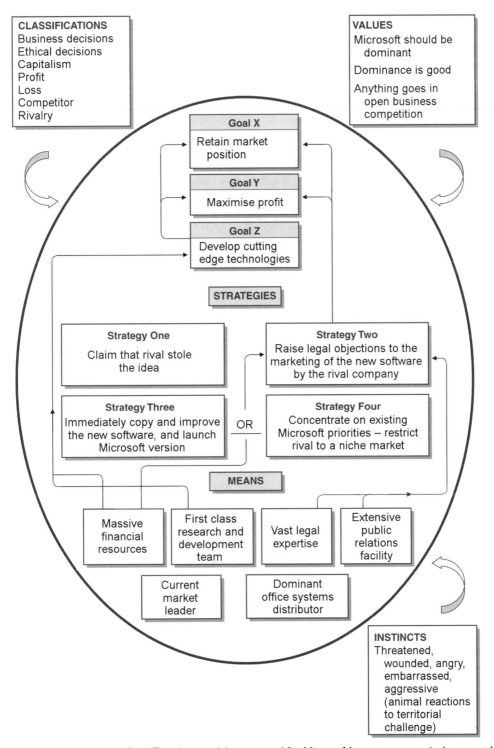

CLASSIFICATIONS
Business decisions
Ethical decisions
Capitalism
Profit
Loss
Competitor
Rivalry

VALUES
Microsoft should be
dominant
Dominance is good
Anything goes in
open business
competition

Goal X
Retain market
position

Goal Y
Maximise profit

Goal Z
Develop cutting
edge technologies

STRATEGIES

Strategy One
Claim that rival stole
the idea

Strategy Two
Raise legal objections to the
marketing of the new software
by the rival company

Strategy Three
Immediately copy and improve
the new software, and launch
Microsoft version

OR

Strategy Four
Concentrate on existing
Microsoft priorities – restrict
rival to a niche market

MEANS

Massive
financial
resources

First class
research and
development
team

Vast legal
expertise

Extensive
public
relations
facility

Current
market
leader

Dominant
office systems
distributor

INSTINCTS
Threatened,
wounded, angry,
embarrassed,
aggressive
(animal reactions
to territorial
challenge)

Figure 43 The Rational Field Template crudely expressed for Microsoft's response to a rival company's revolutionary software (this is a manufactured rational field)

THE RATIONAL FIELD TEMPLATE AND THE FLUORIDATION CASE STUDY

Recall the conflicting positions on fluoridation described in Chapter Nine:

> If you are of the view that health promotion is a:
>
>> ...descendant of the great old regulatory public health measures which have had such an impact on the population's health over the last century[6]
>
> and if you believe that it is fundamental to the functioning of a stable society that well-established institutions should be supported and maintained (even if these are plainly unjust when seen from alternative points of view), then it is highly unlikely you will even think to challenge conventional, established wisdom. Indeed, you will simply take for granted that:
>
>> ...[f]luoridation of water supplies [can] prevent dental caries (and possibly also osteoporosis)[6]
>
> and mention this casually, without reporting any counter-evidence or difference of opinion. Equally, if you are of the view that capitalist systems encourage the exploitation of citizens by other citizens in the interests of private profit, then you are likely to be suspicious of fluoridation – at the very least because someone will certainly be profiting from the process, and because most people will have no say in the matter. If you are of this persuasion then you may even arrive at the conclusion that:
>
>> ...the fertilizer and aluminium industries promoted fluoridation initially because they were finding it very difficult to dispose of this toxic by-product. Research money from them and the sugar industry ensured the answers they wanted.[129]

Assuming that these are accurate accounts of two ways of thinking about fluoridation, they might be converted into potentially informative rational field templates like Figs 44 and 45.

The following template (Fig. 46) incorporates the basic elements of the foundations theory of health (which constitute the MEANS in Fig. 47).

Of course, each of these templates is a gross simplification of reality, and offers at least a partial guess about the field-forming classifications, values and instincts. Nevertheless, the unquestionable value of rational fields for health promotion is that they make decision-making honest. Once the basic templates for each possible rational field have been initially spelt out (as in the four following figures) it is up to their proponents to correct them. So, for example, if 'it is good to act in people's best interest' is not a field-forming value for the pro-fluoridation camp, the fluoridation advocate can erase it. But then the question becomes: what really *are* the field-forming values? There must be some values, clarifications and instincts in play since (as this book shows) health promotion does not spring from thin and neutral air – all health promotion is prejudiced and is therefore created out of a combination of human classification, instinct and value. The key question is 'which?'

HOW TO USE RATIONAL FIELDS TO PROMOTE HEALTH

The final dialogue – Dialogue Seven – demonstrates an extended example of rational field health promotion, devised by Diane Grant's and James Campion's *Rational Field Health Promotion Ltd*. The benefit of seeing the world as an indefinite set of rational fields is made plain, as is the practical (and ethical) advantage of placing the foundations platform within an explicit rational field.

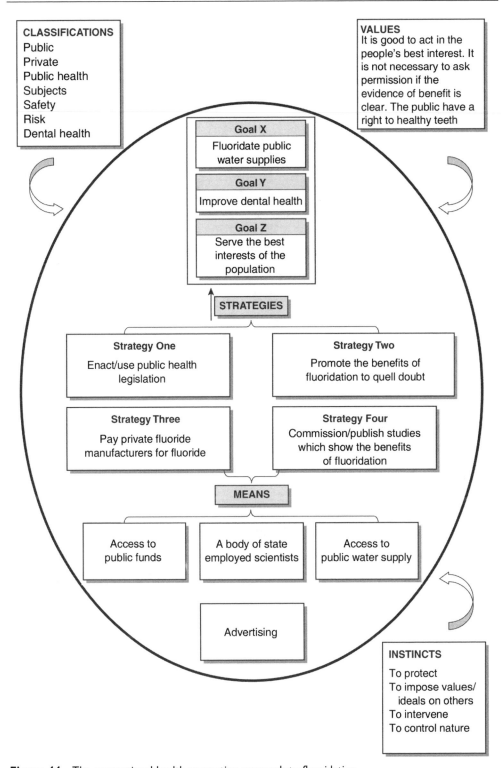

Figure 44   The conventional health promotion approach to fluoridation

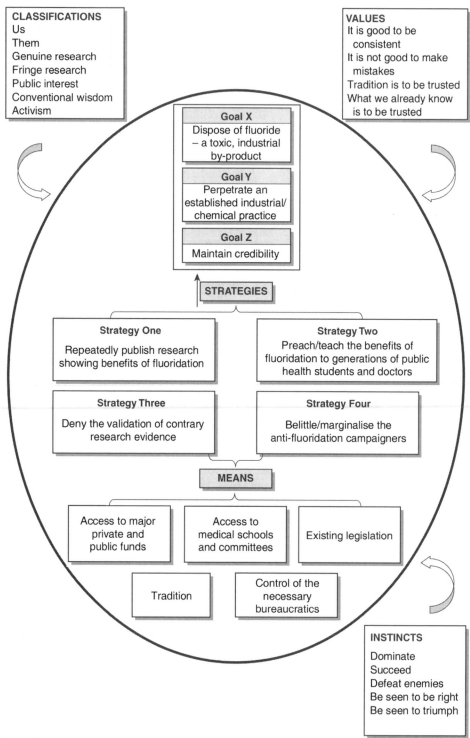

Figure 45 A possible approach to the fluoridation debate created by an anti-fluoridation campaigner, meant provocatively to represent the reality of the pro-fluoridation position

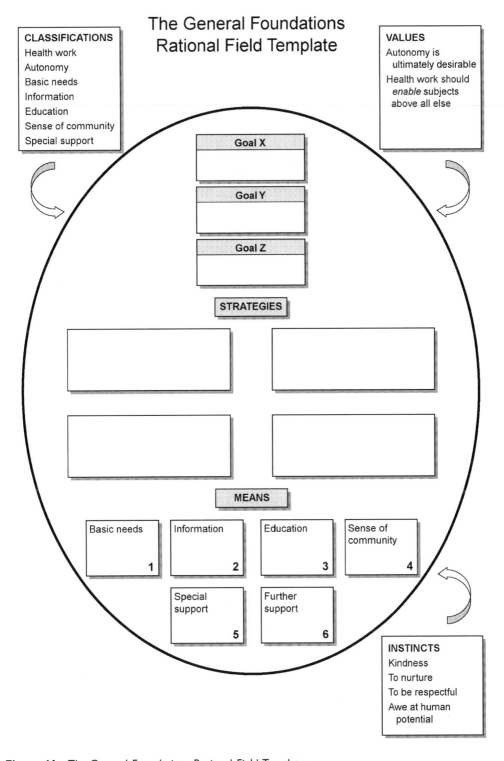

Figure 46 The General Foundations Rational Field Template

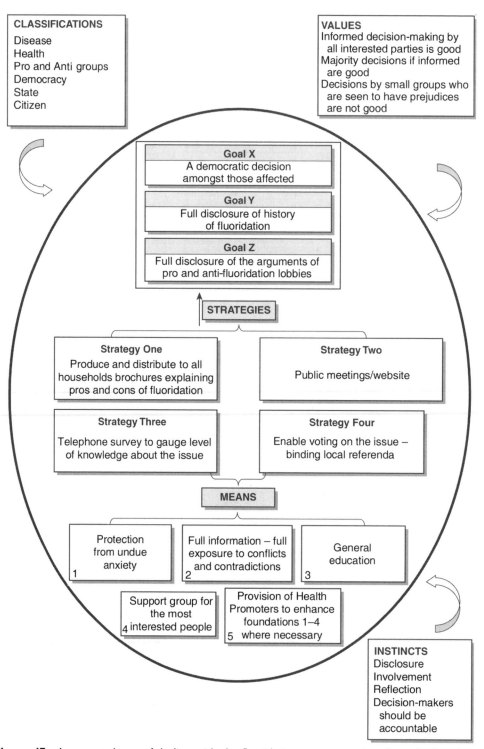

Figure 47 A suggested way of dealing with the fluoridation controversy based on the foundations theory of health

EXERCISE ELEVEN

USING THE RATIONAL FIELD TEMPLATE

ONE

1. Take a blank rational field template.
2. Consider any health promotion activity you have undertaken or read about.
3. As best you can, fill in the template. Begin with the goals, strategies and means within the elipse.
4. As honestly as you can, fill in the classifications, values and instincts boxes.
5. Show your completed rational field template to a colleague.
6. Ask her if she agrees that this is an accurate picture of your health promotion activity.

TWO

1. Take a blank general foundations rational field template.
2. Reconsider the health promotion activity bearing in mind the foundational platform which now makes up the means.
3. As best you can, fill in the new template.
4. As honestly as you can, fill in the classifications, values and instincts boxes.
5. Show your completed rational field template to a colleague.
6. Ask her if she agrees that this is an accurate picture of your health promotion activity.
7. Are your two templates the same? If not, why not?

Teaching notes for: Using the Rational Field Template

This is a very difficult exercise to do. It demands imagination (to complete the boxes, especially the field-forming ones), it demands honesty about one's feelings as a health promoter engaged in working to promote other people's health, and it demands disclosure and openness about a subject that is commonly assumed not to need it (the conventional thinking is that if health is objectively good its pursuit is obviously good, and consequently does not require this honesty and disclosure).

Students may react in many different ways, including being unable to or refusing to complete the templates' boxes. However, assuming your students are willing and able to take a stab at developing templates for discussion, your most likely role will be to suggest simple goals and strategies and then – possibly in group discussion – to help students tease out their prejudices. Since this will very probably be a considerable challenge you ought to demonstrate to the group that it is just impossible to formulate *any* problem-solving strategy without instincts, classifications and values (Fig. 42 – which shows the lost travellers' rational field – is as good an illustration as any of necessary prejudice).

Time to Face the Music

James and Diane are moving slowly along a frost-covered path beside a lake, steel grey despite the sharp blue sky. Ice is forming along the lake fringe. The hum of Saturday morning traffic, headed for Willesville's pre-Christmas free-for-all, is a distant though unnoticed background. Otherwise there is nothing other than the crunch of their boots, and their earnest conversation.

JAMES: Don't you think you should reconsider? I mean, is this really something you should resign for?

DIANE: Yes. It is. And it's done now in any event. Rutherford wouldn't have me back even if I begged him.

JAMES: Are you sure? You're a good writer and you've got guts. I'm sure he rates you very highly really.

DIANE: I doubt it. He dislikes me I think. I'm much better than him, his career's almost over, he feels threatened by my energy – come on – he's well rid of me isn't he? And what about my pride? He completely overrode everything I'd written and included some incredibly dumb stuff under my name, and he couldn't see what I was complaining of. Where would it end?

JAMES: Yes, I'm sure you are right about making some stand. But...don't you think you might be overreacting to the suicide? Tell me I don't know what I'm talking about but isn't it possible you are blaming yourself – and the *Chronicle* – for Andrew Wilson's death?

DIANE: Yes.

JAMES: But his death had nothing whatsoever to do with any of you. It was quite beyond your control. It was beyond anyone's control, except maybe Wilson's himself.

Think about it coldly. Get it clear. (*Looking up*) It should be easy on a day like this. You wanted to turn your daily work into something to get you noticed, and to get you away from the *Chronicle* – to a *better* job. You had a good go and got yourself to a level of understanding about health promotion that most health promoters – and I'd include myself – don't often have. Now you've got some good stuff ready for a quality paper, or perhaps for specialist magazines and journals, and this is going to help you make a name as a serious journalist. During the process you happened to meet Andrew Wilson.

Health Promotion, Second Edition: David Seedhouse
© 2004 John Wiley & Sons, Ltd: ISBNs 0 470 84732 8 (HB); 0 470 84733 6 (PB)

Inadvertently he helped you understand more about health promotion, especially its ethics. I think you're grateful to him for that. You wish you could've helped him in return. And you feel guilty for not noticing how fragile he was. You think Rutherford insulted him by running that pathetic piece on health promotion. You can't help Andrew now but you feel you must do something. So you have to make a protest at the *Chronicle*. Now, I ask you, does this really make sense?

DIANE: You could be right. Maybe I am doing too much reacting and not enough thinking. I don't know. But even if you *are* right I still think it is worth resigning.

JAMES: But there's no connection. What are you resigning for?

DIANE: There is a connection. I don't want to work for a newspaper that trivialises people's lives. Andrew – what he said and what he did – has made me realise – or made me remember – the complexity of people and the range of options we have if we are strong enough...I know what you're thinking. I'm not romanticising Andrew Wilson. It was a brief encounter and he didn't deliberately make me think. But now I have thought I think he was brave.

JAMES: You think suicide is a brave thing to do?

DIANE: Yes.

JAMES: I think it is cowardly, weak and selfish. How much better for you, for instance, if he had just taken a labouring job instead. How much better for other people too if he'd stayed alive – especially if he was as interesting as you say he was.

DIANE: I think it was brave because he could easily have continued. He could have found a niche here and he could have put up with it after a fashion. But that would have been an absolute failure for him, so he said 'no' in the only way he had open to him.

JAMES: Nonsense. There were hundreds of other options he could have taken. He took the easy way out.

DIANE: I don't think so. I don't think there was any choice other than what he saw as futile and leaving it all. And I think it takes courage to throw yourself off a cliff...We'll never agree, will we? But one thing I have learnt is that just because we disagree it doesn't mean that one of us must be wrong.

JAMES: Explain please.

DIANE: Through thinking about health promotion – and the Outsider problem – I've come to realise that what seems to be obviously factual is actually first a matter of opinion. This means that if I think that smoking is *good* for someone I am not automatically wrong – if I've thought about it and I have an alternative account of health then there is not a right account and a wrong one – there are two accounts. And it is just the same with suicide.

JAMES: In that case how can we ever decide anything?

DIANE: In all sorts of ways so long as we both have *thoughtful* accounts of health or suicide. If we have then we'll be able to talk about justifications – I could say when I think suicide is worthy and when I think it isn't and we could also talk of contexts and consequences and the like.

JAMES: And could we also talk about the role of health promotion in all this?

DIANE: Of course.

JAMES: Then please tell me what you think health promotion should have done for Andrew.

DIANE: It depends what sort of health promotion we're talking about.

JAMES: But isn't this where we came in? You're saying it depends what model I adopt.

DIANE: That's the last thing I'm saying. I've been persuaded by my philosopher friend that health promotion models are superficial as far as health promotion purpose is concerned, which is why I can only say what *one* sort of health promotion would have done for Andrew Wilson – I don't know enough about the other sorts.

JAMES: Surely you're wrong. Surely we can say a lot about several alternative approaches: all those different models the textbooks go on about.

DIANE: Not really. You'll very quickly hit a dead end if you try. Of course you'll be able to talk about all sorts of methods and techniques that might have been applied to save Andrew, but all the important questions: What is the ultimate goal for health promotion here? Is it enough just to rescue Andrew, or must we also try to shape his life? Which life goals are to be preferred? Why is one aim more moral than another? When should you stop promoting Andrew's health? All these you'll find hanging in the air.

JAMES: Really?

DIANE: Really. Take the good life form of health promotion for instance. It utterly fails to address the Outsider problem. All it does is insist that a moderate way of living is right and an immoderate one is wrong, without ever seriously considering that 'moderate' and 'immoderate' might be relative terms – and without ever attempting to explain why a moderate life is *objectively* best.

JAMES: But if Andrew had lived moderately I don't suppose he would have killed himself.

DIANE: How can you say that? A moderate life wouldn't have been Andrew Wilson's life and Andrew Wilson's life was valuable – to his mother, to his friends, to his lovers, to me. And surely you of all people know that people who live moderate lives kill themselves too, and often just because their lives *are* so humdrum.

JAMES: Yes, I suppose I'm still trying to come to terms with your friend's foundation theory of health – it seems to undermine so much that I'd taken for granted, yet I also agree with much of it. It is very unsettling.

DIANE: I know. I think that is because it is honest. Other health promotion approaches seem to stop when they reach uncomfortable questions. 'Why is *this* the good life?' It just *is*, says good life promotion. 'If health inequalities are unjust why aren't all inequalities unjust, including genetic inequalities, inequalities caused by extra effort, and inequalities created by special talent? Why aren't these unjust too?' 'Why is equity in health more vital than equity in income?' Social health promotion just stops here. It basically refuses to answer and just gets on with trying to close the morbidity gap – hopelessly, I reckon, until it sorts out the other questions. And these other questions really do need to be answered if social health promoters are to have proper theories about what they advocate.

And, the way I see it, medical health promotion just looks silly when I think of Andrew Wilson.

JAMES: Look. Come on. He was probably thoroughly drunk when he jumped. And if he'd not been he'd probably still be alive now. Alcoholism can cause depressive disorders, a solitary life drinking, smoking, gambling is a miserable life. If a medical health promoter could have got to grips with Wilson we could have been looking at a reformed character in a few months. You're completely off-beam here Diane. Aren't you?

DIANE: I'm not you know. Medical health promotion looks silly with Andrew. It looks silly with anyone who believes life is a rich and dicey thing – because it thinks that all that matters is the evidence. And that idea is so naïve it is ridiculous. Medical health promotion tells people that it is a fact that smoking is bad, that exercise is good, that too much rich food is bad as if the figures produced by science and epidemiology are somehow finally conclusive. But this ignores everything that makes human life important – what people value, what people choose, how people reason and make trade-offs. What is silliest about medical health promotion is that it seems to think that the evidence makes ethics redundant – that the evidence that drinking is bad in certain ways implies that it is morally correct that all sorts of efforts be made to stop it. But – just thinking of Andrew – whether to tell him to cut down, how to tell him to cut down, when, and where – these are all ethically complex matters which require full reasoning and defence – not just morbidity statistics. If it is conceivable that a hedonistic life is worth living then it is *inconceivable* that medical health promotion is objectively correct. And that isn't to say that medical health promotion is utterly misguided and can do no good. Not at all. But it does need to become much more thoughtful to do as much good as it could.

JAMES: I can see you're a real convert. You think foundational health promotion is clearly the best, don't you? (*Diane nods*) But how can you say that? If everything is so ethically complicated, how can you be so sure about the foundations theory?

DIANE: I'm not sure about it, though I admit it appeals to my politics – and I admit that it is the only form of health promotion that explains itself in a way I can make sense of.

JAMES: It suits your prejudices.

DIANE: Of course. And because of that I obviously can't say that it is *objectively* the best theory. That would be silly too, and a misconception, because health promotion is not something that can ever be spoken of entirely objectively. Health promotion takes place where human values exist and conflict, and so any form must be judged on its moral merits as well as on its practical effectiveness. What is good, for me, about foundational health promotion is that it can make use of all sorts of practical techniques to improve people's lives but as it does so it says 'this is an openly prejudiced approach – you can reject it' *and* it tries to get people into positions in their lives where it *is* open to them to reject health promotion if they want. Foundational health promotion is ethically thoughtful health promotion.

JAMES: But that means, in Wilson's case, that it is useless, despite all its theorising, doesn't it? If Andrew Wilson tells the health promoter to sod off then the health promoter must sod off, isn't that right? What on earth can a foundational health promoter do for the likes of Andrew Wilson?

DIANE: A great deal actually. Though you are right that if Andrew – if anyone who is even temporarily an Outsider – is informed and competent then – *in the name of work for health* (and that's a very important qualification) you have to leave him alone even if you feel that what he is doing to himself is abhorrent. But that's not the whole story by any means – a great deal hangs on how the health promoter conceives of her work.

I've thought about this a lot...

JAMES: I can see that. And you've arrived at your views so quickly. You are wasted at the *Chronicle*. Maybe you could go into health promotion yourself. You'd certainly ruffle a few feathers, but with your intellect, and your communication skills...it could be you Diane.

DIANE: That's nice of you, but I think I'm too much of an Outsider myself. I think I'll see if I can make a go of freelance. I might get an ulcer or two but it is hardly ever boring if you get the right contacts...(*startled by their footsteps, a family of geese make an agitated escape from the nearby reeds*).

JAMES: Good luck then, but if you want any help you know...

DIANE: Yes, I know. Thanks. But don't you want to know how I think foundational health promotion could work for Outsiders?

JAMES: Of course I do. Though I think I know what you'll say. I like the foundations theory too, but it is too broad – and too political – for me to be able to espouse it in my official work. I know I'm in a Magpie Profession but I'm not strong enough to make a stand. It'll be 'mix 'n match Campion' until I retire I'm afraid, though I still think I will do some good along the way.

DIANE: You'd do a lot more if you'd be consistent and if you'd openly *tell* people that you are a theoretically informed foundational health promoter. How is the Magpie Profession to become a Reflective Profession unless people like you – insiders – work to improve it?

JAMES: But I'll be accused of being a woolly intellectual, or of being a lefty, or of becoming senile, of rocking the boat, of not being committed to founding principles, or of forgetting my responsibilities...

DIANE: Of course. But you'll know that what you are doing will be worth all that nonsense. You'll be helping to forge a real profession.

JAMES: Well...I don't know...tell me how a foundational health promoter could do something for Andrew Wilson.

DIANE: Gladly. As I say, it all depends on how the health promoter conceives of what she is doing. And I think it helps very much if, before she begins to do anything practical, she asks herself some clear questions. I've come up with a list...it's nothing much, and totally cribbed from my friend's work, but it's meant as a small contribution from me...here (*she takes a sheet of paper from her bag and hands it to James*).

JAMES: (*Reading*)

OPENING QUESTIONS FOR FOUNDATIONAL HEALTH PROMOTERS

Where you have a practical idea in mind, ask yourself 'what is my *priority*?' and 'what is my *authority*?' Choose either Y or Z:

> Y. I will be working *first* to provide or improve foundations for everyone.
> Z. I will be working *first* to provide or improve foundations for a group or an individual.

Then choose either 1 or 2:

> 1. My intervention has been requested by an informed potential recipient, or recipients.
> 2. My intervention is to be done in what I regard to be the interests of one or more other people, even though they have not requested it.

> Finally, list as many likely *harms* and *benefits* as possible and note that this list is based first on your values – not on evidence *per se*, but on evidence as you have interpreted it.

This will give you an initial understanding of the size and social importance of what you propose to do. You will also have a basic hold of the ethics of the task ahead. That is, you must have selected one of:

> Y 1
> Y 2
> Z 1
> Z 2

It is possible to select any of these combinations without a practical idea in mind. That is, you may also decide, *in principle*, if you wish to work broadly; should I work first to provide or improve foundations for everyone – Y? or should I practise more narrowly – Z?

That's very clear Diane, as usual. But it's hardly comprehensive is it? It leaves all sorts of questions unanswered.

DIANE: I prefer to think it *opens up* all sorts of questions. If you begin by asking these questions *I don't think you'll be able to stop*, and that's the way forward for health promotion.

JAMES: I can see that. It obviously makes a big difference which combination you choose.

DIANE: Exactly, and that's why foundational health promotion can do either a lot or nothing for people – depending on the answer and depending on the situation.

They reach a bar fence and cross-bar gate. They climb the stile at the side. James almost slips on the icy surface, but recovers. They head away, through petrified meadow grass, toward the sounds of town and the familiar smell of petroleum.

JAMES: We'll be back in a minute, but could you just take me through your checklist with Wilson in mind. Would you? If it makes sense maybe I *could* become a pioneer.

DIANE: (*Smiles*) I know you could. But it isn't a checklist James. It's just an intelligent start.

JAMES: Of course. I've got to be very careful what I say when I'm with you.

DIANE: Naturally! (*She laughs*) Anyway, take the combinations in order. Let's say you haven't decided exactly *what* to do yet but you think Y1 is the best starting point for your work. If so you will be aiming *first* to provide or improve foundations for everyone and your help will have been asked for in some way by those who are to receive it.

This, because it is work for everyone, and because a foundational health promoter will be likely to offer *generally* enabling conditions, should not create an Outsider problem (though it might if the majority view is to have you close down some opportunity enjoyed by the Outsider – in the interest of health). Perhaps there has been a local election, or a referendum, and most people want to see more 'speed bumps' – devices to slow cars down – in all built-up areas. This is thought to be a health promoting task, you see it as part of the foundations – probably Box 1 – and so you go ahead. This will be helpful to most people if it reduces accidents – and should not impede the Outsider – even the risk-taker – since there will still be an endless list of risks he can take if he wants to.

JAMES: Yes, but . . .

DIANE: James, it is a *summary* of an opening strategy . . . that's all. When further practical complexities and philosophical controversies arise they too have to be solved, and can only be solved by having a theory . . . but you'd need to ask the philosopher about that . . . (*James says nothing*).

OK. Y2. You want to promote foundations for everyone but they haven't specifically requested your help.

JAMES: That's mostly what health promotion is like anyway. The public don't ask us to inform them about the dangers of smoking and unprotected sex. We do it because we think they need to know.

DIANE: Yes. But you only *know* what's needed and what isn't, and when to start and stop promoting those ideas and information, if you have a background theory to help you. And if you don't things can get out of hand – as they have done in the past (you know, all that controversy over funding for HIV education, about the realism of the anti-drug campaigns, about whether health promotion is cost-effective, and so on?). When Y2 is the combination health promotion is very definitely soaked with moral questions – and any health promoter who denies this is, in my opinion, a very stupid and dangerous person. Y2 always requires sustained and open defence – and it always should be open to revision. Y2 can very quickly damage Outsiders, and others too.

JAMES: Z1?

DIANE: That's usually easy – so long as you have good evidence to believe you can do some practical good and the potential recipient understands what she is asking for, and its implications. If Andrew had said 'yes, I am drinking too much, can you help?' or if he'd said 'I'm a bit worried about something...could I see you at work?' and mentioned suicidal thoughts then things would have been very different. I wouldn't have belittled him by handing him those leaflets for one thing.

Of course, if you choose Z1 that doesn't mean you can't do other things as well, i.e. Z2. For instance, you can offer other enabling information and if it is welcomed you can proceed further. But if it is not welcomed and you are asked to stop – or if it seems more damaging than it is worth (maybe the recipient becomes excessively worried about cancer and you'd rather avoid that becoming an obsession) then you should stop.

If you didn't stop, you'd then introduce a further category and combinations. You'd have to ask DO I HAVE AUTHORITY? Call it 3, 'My intervention is to be done in what I regard to be the interests of one or more other people, even though they tell me they don't want it.' This would give you the additional options Y3 and Z3.

You get the picture, don't you? Generally, if you are working with willing recipients you use the foundations to help you decide on agreed practical priorities. If you are working with uninformed recipients you use the foundations to help you meet the most broad needs, in the best way you can, but you know you are trying to enable both physical and mental fulfilment (and therefore, possibly, alternative prejudices) and so you draw a clear line. And if you are working with unwilling recipients you acknowledge this and restrict yourself only to those activities that allow them to continue to be free to be unwilling – you may offer them rich information rather than single-minded information, for instance. And where it gets more complicated then you need to think harder and apply the theory as you can – and so, eventually, develop the theory further.

I don't think my philosopher friend would approve of me, but perhaps it isn't too mischievous to suggest that good health promoters should be *ethical* health promoters. In fact I'd say this:

An **Ethical Health Promoter** should:

- have a theory of health

- have a clear definition of health (she should be able to state and defend the goals of health promotion)

- acknowledge that all health promotion begins with values – that all health promotion must be prejudiced

- be continually willing to reflect both on her priorities and her authority

- have an understanding of the limits of health promotion – be able to state the point at which health promotion becomes *not* justified (in her opinion)

- make explicit public declarations of the above.

JAMES: But for Andrew specifically?

DIANE: I can't be specific. I don't know enough about him. But if you are a broad Y type of health promoter then you will be looking to create social conditions – a social climate – in which people do not become so quickly desperate. You will be looking to create meaningful work, to create empathy, to minimise crises where you can – to do all those things implied by your belief in the importance of foundations 1–4. And if you are a more specific, type Z, health promoter then you'll be seeking out people like Andrew where you can, and you'll be doing what you can to provide a basis to allow them to live fulfilling lives on their terms, and to avoid obstacles – even to pre-empt them if you can. If you thought Andrew was at risk and you heard about the Adams' closure you would be working very quickly and very hard on foundation maintenance. And yes, there *could* come a point where you would stop. There could be a time when you would let him walk away – at least on the foundations theory of health promotion, though perhaps not. It all depends on the condition of his foundations.

JAMES: (*Turning to face her as they reach the street door to the health promotion office, on the outskirts of Willesville*) You have the answers to everything after a few weeks! (*Reddening*) I'm sorry. I know you don't. I'll be honest with you... after all that's what you think health promotion should be about isn't it?

DIANE: Yes. And journalism.

JAMES: (*Smiling*) You do still have a lot to learn about some things. (*Diane pushes her hands a little more deeply into her coat pockets*) Diane, I've truly enjoyed your time with us but it has not been easy for me. (*He breathes in deeply, then exhales a slow cloud into the frozen air, as he speaks*) You see you've made me feel a fool. I've been struggling with health promotion as a foreign language for years – and I more or less gave up trying to work it out – and then you and your friend come along and it all makes much more sense. And that... well, I resent that a bit. My job has become much harder now I've listened to you. And I don't know if I want that or if I'm capable of meeting the challenge. I'm afraid I'm too set in my ways – and my colleagues, you've seen how adamant they are. How can I show them that they are *all* prejudiced? The easy life is the one I had – the one where I balance it all up and hope that we do some good, or at least don't completely waste taxpayers' money. (*He pauses*)

But I don't think I can go back to that because now I know I would be a... charlatan. I thought before I was perhaps playing a game. I know now that I would be, so in a way I wish this – you – hadn't happened.

DIANE: Philosophy changes you. Once you open the door to it you're never the same again. And you're never a fool. Not if you are stirred by philosophy.

Why should you resent me? I haven't thought for you. You know you've come to your own conclusions, as we've worked and talked together. There's no going back for either of us. I see that as good. I see that as what life is for. It's for reflection, for development, and for application – for making a difference when you can. And you think so too.

JAMES: Part of me doesn't want to. Part of me says that life is about... fitting... about finding a comfortable place. But yes. I *do* think so. I think it must be the future for health promotion. I will do what I can.

Strategies for Health

SCENE ONE

Several months later.

A hospital ward. Surgical cases. Bandages. Beeps. Buttons. Groans.

A nurse is standing over an injured man. He is in traction. His head is heavily dressed and his left arm is wired and in plaster. He talks briefly with the nurse, who is holding a mobile 'phone. She nods and presses a couple of buttons. She listens for the ring, and then passes the phone to the man. Gingerly, he holds it against his right ear.

JAMES: *(Rasping, dry)* Diane, is that Diane Grant?

DIANE: *(Puzzled)* Yes, this is Diane Grant. Who's speaking please?

JAMES: It's me. James. James Campion.

DIANE: Oh, James. Good to hear from you. But you sound strange. What's wrong?

JAMES: *(Beginning to weep)*...God...I'm sorry...God Diane, it's good to hear you...I'm sorry to sound like this...I had an accident, a bad accident...a few weeks ago...I'm pretty messed up...

DIANE: Where are you?

JAMES: *(Trying hard to keep his emotions under control)* Diane, I'm sorry, I have no right to come out of the blue and blub to you. I'm so sorry. Give me a second, won't you...

DIANE: What happened?

JAMES: I was driving home one evening, just an ordinary day. I don't know where my mind was, not on the road I guess...Anyhow, out of nowhere, a car came across a T-junction as I was crossing. It smashed into the near-side of my car. Hard. Really hard. A write-off apparently. Then I woke up, but I'd missed some days, nearly two weeks, in a coma...

DIANE: What's wrong with you James? How bad is it?

JAMES: *(Forcing back his distress once more)* It's bad. Really bad. I can't walk. Very likely I'll never walk again. And my memory is affected. And my arm too. My left arm is smashed

Health Promotion, Second Edition: David Seedhouse
© 2004 John Wiley & Sons, Ltd: ISBNs 0 470 84732 8 (HB); 0 470 84733 6 (PB)

and numb. Maybe it will never work again either... Diane, I'm sorry I called you, it isn't your problem. It is just that I...I...(*he speaks in a rush*) I've been thinking of you and wondering how you are...

DIANE: So, James, shall I see you?

JAMES: Yes, yes please.

DIANE: Where are you?

JAMES: Morton Street General, Ward 12...

SCENE TWO

It is several weeks later. James is sitting up in his bed. His arm is still in plaster, but otherwise there are no longer any outward signs of his accident. Diane is seated by James' bedside. She is leaning forward. Her elbows are on the bed. James is looking away from her.

DIANE: Ok, there is no denying that it is bad.

JAMES: Bad? It's devastating. A few weeks ago I had everything ahead of me. 20 years or more left in work, promotions almost certainly, lots of friends, a house I could manage. A bit late maybe for a wife and kids but not THAT late at 45. And I could run, and ride...and ...and just get up when I wanted to and walk outside and smell a rose. I had everything and now I have nothing, I am ruined. I am broken. It isn't bad, it is the end.

Painfully James lays down, squeezing his eyes shut.

DIANE: James, you will get over it. You must do. Yes, your life has changed and yes there is no going back, but there is no going back for any of us, is there? Nothing stays the same and we just have to cope with that. We all have to move on and we all have to play with the cards we are dealt.

James is silent.

DIANE: And yes, you have a lousy hand just now. But you aren't totally bust like you think you are.

Further silence.

DIANE: (*Angrily*) What will you do then? Lie here forever?

JAMES: (*Opening his eyes, staring fiercely at her*) What's it to you?

DIANE: (*Gasps slightly*) I don't know what it is to me. You called me. I've been visiting you these past six weeks and to be honest I don't know why. I don't even know if I should have been. I don't seem to be helping you. In fact you seem to use me as a place to unload all your resentments. You used to be...I mean...I admired you. I thought you did an amazing job with your Health Promotion Unit. You were calm, in charge. You moved things on, despite all your reservations and your need to find answers to fundamental questions. You moved things on and you took others with you and you made a difference. I really did admire you. To me you seemed to be a thoroughly healthy man.

JAMES: And now? I'm hardly healthy now am I?

DIANE: No, you aren't healthy now.

JAMES: Correct. And all that philosophical bullshit you were so fond of to one side, the reason I'm not healthy is that I'm a cripple. I'll never walk again. I've lost feeling in my left arm. You know I cut it on a broken glass yesterday and I didn't notice until I saw my trouser leg covered in blood? Of course I'm not healthy. I'm permanently wounded.

DIANE: Yes, in some ways, you are permanently wounded. But in other ways don't you think you are only temporarily wounded?

JAMES: No. I'm permanently damaged. That's the reality, whatever spin you try to put on it. And you haven't seen this have you?

He pulls an envelope out from under the sheets and tosses it to her.

DIANE: What's this?

JAMES: My redundancy notice.

DIANE: What?

JAMES: Read it.

Diane carefully reads the letter.

DIANE: Can they do this?

JAMES: Presumably yes.

DIANE: But that's so unfair. Even if you can't walk you can still do your job, at least once you recover.

JAMES: Not if I'm a mental wreck too. That's the bit about 'continuing psychiatric morbidity'.

Diane re-reads the letter.

DIANE: But you're sick.

JAMES: They can't wait forever.

DIANE: The bastards. They are supposed to be a Department of Health for Christ sake.

JAMES: Ironic, isn't it?

DIANE: Will you fight it?

JAMES: No. Of course not. I'll do nothing. There's nothing I can do. I'm finished. I've had to put my house on the market. I'm getting fewer and fewer visits. It's like I'm vanishing from the world . . . There was this 50s movie – it was called *The Incredible Shrinking Man* I think, something like that. It was about a man who went through some radioactive fog and began to shrink. After a while he became so small he had to live in a doll's house, and then a matchbox. In the end he just disappeared. That's me. I feel like I'm in an unreal swirl, falling faster and faster into the plughole. One day soon . . . whoosh . . . I'll be gone Diane. And I hope it comes soon. I don't care any more.

James closes his eyes and turns his head away from Diane. She puts her hand on his shoulder. James pulls away.

Diane brushes a tear from her eye.

DIANE: James, it will get better. There is a future for you. I can help you make it a positive future if you'll let me. But I can't keep on being punished by you. The accident was nothing to do with me.

JAMES: (*Mumbling*) Wasn't it?

DIANE: What? What are you talking about?

JAMES: (*Still facing away*) Who do you think I was thinking about at the crossroads?

DIANE: What!? What? Oh. Oh, I see.

Silence.

DIANE: James, I deliberately didn't keep in touch with you. But not because I didn't want to deep down.

JAMES: Why then?

DIANE: You are much older than me. You're a mature man. I didn't want to mess up your stability, and I didn't want to make a fool of myself either.

JAMES: Damn, damn. And now it is worse than ever. Now you are here through pity, duty, all the wrong reasons.

DIANE: Perhaps you're right. I think perhaps I'll leave now James.

JAMES: No. Don't.

DIANE: Why not?

JAMES: Because I need you to help me. I don't have anyone else who isn't paid to help me, and I need voluntary help. That's obvious, isn't it? I don't want to vanish. I don't want to rot in some poky flat somewhere. I want to be back like I was ... but I know I can't be. Whatever happens I have no job, no poise, no assurance. My maturity is not as strong as you thought, is it? I've become a different person. I am a different person. I need you to help me accept this somehow.

James looks down for a moment.

Diane, if you will still visit me, I promise that what we just discussed will not be mentioned again. As the James I used to be maybe there was a chance that we could have got together somehow (*he holds up her hand to stop her interjecting*) but that possibility no longer exists.

DIANE: You are making several assumptions James. I'd like to discuss them with you one day, when you are feeling more settled. But right now I know you need support.

Let me just say this: I have not been here the last six weeks entirely out of pity. Pity doesn't last that long. I've been here because I like you – as you were and, believe it or not, as you are – and because you obviously need me. I hope I can support you as a friend. One day you may be able to do the same for me.

Now, please turn back to me. This is a crisis right now. But let's look at the future. Let's begin to look at all those things you CAN do, OK? ...

SCENE THREE

It is two years later.

A telephone rings in a well-presented foyer.

RECEPTIONIST: Good morning. Rational Field Health Promotion Ltd. How can I help you?

CALLER: I'd like to speak to a health promoter please.

RECEPTIONIST: May I ask what your call concerns?

CALLER: Well, there's a group of us who've got together recently. We think we've got a health issue – actually we think our health is at risk – but the Public Health Directorate won't have anything to do with us. They say it isn't a health issue.

RECEPTIONIST: What is your name?

CALLER: Eve Parsons.

RECEPTIONIST: One moment please, I'll put you through to Ms Grant, our community health specialist.

The receptionist transfers the call.

DIANE: Hello, Diane Grant speaking. How can I help you?

EVE: Hello, my name is Eve Parsons and I think my friends and I have a health issue.

DIANE: What sort of health issue?

EVE: Well, it is rather unconventional.

DIANE: That's fine. That's mostly what we deal with here.

EVE: Yes, I heard that. Look, can you briefly confirm what you actually do before I go into too many details? It is a rather sensitive issue.

DIANE: Certainly. I'll have our administrator send you some background information. Our website is www.rationalfields.com if you want to look it up immediately.

But in a nutshell our small company takes the view that while conventional health promotion can often produce desirable results, it is too limited in its scope, it can be coercive, and it tends not to help people who have needs not directly related to clinical outcomes. If you want help to quit smoking, or if you need advice and support to alter your eating patterns, or if you want a campaign aimed at reducing a certain type of disease, then conventional health promotion does that pretty well. However, if you want support to achieve your broader potentials, or if you think that conventional health systems are impeding rather than enabling you, or if...

EVE: That's it, that's it exactly.

DIANE: In what way?

EVE: We have been damaged by conventional health promotion.

DIANE: I see. Well, there are many ways that that can happen. How have you been damaged?

EVE: We are all children conceived by donor insemination, a service offered by the state health system. We are supposed to be 'health outcomes' — somebody actually told me that once – and yet we don't feel healthy. We feel incomplete. We feel we are items, traded products. We've been bought and sold.

DIANE: I see.

EVE: Do you? I doubt it. Most people can't see what the problem is, they say we're ungrateful.

DIANE: Of course. That's because they see your situation from within only one very limited rational field. Part of our job here is to reveal other rational fields. We show to anyone who'll open their eyes that there is much more to any situation than it seems. Then we use these rational fields to help create health promoting strategies for our clients.

EVE: What's a rational field?

DIANE: Good question. It's a bit complicated to explain over the 'phone. But, essentially, a rational field is a system that has at least one purpose.

A pause.

EVE: But you're describing any system, surely?

DIANE: Any live system, yes. But that's not a problem. That's just the way things are. The real problem is that rational fields are everywhere, and yet most of us can see only a very few of them. Our health promotion challenge is to reveal all relevant, hidden rational fields to our clients. And then we help them create their own rational field strategy to maximise their future health.

EVE: So do you think can you help us?

DIANE: I don't know enough about your case to be sure, but it sounds to me like your situation is well suited to rational field health promotion. Would you like to make an appointment to come and see my colleague and I? And would you also like to bring along some of your colleagues?

EVE: What will that cost us?

DIANE: The first hour of any consultation is free, with no obligation. After that our fee is $300 per hour, plus any expenses incurred and plus materials. Our minimum charge for groups is $1000. We make a point of accessing whatever state benefits are available to our clients. Sometimes our clients even end up better off. However, this is what you may have to pay. Is that acceptable to you?

EVE: (*Lightly*) That will be fine. Fortunately, many of our families are quite well off. And we're all pretty smart, so some of us have good jobs.

Can we set up a time to see you for an hour one day next week?

SCENE FOUR

Diane and James are sitting in a comfortable, carpeted meeting room. James is in a wheel-chair. They are both sipping coffee. There are sofas and easy chairs casually arranged about the room. In the corner there is a large electronic whiteboard, the surface of which has been wiped clean.

DIANE: I think this is going to be really interesting.

JAMES: (*Smiling*) I'm sure you're right.

DIANE: Of course I'm right. You know I'm always right don't you? (*She winks*)

JAMES: Yes, yes, what can I say?

DIANE: (*Suddenly serious*) You're okay now, aren't you? There've been a lot of changes over the last two or three years. Now it feels like you're back, but you're different too. I think you're in a very different place these days.

JAMES: Yes, it feels like that to me too. You know, when you first came to see me I was secure in a socially useful job for life, or at least I thought I was. Mind you, I wasn't absolutely clear *what* use it was, but I was sure it was valuable.

He pauses.

When I say 'thought', I know now that I didn't think very deeply. I didn't really know how to. I knew there was a problem somewhere – like hearing a foreign language and not being able to translate it, not even knowing if it is translatable, remember? But I just skipped over it and got on with mixing 'n matching.

DIANE: And now things are different.

JAMES: Yes, they are completely different and yet not different.

DIANE: Go on.

JAMES: I mean, I'm still a health promoter. I can still promote health in the ways I used to. We get people here who want to stop smoking, who reckon they drink too much, who want exercise plans, who need to diet in safe ways – I do all that stuff, and achieve some good results, sometimes the same level of result I would have done in my old job. But I go about my work differently. I think of it in different ways, and of course I get involved in doing some things I would never have dreamed of doing in the past.

DIANE: Do you think it's right to call what we do here 'health promotion'?

JAMES: Oh yes, certainly, much more so than before. Now we actually *know* what we are doing, don't we? I mean, we have clear reasons, a clear framework, ways of organising our priorities, ways of expressing problems differently. We have ways of helping people look for autonomy creating solutions that can begin and end without *ever* having to be fixed to disease issues.

DIANE: (*Smiling*) I like it when you talk like this. You've become an enthusiast. You've never been an enthusiast before.

JAMES: You're right, I have. I'm excited by what we do here. We're expanding the horizons of health promotion, and doing it meaningfully. We have David's theoretical insights and structures to base our work on, we have all sorts of practical methods we can take at will from mainstream health promotion, and we have a growing list of practical successes and satisfied clients. Sure I'm excited, who wouldn't be excited?

DIANE: You're about as healthy as you can get now, aren't you?

JAMES: Yes. I can't walk and I can only use one hand properly. I'm half the man I was and yet I am much more than I was. There is so much I can do now, and so much I want to do now.

There's a knock on the door. Diane gets up to open it. As she passes James she squeezes his shoulder.

DIANE: Come in. Come in. Hello, you must be Eve?

EVE: Yes, pleased to meet you Diane. This is Charles and this is Petra. They are both DI offspring too.

DIANE: Welcome to you all. Let me introduce you to my colleague, James Campion.

They all shake hands. Eve, Charles and Petra make themselves comfortable. Eve sits in an armchair while Charles and Petra share a sofa.

JAMES: We're pleased you came to us. We consider that we may be able to help you. In this first session we hope you will be able to tell us the nature of your problem. We will then ask you some questions and feed back our first impressions to you. If you think these make sense we can arrange further sessions. In the end we will present you with a rational field strategy we consider best suited to the promotion of your health. Does that sound acceptable to you?

EVE: Yes.

Charles and Petra nod.

DIANE: Eve, perhaps you can begin by explaining what brought you to us?

EVE: I'll do my best. The others can fill in if I leave important material out. I'm 25 years old and Charles and Petra are 26. We were each conceived artificially. That means we are not the result of sexual union in the normal sense. Our mothers and social fathers were unable to have children of their own – shared children – because our social fathers were infertile, or maybe sub-fertile. Whatever the case, they decided to seek help and eventually concluded that the best way forward was to buy sperm from an anonymous donor and to get a doctor at a clinic to inject that sperm into the neck of our mothers' cervixes. Obviously, it worked. We are the proof of that.

She picks up a cup of coffee from the table in front of her. She takes a welcome sip.

These donations, just as much these days as at the time, were promoted to our parents as a health initiative. Here's how it went: first, our parents were told that infertility is a disease, something that could perhaps be cured by medicine, and if not, a disease that could be overcome in another way – like DI. They went to health clinics with a health problem and they got it fixed – or so they thought. Second, even now there is an idea about that not having kids is 'unhealthy'. The ideal family, the truly healthy family unit, has a Mum and a Dad and a couple of kids at least. Third, our parents were definitely suffering. They really wanted kids, they really wanted to be a normal family. They were upset, embarrassed, often repressed and upset in social situations where children were around or were discussed – it was quite a mess and we were the solution. The solution, note.

So, if people have a health problem and they get it fixed that has to be health promotion, doesn't it? Okay, it wasn't explicitly sold as health promotion, but our parents were definitely led to believe that their lives would be immeasurably improved by the service offered by the clinic.

CHARLES: I'd put it strongly and simply. Infertility is clearly regarded as a health issue. There are private and State clinics all over the place, and doctors can study to be infertility specialists at state sponsored medical schools.

DIANE: (*Nodding*) I think we can grant that infertility is generally considered to be a health issue. In fact (*looking at James*) the way you put it I'd say infertility is – or certainly can be – a health problem for the couple concerned according to the theory of health we use as well. I would have thought infertility could be seen as a real impediment to autonomy, both with respect to a basic biological impulse and with regard to the importance of having a sense of community, a sense of belonging. You'd agree, James?

JAMES: Absolutely. Potentially devastating health effects can result from infertility. There are lots of journals around that report them. (*He looks at each visitor in turn*) But it isn't the health problem for your parents that you're concerned about, is it?

PETRA: (*Looking down*) No. Of course we are here basically to get help with our own health problem. However, I think we would all agree that our parents too are in need of health promotion, despite their thinking that they had fixed the problem with DI. It seems to us that as soon as we were conceived our parents' health status became fragile. Effectively the DI made their health more vulnerable.

DIANE: That's really interesting. How about you tell us how you see your own health problem first, as things stand with you?

EVE: Shall I do that?

Her friends nod.

EVE: Most of the words I will use to describe our problem are not medical ones, is that alright?

JAMES: Of course.

EVE: Right, first things first. I don't know if Charles is my brother or if Petra is my sister. We might have the same father and not know it. (*Diane is shocked. Eve looks her in the eye.*) We all come from the same area, and we are pretty sure that our parents each used the same clinic.

JAMES: Can't you find out for certain?

EVE: Well, Charles and I know for sure which clinic they used, but Petra's parents won't tell her.

JAMES: I'm sorry to be ignorant of this point, but don't you have rights? Can't you just go to the clinic and find out?

EVE: No, we can't. The clinic's still there. In fact we understand it's doing very well for itself. But if they kept records at all they certainly won't let us have them. The deal for the parents and the donor is anonymity, guaranteed. Bottom-line. They have all the rights. At the moment we're allowed to find out our biological fathers' height and hair colour, if there is anyone who knows. But that's all.

DIANE: That's awful.

EVE: Yes, it is. And there is also a very obvious medical issue here. Nevertheless, it doesn't seem to make a difference to anyone.

JAMES: What is it?

EVE: Genetic information, medical history. The medical history of my social father is recorded on my medical records, but that is completely irrelevant to me. He might not have a genetic deficiency, but my biological Dad might, and I won't know. And neither will my husband – so we won't know what we might pass on to our kids. And neither will a life insurance company. What do I do about that? Is my insurance invalid if I mention only my social Dad?

PETRA: That is a huge issue. And you know I only just found out last year. They kept the truth from me all this time. So my question is, was my insurance policy valid even though it contained false information? I told the truth as I knew it, but in reality I supplied false information.

JAMES: I see. This is quite a mess.

EVE: It is horrible. And I haven't explained the worst of it yet.

Charles reaches across from his chair and takes Eve's hand.

EVE: I...we...don't know who we are. We don't have a real identity. We don't know – and we never will know – half our biological family. One half of our ancestral line is invisible – it's like it has never been. No one from that part of the family will be at our weddings, at our kids' Christenings. Not one of them will mourn at our funerals, not one of them will even know we are dead. Worse, none of them will even be aware that we have lived. (*She finishes her coffee in one large swallow.*) I might meet my father in the street and never know. I might even marry him and never know.

She puts her cup down on the table and looks directly at James.

I have no photograph albums of half of my family, no memory of their faces, their sounds, their smell, their touch, their laughter. All that is denied me. I have a family already, they say. I have a history with my Mum and my social Dad – why would I want another one? (*Her voice cracking slightly.*) Why would I not, I say? I go to weddings on my Dad's side of the family. Am I with my family? Of course not, I'm with strangers. Total strangers. They don't look like me, they don't have my blood. I'm a cuckoo in their midst.

JAMES: (*Sympathetically*) I can see how deeply you feel this. And I am very sorry you are all so troubled. But...but...can I be devil's advocate for a moment?

Charles groans.

JAMES: I do realise that you will have heard all this before. But you will understand that if we are to help you we need to see the fullest possible picture.

EVE: We understand.

JAMES: Well, there are lots of different conceptions of family, aren't there. Not every family is related genetically. We talk of the family of nations, of extended families, we have step-relatives, relatives-in-law. Many times our friends and colleagues seem much more like family than anyone we're related to. And we usually see a lot more of them; spend a lot more time with them. We are all human beings; we are all descended from a few women who lived in Africa many thousands of years ago. Aren't you being...um...forgive me...too precious, too perfectionist – sorry I can't find the word I want – about the idea of family? Can't you just decide to accept the families you have and get on with life?

CHARLES: We have heard all that, many times. It's a point of view, but it's one that's a lot easier to hold if you are already secure within your own family. You're suggesting that we should deny our feelings and turn our backs on what we believe to be rightfully ours – our histories and our identities. It is a heritage that most people just take for granted – but it is a powerful heritage nonetheless, reassuring, continuous, protecting. Most people know where they come from and where they belong, especially if times get rough. They can wrap their families around them when they need to.

EVE: Yes. What really gets me is that I feel like a product. They didn't want ME – they wanted any baby...

JAMES: (*Interrupting her*) Surely that's true of all parents?

EVE: But at least they have sex. We were deliberately created, and paid for. Don't forget that money changed hands for us. The donors got paid for their sperm and the clinics got paid – a lot more – for inserting it. We're not the result of love – we're chattels, property. That's not hyperbole. It's the truth – we were bought and sold and that's how we feel.

DIANE: I'm very sorry. I really had no idea about all this. You are in a similar situation to adoptees, aren't you?

EVE: In some ways. But at least adoptees were the result of sex. They weren't deliberately created. Adoption is a way to meet the needs of an existing child. DI is only a way to meet the needs of an infertile couple. It can't be anything else. And adoptees have more rights than us too.

JAMES: Just thinking out loud here, but I wonder if this is more a legal issue than a health matter?

Diane looks at him fiercely. James notices.

JAMES: (*Quickly*) I mean...of course that's not to say that it isn't a health issue too – in some profound ways – but I wonder if the way to go is not to try the courts to secure some rights in some way?

EVE: A couple of DI children are trying that. I can give you the details if you like, but at best they will be able to achieve only very limited rights.

She leans forward and places her hands on the coffee table.

Look, we think we have a real health need, but no one will acknowledge it. Either we get offered anti-depressants, or we get some polite attention and then shown the door. Mostly we just get ignored, or accused of being selfish, or of being family wreckers, or worse... But it hurts. It really hurts. It gets in the way of our living normal lives. We feel deeply upset, damaged... damaged goods. We can't get on with growing, we can't settle. Yet we want health – we want to be all we can be. Why shouldn't we hope for that? We've come to you for that. We've come to you to find a strategy that will promote our health – not pills and not platitudes. We want a way to sort this out. Can you help us?

JAMES: Yes, that is a possibility. Yours is certainly quite a complex case. We'd need to think about it for a while...

DIANE: (*Swiftly*) Perhaps not for too long though James. Yes, there's a lot here but I think if we ask some questions now we might be able to get a pretty good picture of the key rational fields, don't you?

JAMES: (*Blinking*) Yes. I agree.

He turns to the clients.

JAMES: You have given us a complex picture. However, all life situations are complex. Because life is so complex, conventional health promotion prefers a simplified set of topics, and therefore excludes sperm donation and many other health issues. We are more inclusive. And yet rational field health promotion is an oversimplification of reality too. But having said that, the first goal of our approach is to try to show the extent to which there are different interests and goals in play in any life situation. Once we have established this we can begin to decide how to proceed more knowledgeably.

DIANE: I don't think you are being quite as clear as you might be...

JAMES: (*Raising his voice a little*) What we CAN see almost instantly is that there is no such thing as THE health promotion strategy. There are no absolutes in health promotion. So when conventional health promotion denies help to you it is denying only a particular sort of help, based on a particular sort of prejudice. But you look puzzled.

EVE: I am. We are. Do you think you could illustrate what you mean with reference to our case?

JAMES: Of course. In your case, as with any other, there are many different rational fields in play. Just remember that a rational field is a system that has at least one purpose – rational fields are formed by any kind of problem-solving behaviour, and are initially created by a value-judgement or an instinct or both.

DIANE: So, for example, when your parents decided to seek 'treatment' at the infertility clinic they instantly created a rational field.

CHARLES: So, how can we find out what this rational field is?

DIANE: There are several ways, though we have to accept that because people's motivations are so multifarious the best we can do is come to some approximation of the make-up of each rational field. Yes, we have to guess sometimes, but so long as we recognise that, our project is not undermined.

JAMES: Let me show you what we mean.

The Rational Field Template

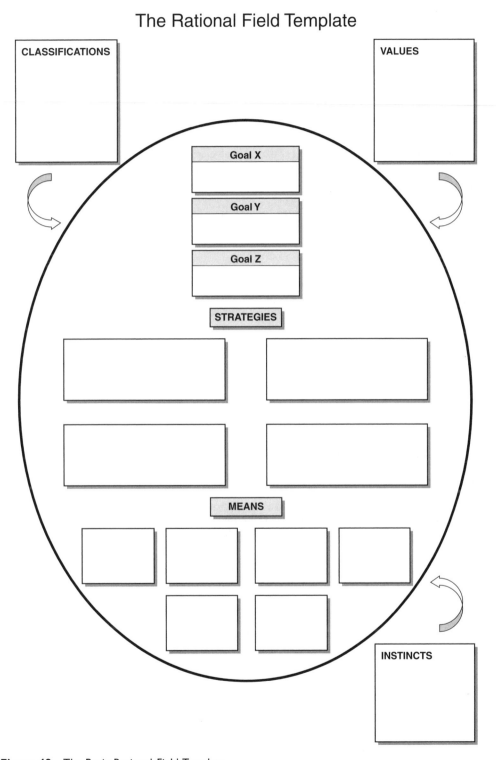

Figure 48   The Basic Rational Field Template

James presses a button on his wheelchair. The lights dim, blinds close and a projector starts up. An image (Fig. 48) appears on the screen behind him. He turns to look at it.

JAMES: This is as simple as it gets. A rational field is contained within the elipse in the figure. A rational field must consist of at least one goal, at least one sort of means, and at least one strategy to link the means to the goal. A rational field comes into being as someone or something tries to find a solution to a problem – which of course means that the field's goals, strategies and means do not exist of themselves. Rather they are defined as goals, strategies and means by a set of classifications, values and instincts that are usually hidden even from a rational field's creator. These classifications, values and instincts are all forms of prejudice because they form a pre-judgement that defines first the goal and then the rest of the rational field.

EVE: That's complicated. I'm not sure I understand all that. How do you know the difference between all those categories you mention, between a 'value' and a 'classification' for example?

James looks across to Diane.

DIANE: These are not absolute categories. We are very aware that we often create distinctions ourselves as we use them to try to understand the interactions between different rational fields. However, sometimes the distinction IS very clear. For example, a CLASSIFICATION of reality is a human decision to divide physical states of affairs into 'diseases' and 'not-diseases', and a VALUE is what lies behind the decision that some physical states are more desirable than others. I know that can sound weird. People often object that it ISN'T a classification to call a painful cancer a disease. A cancer just is a disease because it just is bad, they say. My counter to that is that NOTHING is obvious – human beings classify EVERYTHING.

Diane lifts a book from a bookshelf beside her chair.

Listen to this, for example:

> By the time I saw him, His Holiness had already had many operations, some parts of his body removed, things put inside him, his blood transfused, and so on. Every day the doctors discovered the symptoms of some new disease, only to find them gone the next day and replaced by another illness, as if all the diseases in the world were finding room in his flesh. For two months he had taken no solid food, and finally his doctors gave up hope. It was impossible for him to live, and the doctors thought the life-supporting systems should be discounted.

> But the Karmapa said, 'No, I'm going to live. Leave them in place.' And he did live, astonishing the doctors, and remaining seemingly at ease in his situation – humorous, playful, smiling, as if he were rejoicing at everything his body suffered. Then I thought, with the clearest possible conviction, that the Karmapa had submitted himself to all this cutting, to the manifestation of all these diseases in his body, to the lack of food, in a quite intentional and voluntary way: He was deliberately suffering all these diseases to help minimise the coming pains of war, disease and famine, and in this way he was deliberately working to avert the terrible suffering of this dark age.[138]

She rests the book on the arm of her chair.

For the Holy Man disease and illness are classified as good. He was welcoming something most of us habitually define as unwanted, and this shows that it is not the thing or state itself that is intrinsically good or bad. It is the way we classify it that shapes it.

EVE: That's a lot to take in all at once. It's hard to see what it has to do with health promotion too.

DIANE: I accept that. But let's just take your case first, to give you an accessible example. Then you'll see more clearly what we have in mind, and you will be able to decide whether you want us to work with you.

Look at the template on the screen. It has three notional goals. Let's try to fill these in, in order to gain insight into the rational fields created by your parents as they decided to seek 'treatment'.

EVE: That's easier. Obviously one goal was to have a child.

PETRA: Another was to be a normal family.

CHARLES: Presumably another was to be cured of the disease of infertility.

DIANE: Fair enough. And the means and strategy?

EVE: Also obvious.

DIANE: Okay, but perhaps we should write down a few of the components so we don't forget them?

EVE: Sure.

Diane does so, using her laptop (Fig. 49).

DIANE: Now for the harder bit. What about the instincts, classifications and values?

PETRA: But we aren't sure what you mean by those.

EVE: Can you help us Diane?

Diane reaches for her laptop and begins typing once more. She presses 'Return' and the re-drafted image appears (Fig. 50).

EVE: Wow. I'm beginning to see what you mean. Can you explain a bit more please?

DIANE: Yes, I shall, but I'd rather not go into full detail right now. My suggestions are bound to be arguable and I really just want to show you in general how the rational field idea can be helpful to you. Basically, all I'm suggesting is a general set of classifications and values that most of us take for granted in our present society, and some pretty obvious instincts. Putting these round the very basic rational field we have so far creates a simple hypothesis a) that this is your parents' rational field and b) that the field was created by something like this combination of classifications, values and instincts.

JAMES: What we'll do, if you accept our terms, is create a more detailed set of rational fields for you to think about – in essence these will give you fresh insights into your position – or they will at least consolidate the insights you have already. At the very least you will be able to show these to other people, so that they will properly appreciate the extent of your situation.

DIANE: Yes, and after that we'll work on those rational fields with you, in three steps. First we'll analyse each rational field independently, by asking ten clarifying questions. Second we'll compare and contrast other relevant rational fields, again by asking ten clarifying questions. Then finally we'll feed in the bones of the foundations theory of health

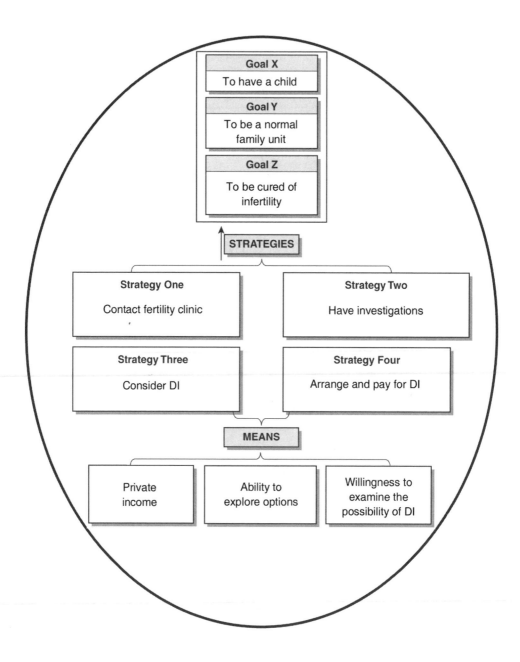

Figure 49   The parents' rational field – opening draft

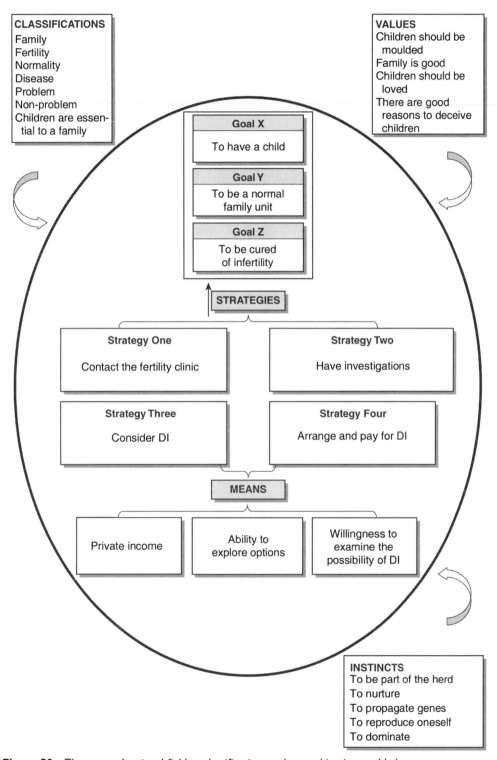

CLASSIFICATIONS
Family
Fertility
Normality
Disease
Problem
Non-problem
Children are essen-
tial to a family

VALUES
Children should be
moulded
Family is good
Children should be
loved
There are good
reasons to deceive
children

Goal X
To have a child

Goal Y
To be a normal
family unit

Goal Z
To be cured
of infertility

STRATEGIES

Strategy One
Contact the fertility clinic

Strategy Two
Have investigations

Strategy Three
Consider DI

Strategy Four
Arrange and pay for DI

MEANS

Private income

Ability to
explore options

Willingness to
examine the
possibility of DI

INSTINCTS
To be part of the herd
To nurture
To propagate genes
To reproduce oneself
To dominate

Figure 50   The parents' rational field – classifications, values and instincts added (our philosophy of health promotion) in order to devise the most health promoting rational field.

To show you what we mean let's work on the example we have on the screen ... Oh, before that you need to see the ten key questions by the way.

Diane presses a button, and the image on-screen changes

TEN CLARIFYING QUESTIONS

1. ARE THE RATIONAL FIELD'S GOALS COMPATIBLE?

2. IF NO, IS IT POSSIBLE TO SELECT ONLY COMPATIBLE GOALS, OR TO CHANGE THE GOALS?

3. ARE THE GOALS REALISTIC WHEN SEEN IN THE LIGHT OF THE PRIMARY SURROUNDING RATIONAL FIELDS?

4. DO THE GOALS CREATE THE MOST AUTONOMY IN THE SUBJECT(S) WHO INHABIT OR WILL INHABIT THE FIELD?

5. ARE THE GOALS DESIRED BY THE SUBJECT(S) WHO INHABIT OR WILL INHABIT THE FIELD?

6. ARE THE STRATEGIES/MEANS APPROPRIATE TO THE ACHIEVEMENT OF THE GOALS?

7. IF NO, WHAT POSITIVE GOALS CAN BE ACHIEVED USING THESE STRATEGIES/MEANS IN CONTEXT?

8. WHAT PREJUDICES HAVE CREATED THE RATIONAL FIELD?

9. IS THE FIELD RIGID, FLEXIBLE OR DISINTEGRATING?

10. IS IT POSSIBLE TO ALTER THE RIGIDITY OF THE FIELD?

THE PURPOSE OF TOTAL HEALTH PROMOTION IS TO WORK OUT HOW TO

DESIGN REALISTIC RATIONAL FIELDS, ABLE TO CREATE THE BROADEST AUTONOMY

Figure 51

DIANE: Now, let's show the basic rational field and the ten questions side by side on screen.

Diane presses more keys on her laptop. The screen changes again to show both the developing rational field and the list of questions (Fig. 52).

DIANE: (*Looking at the screen*) Right. Question 1.

1. ARE THE RATIONAL FIELD'S GOALS COMPATIBLE?

EVE: (*Reading aloud*) To have a child. To be a normal family. To be cured of infertility.

I'd say these are incompatible (*she pauses*) ... but I guess most people don't see it the way we do. I imagine the goals would look compatible to most people. But they'd be wrong. And you know, I'd say that only the first goal was ACTUALLY achieved in our cases. In fact I'd say that only the first goal is actually achievable in ANY instance using DI.

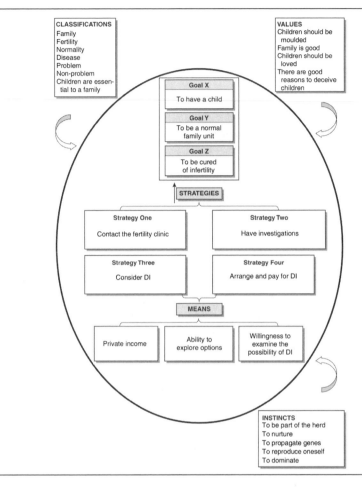

CLASSIFICATIONS
Family
Fertility
Normality
Disease
Problem
Non-problem
Children are essential to a family

VALUES
Children should be
  moulded
Family is good
Children should be
  loved
There are good
  reasons to deceive
  children

Goal X
To have a child

Goal Y
To be a normal
family unit

Goal Z
To be cured
of infertility

STRATEGIES

Strategy One
Contact the fertility clinic

Strategy Two
Have investigations

Strategy Three
Consider DI

Strategy Four
Arrange and pay for DI

MEANS

Private income

Ability to
explore options

Willingness to
examine the
possibility of DI

INSTINCTS
To be part of the herd
To nurture
To propagate genes
To reproduce oneself
To dominate

TEN CLARIFYING QUESTIONS

1. ARE THE RATIONAL FIELD'S GOALS COMPATIBLE?

2. IF NO, IS IT POSSIBLE TO SELECT ONLY COMPATIBLE GOALS, OR TO CHANGE THE GOALS?

3. ARE THE GOALS REALISTIC WHEN SEEN IN THE LIGHT OF THE PRIMARY SURROUNDING RATIONAL FIELDS?

4. DO THE GOALS CREATE THE MOST AUTONOMY IN THE SUBJECT(S) WHO INHABIT OR WILL INHABIT THE FIELD?

5. ARE THE GOALS DESIRED BY THE SUBJECT(S) WHO INHABIT OR WILL INHABIT THE FIELD?

6. ARE THE STRATEGIES/MEANS APPROPRIATE TO THE ACHIEVEMENT OF THE GOALS?

7. IF NO, WHAT POSITIVE GOALS CAN BE ACHIEVED USING THESE STRATEGIES/MEANS IN CONTEXT?

8. WHAT PREJUDICES HAVE CREATED THE RATIONAL FIELD?

9. IS THE FIELD RIGID, FLEXIBLE OR DISINTEGRATING?

10. IS IT POSSIBLE TO ALTER THE RIGIDITY OF THE FIELD?

THE PURPOSE OF TOTAL HEALTH PROMOTION IS TO WORK OUT HOW TO

DESIGN REALISTIC RATIONAL FIELDS, ABLE TO CREATE THE BROADEST AUTONOMY

Figure 52

DIANE: Alright. Let's just hold that thought for a minute. How about we go to Question 3? ARE THE GOALS REALISTIC WHEN SEEN IN THE LIGHT OF THE PRIMARY SURROUNDING RATIONAL FIELDS?

Presumably you also have a problem with this?

EVE: Yes. I'm bound to, aren't I?

DIANE: I think a lot of the help we might give will concern the surrounding rational fields. But let's try to keep it as straightforward as possible while we explain the basic idea to you.

EVE: Fine.

DIANE: OK, Question 4. A big one for our health promotion aims. DO THE GOALS CREATE THE MOST AUTONOMY IN THE SUBJECT(S) WHO INHABIT OR WILL INHABIT THE FIELD?

CHARLES: Would you mind explaining what you mean by autonomy please?

DIANE: Yes, of course. That is essential if you are to understand all this. 'Create autonomy' is the key term for the theory of health we use. Basically it means 'give control to'. In a more extended form it means 'provide protection and purpose; give information; provide education; foster a sense of belonging; and respond to crises in a way that offers the most fulfilling subsequent existence'.

Eve gasps as she hears this.

EVE: Wow. Ouch. Bloody ouch.

JAMES: (*Surprised*) What do you mean, Eve?

EVE: If you look at it like that then it makes it just so obvious how we have been USED. That rational field created autonomy for our makers, our parents, but it almost did the OPPOSITE for us. God.

She shakes her head.

By breeding us THEY got their purposes met. Our parents got all the information they wanted, and all the control over it THEY needed. But not us. That rational field didn't create autonomy for us.

DIANE: Well, that's good. (*Quickly*) I mean, the good news here is that we're seeing things eye to eye in so far as health is concerned. Now, let's just look at the next three questions:

5. ARE THE GOALS DESIRED BY THE SUBJECT(S) WHO INHABIT OR WILL INHABIT THE FIELD?
6. ARE THE STRATEGIES/MEANS APPROPRIATE TO THE ACHIEVEMENT OF THE GOALS?
7. IF NO, WHAT POSITIVE GOALS CAN BE ACHIEVED USING THESE STRATEGIES/MEANS IN CONTEXT?

Answering these questions will take us to the heart of the matter. Can we combine your rational fields with those of your parents, or must we look for more radical ways forward?

If you agree to our exploring these questions with you I'm confident we will reveal some very positive health promoting goals and strategies for you to consider.

EVE: I think what you are saying is very interesting. But in a way you are only telling us what we know already. Are you going to offer us something else? (*She reddens slightly*) I'm sorry, but if we are going to invest in your service we need to know that we're going to get good value.

DIANE: Of course, that's only reasonable. So far we have only shown you how we can begin to analyse one of the very many rational fields that exist in your case. Next we would want to compare a SET of different rational fields. This would give us a fuller picture. And after that we'd try to establish which rational fields might be the most health promoting for you, and of course we'd take a close look at the values and instincts that create them. And then – and this is key – we'd feed in the foundations theory of health. By doing this we would hope to be able to show you the path to the greatest health, or greatest level of autonomy, if you like. It's the same thing in the end.

A pause.

Do you want us to do that?

EVE: Can my friends and I talk for a while?

DIANE: Sure. We'll go get a coffee and come back in a few minutes, if that's OK.

Diane and James leave the room.

SCENE FIVE

The meeting room again. The same characters are present. Diane has the laptop and is showing six different rational fields, one by one.

(They are:

The rational field of the fertility clinic (Fig. 53)

Two possible rational fields of the donor (Figs 54 and 55)

The rational field of the sperm (Fig. 56)

The State's rational field (Fig. 57)

The parents' rational field, as it was presented in the previous meeting (Fig. 50))

Diane puts the six images together on one screen. Everyone stares, transfixed.

JAMES: Now, the question is: can we make sense of these fields?

DIANE: And the question after that is: can we construct a workable rational field for you? We will try to do both in this session. That might be enough for you. Or you might want to come back again. We'll see.

First of all, how do you react to our interpretation of your reality?

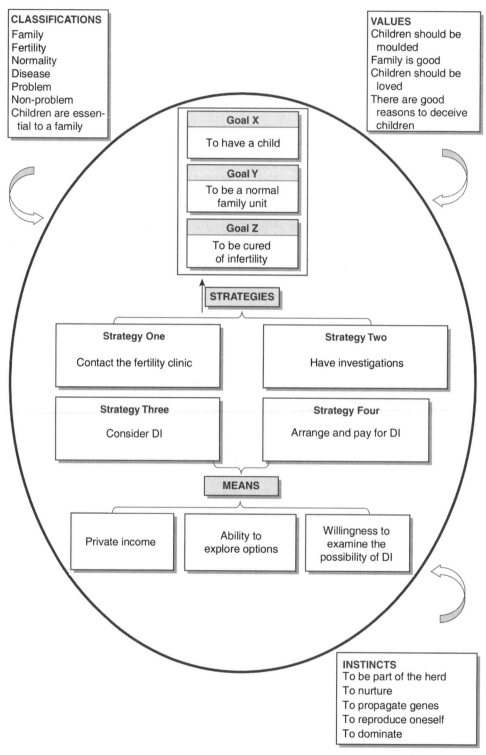

CLASSIFICATIONS
Family
Fertility
Normality
Disease
Problem
Non-problem
Children are essen-
  tial to a family

VALUES
Children should be
  moulded
Family is good
Children should be
  loved
There are good
  reasons to deceive
  children

Goal X
To have a child

Goal Y
To be a normal
family unit

Goal Z
To be cured
of infertility

STRATEGIES

Strategy One
Contact the fertility clinic

Strategy Two
Have investigations

Strategy Three
Consider DI

Strategy Four
Arrange and pay for DI

MEANS

Private income

Ability to
explore options

Willingness to
examine the
possibility of DI

INSTINCTS
To be part of the herd
To nurture
To propagate genes
To reproduce oneself
To dominate

Figure 50 The parents' rational field — classifications, values and instincts added

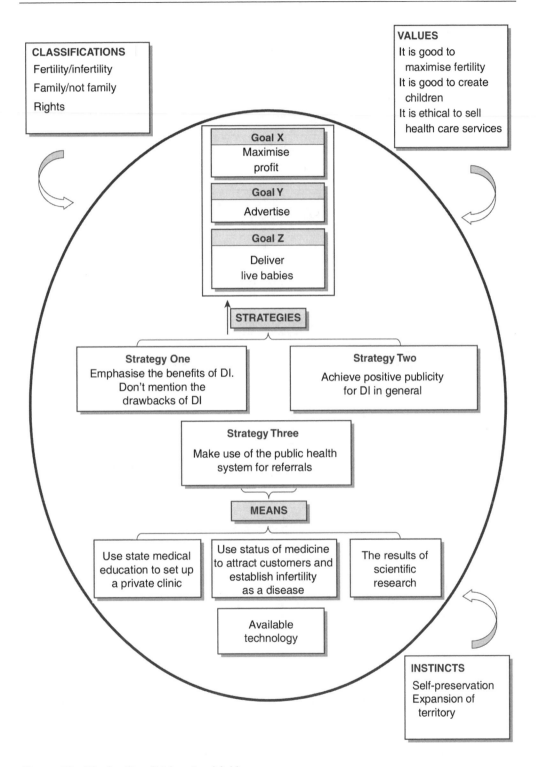

Figure 53 The fertility clinic's rational field

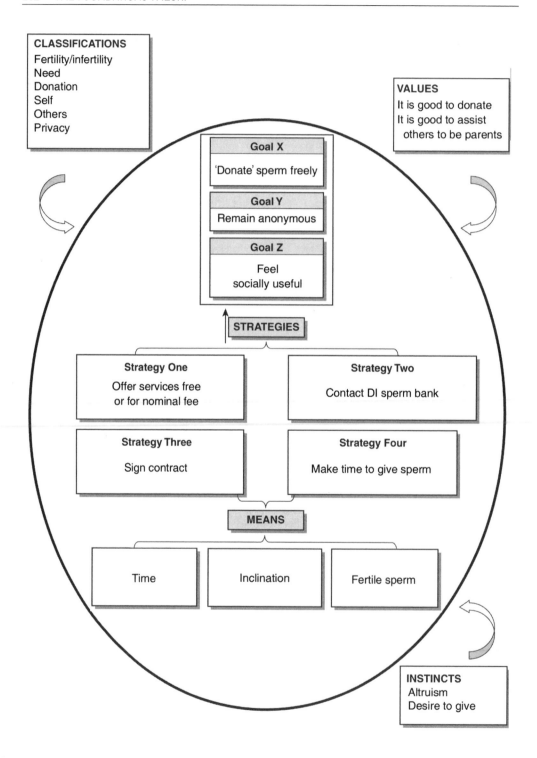

Figure 54   Donor rational field I

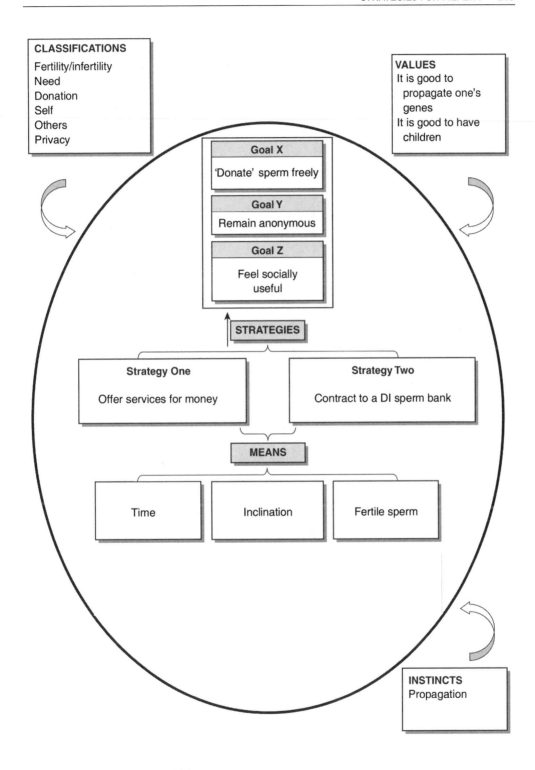

Figure 55 Donor rational field 2

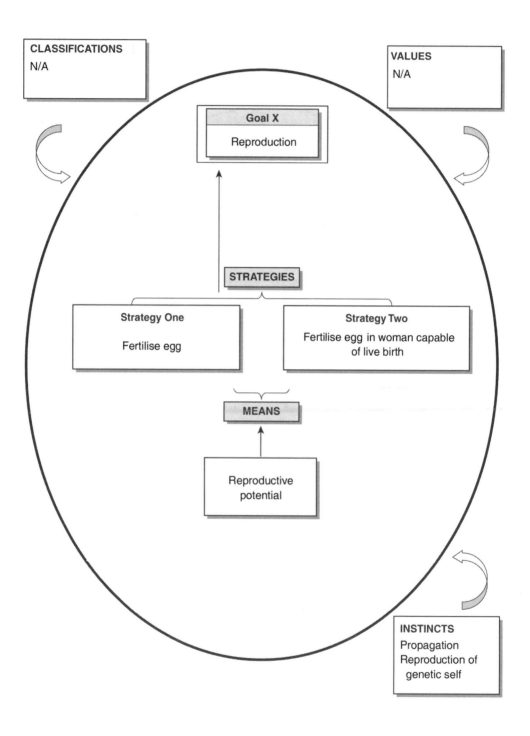

Figure 56   The sperm's rational field

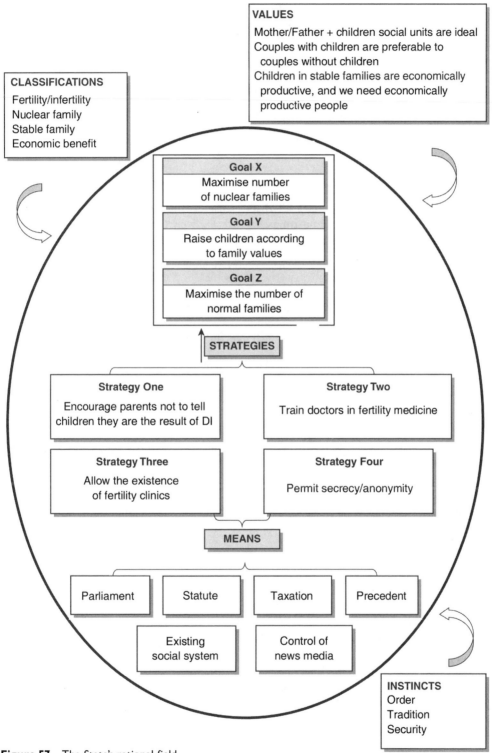

Figure 57 The State's rational field

EVE: It's amazing. Somehow you've articulated everything I've been trying to get out in recent years. It is a shock to see it so plainly, so in your face.

Eve cups her hands over her nose and breathes out hard.

JAMES: (*Directly to Eve*) We understand. It's always a shock to see everything turned inside out. We find this happens a lot with rational field health promotion.

DIANE: What do you think about these rational fields?

EVE: I think...I think they ALL exist. I think they are ALL true. And that isn't easy to deal with, I can tell you.

JAMES: Why not?

EVE: Well, obviously, they don't all make sense. I mean, taken together they are a complete mess. But at the same time they are each part of the truth. Even – perhaps particularly – the two possible rational fields for the donor.

JAMES: (*Encouraging her*) How? What do you mean?

EVE: Well, the way you've got it the two fields are contradictory – one type of donor does it for the good of others, the other type does it for the good of his genes. But then when you start to think about it, you could have both of those fields simultaneously – the donor could be BOTH altruistic and selfish, couldn't he?

JAMES: Hmm. I'd not thought of that. I'd need a little time to digest that.

DIANE: Yes, it's arguable. In the end it might rest on what is meant by 'altruistic' – on whether, for example, you have to be TOTALLY unselfish to be altruistic. I'd have to think about that some more too...

But, whatever the case, and however complex we take any donor field to be, the important thing is that we spell out the possibilities. In your case, since the donors were anonymous we have no idea what their motives were. We know they were paid but we don't know whether they kept the money for themselves, though presumably most of them did. All we know for sure is that there is a range of possible motives AND that until these motives are clear you, the children, will remain damaged.

Is it fair to say that?

PETRA: It is certainly fair to say that.

EVE: Yes...but we CAN be clear about some of the motives. One of them – whether the donor was unselfish or selfish – was NOT to know us, NOT to parent us, NOT to love us. They are motives, aren't they? Can we add those?

DIANE: Yes.

She types in these extra consideration on the relevant RFs (Figs 58 and 59).

DIANE: Now, let's get to work. Let's try out STEP I for each rational field. First, the clarifying questions.

Where shall we start?

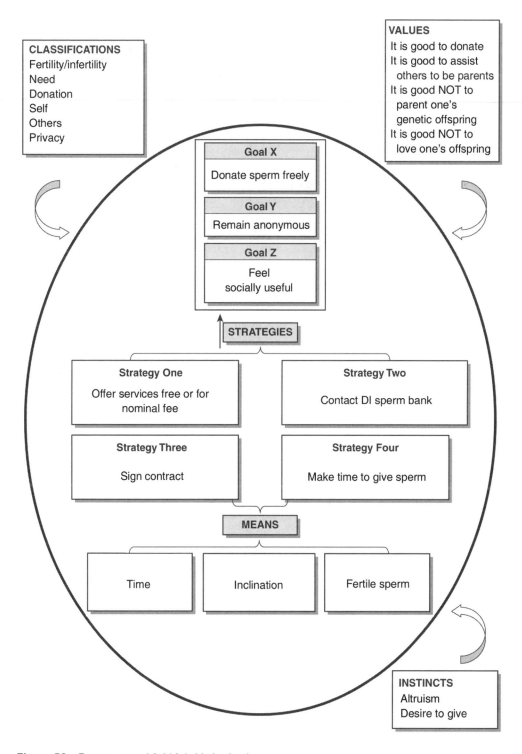

Figure 58   Donor rational field I (added values)

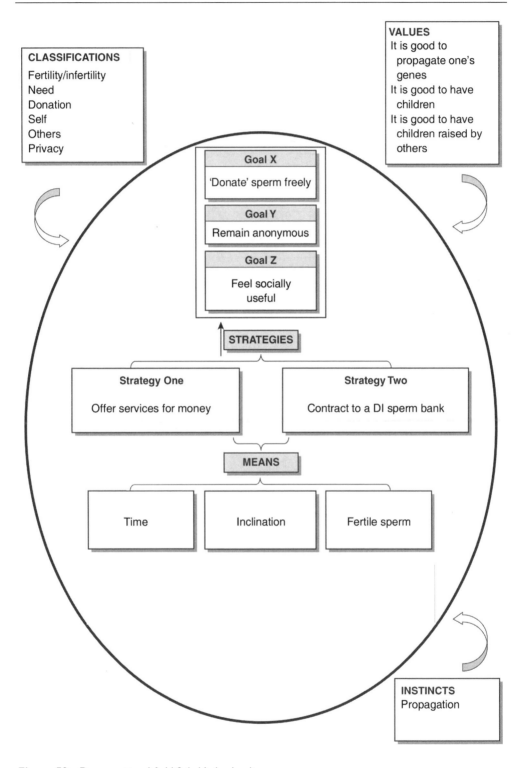

Figure 59   Donor rational field 2 (added values)

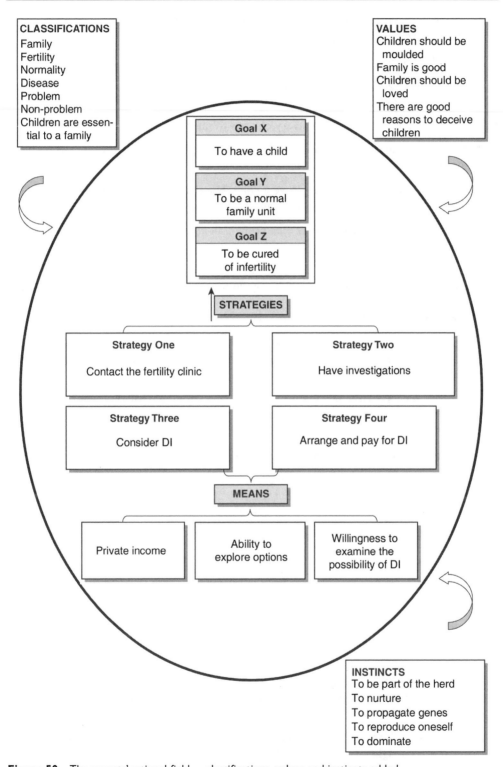

CLASSIFICATIONS
Family
Fertility
Normality
Disease
Problem
Non-problem
Children are essen-
  tial to a family

VALUES
Children should be
  moulded
Family is good
Children should be
  loved
There are good
  reasons to deceive
  children

Goal X
To have a child

Goal Y
To be a normal
family unit

Goal Z
To be cured
of infertility

STRATEGIES

Strategy One
Contact the fertility clinic

Strategy Two
Have investigations

Strategy Three
Consider DI

Strategy Four
Arrange and pay for DI

MEANS

Private income

Ability to
explore options

Willingness to
examine the
possibility of DI

INSTINCTS
To be part of the herd
To nurture
To propagate genes
To reproduce oneself
To dominate

Figure 50   The parents' rational field − classifications, values and instincts added

EVE: Can we revisit the parents' rational field please? I know we looked at it last time but I don't want to miss anything.

Diane selects this rational field only on the screen (Fig. 50).

DIANE: Well, Question 1 asks ARE THE RATIONAL FIELD'S GOALS COMPATIBLE? What do you think?

CHARLES: No they are not. It's very obvious to me that they are not.

JAMES: It isn't so obvious to me. Surely by achieving Goal X they THEREFORE achieve the other goals?

CHARLES: Not at all. Yes, they have a child, but they are NOT a 'normal family unit' because they are not a normal family, they are an abnormal family, a cuckoo's nest.

DIANE: Well, that's what you say but surely it all depends on what is meant by 'normal family unit'?

EVE: (*Smartly*) No, Charles is right, no question. Their goals are incompatible because THEY KNOW they are not a normal family. In particular, the father KNOWS he is not a normal father – he knows deeply and acutely that the appearance of normality is not actually normality. It's with him all the time. There's no escaping it.

JAMES: Hold on a minute. Surely there's evidence that many social fathers are happy with the outcome? Surely it's better for them to have a family like this than not to have a family at all?

EVE: Some men say that, but I don't believe them. Imagine what they are confessing to their child if they say anything else?

JAMES: I have to say that that is speculation. I'm sure not all of these social fathers can be lying. I'm sure some of them love their children...

EVE: (*Interrupting him*) We'll have to agree to differ on this point. I don't think anyone can say for sure what the truth is about the way people feel, but we DO know how many fathers need psychiatric help as a result of their using DI.

DIANE: (*Changing* tack) What about the other fields?

PETRA: Well, at least we can all agree about the sperm field!

There is laughter.

EVE: Don't laugh. I think the sperm field is crucial somehow. There just is something so raw about it. (*She shakes her head in frustration*) I can't explain myself properly. I hope Diane or James can help me.

DIANE: Yes, we see it as a crucial point too. The sperm that made you was itself a natural rational field. It had a single purpose quite outside the realm of human convention. The sperm had no values and invented no classifications of reality – it just was: it existed for a pre-programmed purpose...

EVE: (*Breaking Diane's flow, in her enthusiasm*) Yes. And another point for me – a point that just stands right out when you present it as a rational field – is the State's rational field, which basically promotes a version of 'family values' (Fig. 57).

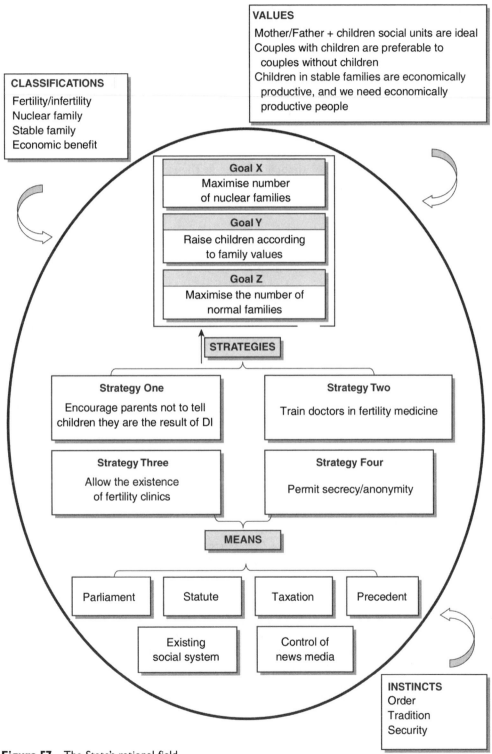

Figure 57 The State's rational field

Diane selects this rational field only on the screen.

Look at Goal Y, where it says 'raise children according to family values'. Of course, your field is only illustrative – there's a lot of room to spell the values out – but I reckon it would be very hard to include gross and continuing deception as part of anyone's set of family values. Families are not supposed to be based on deceit. I doubt very much that even George W. Bush's set of family values would include CONTINUAL BAREFACED LYING to one's offspring. But that is what Strategy I (encourage parents not to tell children they are the result of DI) of that rational field requires. You might also argue that it is NECESSARY for Goal X.

DIANE: (*Thoughtfully*) I'd not thought of that. It shows how spelling out even simple rational fields can be illuminating. What you're saying is that encouraging parents not to tell their children about their DI origins is actually counter-productive to Goals X, Y and Z in this field?

EVE: That's the way it looks to me.

PETRA: But there are so many questions and so many rational fields – do we have to go through them all?

DIANE: (*Smiling*) We could do. But no we don't have to do the lot. We really need to clarify only the rational fields we are uncovering for ourselves. Of course there will always be many possible rational fields that will remain hidden.

CHARLES: In that case, what are we essentially trying to do here?

DIANE: We are painting a picture for you. We don't want a simple, one-dimensional picture – we want to display a rich and conflicting picture to you, because that is how things are. We are trying to show you different layers of a picture – the layers of the reality that are affecting you right now . . . look, tell us, does anything else stand out to you that we ought to include?

EVE: Yes. I want to say that Figures 50 and 55 are TERRIFYING when you put them side by side.

JAMES: Explain please.

Diane types. The screen displays the two figures (the parents' rational field (Fig. 50) and the donor rational field 2 (Fig. 55), side by side). Everybody looks, trying to take in the implications.

EVE: Surely this is an obvious point? It is necessary for the parents that the donor – I'd put quotes round donor actually – is NOT a part of this. He has to be nothing: in the end the best thing for the family is that they convince themselves he never even existed. Failing that they have to think he has disappeared forever, perhaps left the country or died. BUT, if the non-altruistic donor rational field is to succeed, the donor must be a large presence forever. The point of donating sperm within this rational field is NOT anonymity, not at all. I can imagine this sort of donor secretly seeking out and protecting his offspring, waiting for them after school, putting money into their bank accounts, smoothing their path through life if he has social power . . .

She leans forward and holds her head in her hands.

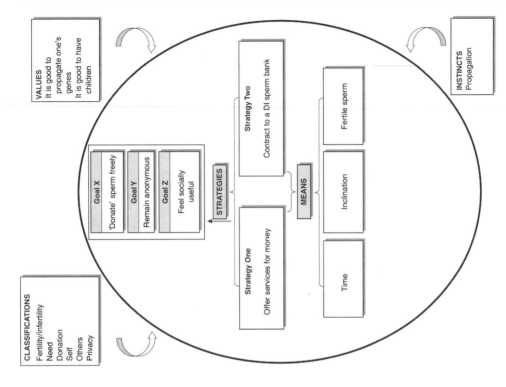

Figure 55 Donor rational field 2

Figure 50 The parents' rational field – classifications, values and instincts added

I'm sorry. Maybe that's going too far. But it's just such a horrible mess. There's supposed to be secrecy but – apart from some of the children – everybody knows what's going on and yet no one wants to front up to it.

JAMES: Perhaps that is a bit over the top.

DIANE: (*Swiftly*) No, no, I don't think it is. In any case, it's what Eve feels and that has to be valid, right James?

JAMES: Oh, of course, I didn't mean . . . um . . . to degrade you Eve. I'm just trying to keep matters balanced. There are many rational fields in play here. We need to be careful not to get carried away just with those that seem the most obvious to us.

EVE: Oh?

JAMES: (*Weakly*) Basically it might be that it isn't all quite as sinister as we are making out.

EVE: I think it is. And I think these rational fields make this as clear as can be.

There is an uncomfortable pause, which Diane eventually breaks.

DIANE: I'd like to return to the sperm if I may. Remember that the sperm had a single purpose quite outside the realm of human convention. The sperm had no values and invented no classifications of reality – it just was: it existed for a pre-programmed purpose. I'd like to spell out the implications of this . . . There are layers here, you see. Once you recognise this the whole matter becomes open to debate, which is what I think you need. Let me see if I can picture this for you.

Diane opens a blank page on her laptop and begins to type. Eventually she posts a simple description of four layers (Fig. 60).

LAYER ONE (outside the world of human classification, value and instinct):
The sperm's natural purpose.

LAYER TWO (one human interpretation of the function of the sperm):
The sperm has no role other than to fuse with the mother's egg to create a baby who will then be part of a normal family – the sperm is wholly INSTRUMENTAL to the needs of the family.

LAYER THREE (another human interpretation of the function of the sperm):
The sperm's role is to create a baby that will perpetuate its genetic material. While this role is inevitably accomplished at fertilisation, it is of minor importance when placed against the nurturing and socialisation provided by the family in which the baby will be raised – in other words the sperm is HIJACKED by the family: like all hijackers, the family continually attempts to change the course of the process originated by the sperm.

LAYER FOUR (another human interpretation of the function of the sperm):
The sperm's role is to create a baby that will perpetuate the genetic material carried by the sperm. This is successfully achieved at fertilisation, and there is nothing anyone can do to change that – the family is INSTRUMENTAL to the needs of the sperm.

Figure 60

The others read what Diane has written. Everyone sits back, a little shocked.

DIANE: The point is that WE place the sperm within the rational fields we manufacture. And as we do this we COLOUR or ADD TO the raw sperm. We take what just is, and we make it something else as we respond to it instinctively, as we value it, and as we classify it. What I'm trying to say is that we LAYER the sperm and its basic purposes with our HUMAN meanings. If we feel that the need for a normal family is more important than anything else, we will use something like LAYER TWO – we will think of the sperm as merely instrumental to us. But if we see things differently, if we feel used as you feel used, then we might apply something like LAYER FOUR instead.

CHARLES: Yes, that's right. I think LAYER FOUR is getting there – that reflects the reality of this.

DIANE: I don't think we can say that. There are different realities in play. I wouldn't want to say that one of them alone is the TRUE reality.

EVE: *(Anxiously)* What do you mean? I thought you were working to help us?

DIANE: We are. But we need to be logical about it. The alternative is for us to side with you on an emotional level, and that really isn't the help you are paying for here.

EVE: But aren't you saying that our parents' truth and our truth are EQUAL truths?

DIANE: Yes, but that isn't the whole story. Look, you must agree that there are the raw data here – the sperm, the fertilisation, the pregnancy, babies, children growing up... How these data are seen differs according to who is observing, and it is impossible to say definitively that any of these ways of seeing the data are more and less true. It is only the data that are true – only the raw facts. Interpretations are just that, interpretations.

EVE: So we don't have a case, then? Is that what you're saying?

DIANE: No. No. Not at all. You do have 'a case'. Your case is that you have been severely and thoughtlessly damaged by an apparently simple procedure intended to be for everyone's benefit. Your parents have probably been seriously damaged too. Your 'case' is that your health is suffering and you need a way to bring it up to the very optimum level.

EVE: Yes, we badly need that.

DIANE: I think the best thing to do now will be to work out the most health promoting rational field for all concerned, or we could do fields for the three of you individually if you like.

PETRA: Personally I'd prefer for us to work on a shared rational field.

JAMES: We can try but we may have to hide some incompatibilities, and this isn't always a comfortable thing to do.

DIANE: Let's try anyway.

She projects a blank General Foundations Rational Field Template on the screen (Fig. 46).

DIANE: I'd like us to take for granted the means and the walls, since these are the basis of our form of health promotion. However, we need to fill in the specific meanings of the means as we try to create the most health promoting rational field for you.

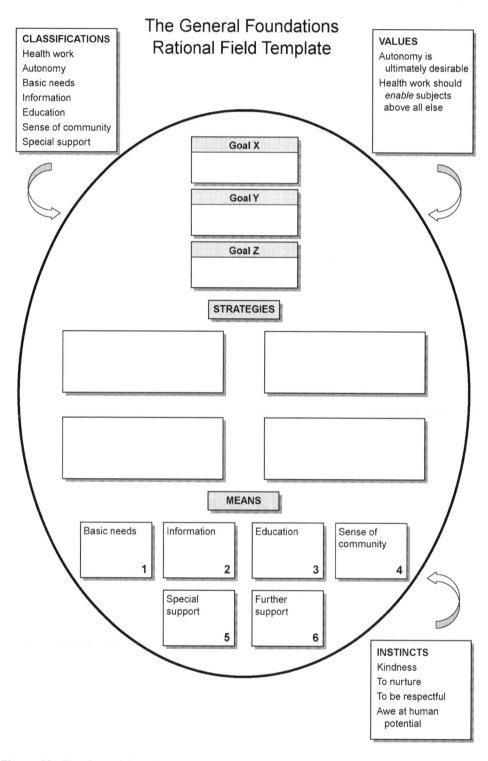

Figure 46   The General Foundations Rational Field Template

Now, bear in mind that the purpose of total health promotion is to work out how to design realistic rational fields, able to create the broadest autonomy. Given this I guess the place for you to begin is your goals, and of course you can have more than three if you like, or less, it's up to you.

What goals do you think would most promote your health?

EVE: Well, on a personal level I don't think there's much more I can do. My relationship with my mother and social father seems to have been damaged beyond repair.

DIANE: Maybe. Let's try to establish some health promoting goals, remembering that they need to be realistic goals.

EVE: I'll try.

Eve takes a stab at some realistic goals. Diane types. Eventually the screen shows this image (Fig. 61).

DIANE: Do you all agree that these are realistic goals?

PETRA: Yes, I do. I can see that other DI children might choose other goals, but I think these work for us.

DIANE: What other goals?

PETRA: Well, some people I know have already done it. They have decided to ignore the issue and just get on with life...

EVE: (*Quickly*) But that is just denial Petra, you know that...

JAMES: (*Raising a hand*) Please. We need to focus on just the one field for the three of you.

DIANE: James is right, you know. Shall we consider the means and strategies boxes?

There is considerable discussion. Finally the group agrees on an image (Fig. 62).

JAMES: I like this. We are really getting somewhere now. This rational field is proposing revelation and reconciliation.

CHARLES: But what if our parents won't come? And which parents do we mean – all of them?

EVE: I guess they may not come and I think we ought to invite both social and biological parents if we can – I think this is what rational field health promotion is all about: openness. Probably most of them won't come but then at least we will have tried. And we have other strategies – the more we get into working out different rational fields the more we may understand about our situation. And we also want to set up a charitable trust, which may help us and others. I think this is a way forward, and perhaps we can ask James and Diane to assist us to get it going?

JAMES: Yes, certainly. I think independent moderation will be crucial, at least in the early stages.

DIANE: Good. But what about the instincts, values and classifications? We don't want to fall into the trap of forgetting about these. All the trouble STARTS when we think of our rational fields as concrete.

Figure 61   Eve's goals

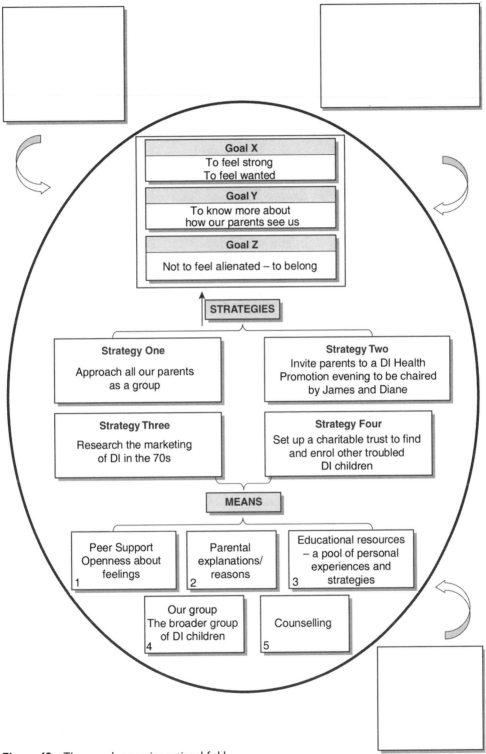

Figure 62   The group's emerging rational field

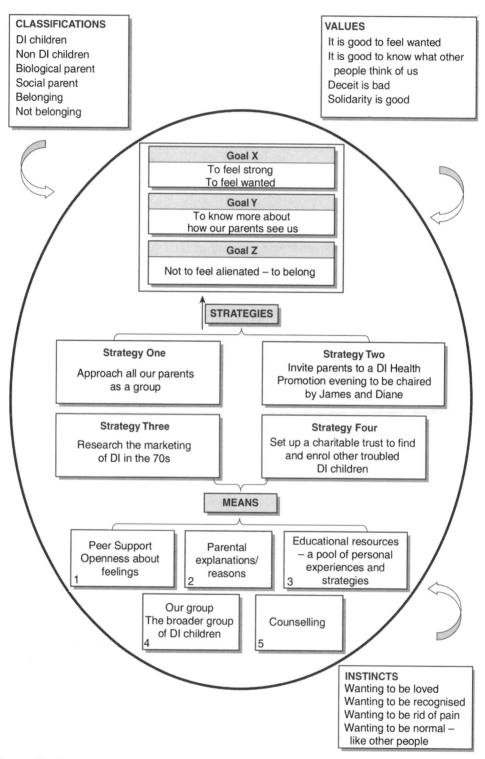

CLASSIFICATIONS
DI children
Non DI children
Biological parent
Social parent
Belonging
Not belonging

VALUES
It is good to feel wanted
It is good to know what other
  people think of us
Deceit is bad
Solidarity is good

Goal X
To feel strong
To feel wanted

Goal Y
To know more about
how our parents see us

Goal Z
Not to feel alienated – to belong

STRATEGIES

Strategy One
Approach all our parents
as a group

Strategy Two
Invite parents to a DI Health
Promotion evening to be chaired
by James and Diane

Strategy Three
Research the marketing
of DI in the 70s

Strategy Four
Set up a charitable trust to find
and enrol other troubled
DI children

MEANS

Peer Support
Openness about
feelings
1

Parental
explanations/
reasons
2

Educational resources
– a pool of personal
experiences and
strategies
3

Our group
The broader group
of DI children
4

Counselling
5

INSTINCTS
Wanting to be loved
Wanting to be recognised
Wanting to be rid of pain
Wanting to be normal –
  like other people

Figure 63   The group's emerging rational field (classifications, values and instincts added)

EVE: Perhaps you could suggest these for us? We are becoming rather tired.

DIANE: Okay, I can make some suggestions.

She types again and posts an amended image (Fig. 63).

EVE: Phew, those are some suggestions. They are REALLY controversial.

DIANE: Don't you accept them?

EVE: I'd want to think very carefully about them . . . I mean, for example, that 'classification' between a 'social' and 'biological' parent – that's just a reality, surely.

DIANE: Maybe. Or maybe there's more to discuss even here? Sure, only one man's sperm and one woman's egg created each of you, and your social fathers are not the men who provided the sperm. That's a fact. BUT your taken for granted classifications are not themselves necessary. You could, instead, merely have a classification of 'parent' and 'non-parent' and define parent as 'a person responsible either for our nature or nurture or both'. And if you did that you could all have THREE parents, or even more if you also have step-parents and grandparents. It really DOES depend on how you look at it.

EVE: No. I don't accept that.

JAMES: Can I suggest that this isn't the time to debate this particular subject. Can we instead think about the internal aspects of the template onscreen? I mean, do you think that the means, strategies and goals fit together?

PETRA: Basically yes.

JAMES: We should try out our ten clarifying questions.

DIANE: *(Checking her watch)* We are way over time for this session. Perhaps we should take this draft rational field away with us and think about it some more, along with the clarifying questions. I can print out copies for each of us. Then we could reconvene in say a week to iron out these other issues?

CHARLES: I think that would be an excellent idea. *(He looks briefly at his two colleagues)* Speaking for myself, I find what you are doing immensely helpful. I feel I understand my situation – and other's people's points of view – much more clearly and simply now. I can see that this isn't a matter of absolute rights and wrongs, but of finding workable ways to give more control and confidence – I think even acceptance – to everyone involved. If we can actually achieve this then you really will have promoted our health for us. And if we can then help other DI children and parents then, well, that would be significant wouldn't it?

JAMES: Well, we'd like to think so. Thank you for coming. If you go outside with Diane we can fix up the next appointment at reception.

They all leave, apart from James. After a few minutes Diane returns.

DIANE: That was fascinating, wasn't it?

JAMES: I thought you did brilliantly. You got it straight away and you were so empathic.

DIANE: Thank you. I felt empathic. They really are suffering.

JAMES: Tell me, do you still believe in this rational field health promotion idea as much as when we first set up this business?

DIANE: (*A little surprised*) Yes, of course. Why do you ask?

JAMES: Some of the things they said. In a way it really is just commonsense, isn't it? And the rational fields we show people are extremely simple – they don't reflect life's complexity, do they?

DIANE: James, James, not again!

JAMES: I know you can convince me otherwise but I can't fully shake off this feeling that we aren't really doing anything ... well ... specialised or professional.

DIANE: But that's just it. We aren't doing anything other people can't do. Basically all we do is use a simple idea to draw out different ways of looking at the world, and then we leave it up to the subjects to work out how to move forward. I don't think we should apologise for that. I think we should be proud of our simple approach. And yes, reality is more complex. We could offer complicated, quantified decision trees. We could offer complex decision support systems – there's plenty of software out there capable of that. But this isn't what the people who come to us want, and it wouldn't be particularly useful to anyone either. That sort of fine detail can be done once the health promoting rational field has been decided on by our clients – what we are doing is showing the choices they have, showing the rational fields of other interested parties that inhabit social reality, and showing that each of these fields has been created by other vulnerable human beings. I think that is wonderfully liberating.

She pauses.

And look at the alternative. Conventional health promotion advice is offered within ONE rational field considered, by the conventional health promoter, to be the ONLY TRUE WAY OF LOOKING AT HEALTH. And that is ridiculous and belittling. And not only that, it is bad for the conventional health promoter too. You see, he can't see over the self-created walls of his supposedly health promoting rational field – so he is blind to all the other ways of striving for a healthy life. There is a sea of rational fields beyond his apparently objective fortress, and he can't see them because he is already certain what health is.

JAMES: Okay. I know. I do know. But if you break down the conventional walls, what are you left with?

DIANE: A realistic view of the social world – a world where there are so many different values and goals that the observer is left humbled and excited. The alternative – as I've said – is either to be blind through ignorance or blind through arrogance that only your way of being rational is healthy.

JAMES: You are so passionate about your work. What would I have done without you?

DIANE: Who knows? Maybe you'd be happy and settled with those kids, beginning to think about a pension as a health promotion specialist?

JAMES: (*Looking rueful for just a moment*) But that's not real now is it?

DIANE: No it's gone. But I'm here. Let's go home. Are you ready to go home?

JAMES: Yes. Please.[139]

References

1. Lalonde, M. (1974). *A New Perspective on the Health of Canadians*, Information Canada, Ottawa.
2. Winter, G.H. (1988). *Complete Guide to Vitamins, Minerals and Supplements*, Fisher Books, Tucson.
3. Lado, R. (1964). *Language Teaching, A Scientific Approach*, McGraw-Hill, New York.
4. Tonias, D.E. (1995). *Bridge Engineering: Design, Rehabilitation, and Maintenance of Modern Highway Bridges*, McGraw-Hill, New York.
5. Bronnitt, S. (1996). Health Care Law: Fracturing the criminal law: disease control and the limits of law-making. *Health Care Analysis* **4**(1), 59–63.
6. Downie, R.S., Fyfe, C. and Tannahill, A. (1990). *Health Promotion: Models and Values*, first edition, Oxford University Press, Oxford.
7. Fitzpatrick, M. (2001). *The Tyranny of Health: Doctors and the Regulation of Lifestyle*, Routledge, London. See especially Chapter Three: The Regulation of Lifestyle.
8. Green, L.W. and Raeburn, J.M. (1988). Health promotion. What is it? What will it become? *Health Promotion* **3**(2), 151–159.
9. Ashton, J. and Seymour, H. (1988). *The New Public Health*, Open University Press, Birmingham.
10. Tones, K., Tilford, S. and Robinson, Y. (1990). *Health Education: Effectiveness, Efficiency and Equity*, first edition, Chapman and Hall, London.
11. Tones, K. and Tilford, S. (1994). *Health Education: Effectiveness, Efficiency and Equity*, second edition, Chapman and Hall, London.
12. Yeo, M. (1993). Toward an ethic of empowerment for health promotion. *Health Promotion International* **8**(3), 225–235.
13. See: http://www.who.dk/eprise/main/WHO/Progs/HPA/Targets/20020319_1 for the latest on WHO Targets at the time of printing. The European targets were updated in 1998, in a document called *Health 21*, http://www.changenet.sk/azms/publications/ health21.htm Exactly the same criticisms apply to these targets as apply to the 38 targets. The only difference is that 'health for all 2000' has now become 'health for all in the 21st century'.
14. Rootman, I. (1994). How is Quality of Life Related to Health and Health Promotion? In *Health Promotion and Prevention: Theoretical and Ethical Aspects*, ed. P-E. Liss and N. Nikku, Forskningsradsnamnden, Stockholm.
15. Earp, J.A. and Ennett, S.T. (1991). Conceptual models for health education research and practice. *Health Education Research, Theory and Practice* **6**(2), 163–171.
16. Jones, G.W. (1975). *Population Growth and Educational Planning in Developing Nations*, Irvington Publishers, New York.
17. Morse, D. (1971). *Motown and the Arrival of Black Music*, Studio Vista, London.
18. Popper, K. (1979). *Objective Knowledge: An Evolutionary Approach*, revised edition, Oxford University Press, London.
19. Green, L.W., Glanz, K., Hochbaum, G.M., Kok, G., Kreuter, M.W., Lewis, F.M., Lorig, K., Morisky, D., Rimer, B.K. and Rosenstock, I.M. (1994). Can we build on, or must we replace, the theories and models in health education? *Health Education Research* **9**(3), 397–404.
20. McLeroy, K., Bibeau, D., Steckler, A. and Glanz, K. (1988). An ecological perspective on health promotion programs. *Health Education Quarterly* **15**, 351–377.

Health Promotion, Second Edition: David Seedhouse
© 2004 John Wiley & Sons, Ltd: ISBNs 0 470 84732 8 (HB); 0 470 84733 6 (PB)

21. Blaikie, N.W.H. (1991). A critique of the use of triangulation in social research. *Quality and Quantity* **25**, 115–136.
22. Wright, J.J. and Liley, D.T.J. (1996). Dynamics of the brain at global and microscopic scales: neural networks and the EEG. *Behavioural and Brain Sciences* **19**, 285–320.
23. Seedhouse, D.F. (2001). *Health: The Foundations for Achievement*, second edition, John Wiley and Sons, Chichester.
24. Tannahill, A. (1985). What is health promotion? *Health Education Journal* **44**, 167–168.
25. French, J. and Adams, L. (1986). From analysis to synthesis: theories of health education. *Health Education Journal* **45**(2), 71–74.
26. Tones, B.K. (1979). Past Achievement, Future Success. In *Health Education Perspectives and Choices*, ed. E. Sutherland, Allen and Unwin, London.
27. Seedhouse, D.F. (1992). Avoiding the myths: a prerequisite for teaching ethics. *Postgraduate Education for General Practitioners* **3**, 117–124.
28. Pellegrino, E.D. (1981). Health promotion as public policy: the need for moral groundings. *Preventive Medicine* **10**, 371—378.
29. Doxiadis, S. (1990). *Ethics in Health Education*, John Wiley and Sons, Chichester.
30. Moreno, J.D. and Bayer, R. (1985). The limits of the ledger in public health promotion. *Hastings Center Report* **15**, 37–41.
31. Tobacco Institute of New Zealand (1989). *The Smoking Debate*, Auckland, New Zealand.
32. Accident Compensation Corporation (1994). *Tackling Rugby Injuries*, Wellington, New Zealand.
33. *Sunday Star Times*, 4 December 1994, New Zealand.
34. http://www.acc.org.nz/injury-prevention/safe-in-sport-and-recreation/sports-codes/rugby/ background/ According to the ACC in 2002 things seems to have improved. Following an extensive safety campaign, injuries have halved. However, the overall cost to New Zealand in 2001 was over $20 million (and note that this figure is for only the rugby union code).
35. Menzel, P. (1994). Risk perception, addiction and costs to others: an assessment of cigarette taxes and other anti-smoking policies. *Health Care Analysis* **2**(1), 13–22.
36. Health Education Authority (1993). *The Health Guide*, HEA, London.
37. For a 21st century official anti-smoking publication go to: http://www.hda-online.org.uk/ html/research/smoking.html
38. Dawber, T.R. (1980). *The Framingham Study*, Harvard University Press, Cambridge MA.
39. Seltzer, C.C. (1989). Framingham Study data and 'Established wisdom about cigarette smoking and coronary heart disease'. *Journal of Clinical Epidemiology* **42**, 781–788.
40. Viscusi, W.K. (1992). *Smoking: Making the Risky Decision*, Oxford University Press, New York.
41. Newsome, E.L. (1977). *The Trade Descriptions Acts and the Motor Vehicle*, Rose, Chichester.
42. Thomas, E. (1986). Informed consent. *Lancet* **ii**, 1280.
43. Women's Health Action (1993). *Unfinished Business: What Happened To The Cartwright Report?*, Auckland, New Zealand.
44. Goehring, B. (1993). *Indigenous Peoples of the World: An Introduction To Their Past, Present and Future*, Purich Pub., Saskatoon.
45. Plummer, D. (1995). Homophobia and health: unjust, anti-social, harmful and endemic. *Health Care Analysis* **3**(2), 150–156.
46. Le Fanu, J. (ed.) (1994). *Preventionitis: The Exaggerated Claims of Health Promotion*, St Edmundsbury Press, Suffolk, UK.
47. Skrabanek, P. (1994). The ethics of prevention. In *Preventionitis: The Exaggerated Claims of Health Promotion*, ed. J. Le Fanu, St Edmundsbury Press, Suffolk, UK.
48. Caplan, R. (1993). The importance of social theory for health promotion: from description to reflexivity. *Health Promotion International* **8**(2), 147–157.
49. Armstrong, D. (1983). *An Outline of Sociology As Applied To Medicine*, Arnold, London.
50. Taussig, M. (1980). Reification and the consciousness of the patient, *Social Science and Medicine*, 14b, 3–13.
51. Young, A.A. (1980). The discourse on stress and the reproduction of conventional knowledge, *Social Science and Medicine*, **14b**, 133–146.
52. Stainton-Rogers, Wendy (1991). *Explaining Health and Illness: An Exploration of Diversity*, Harvester Wheatsheaf, Brighton, pp. 19–20.

53. Stacey, M. (1988). *The Sociology of Health and Healing: A Textbook*, HarperCollins, London, p. 12.
54. Hollis, M. and Lukes, S. (eds) (1982). *Rationality and Relativism*, Basil Blackwell, Oxford.
55. Ewles, L. and Simnett, I. (1985). *Promoting Health: A Practical Guide to Health Education*, Baillière Tindall, London.
56. Seedhouse, D.F. (1991). Ethics as Health Promotion. In *Health Education at University*, ed. by J. Falk-Whynes et al., HEA Publications, London, pp. 98–110.
57. Ottawa Charter (1986). World Health Organization, Geneva.
58. Spicker, S. (1993). Going off the dole: a prudential and ethical critique of the healthfare state. *Health Care Analysis* 1(1), 33–38.
59. Whittington, C. and Holland, R. (1985). A framework for theory in social work. *Issues in Social Work Education*, Summer, 1–54.
60. Fukuyama, F. (1992). *The End of History and the Last Man*, Free Press, New York.
61. *The Health of the Nation: A Consultative Document for Health in England* (1991). Cm 5523, HMSO, London.
62. The medical-based understanding of health is perpetuated exactly in the later document: *Our Healthier Nation* http://www.archive.officialdocuments.co.uk/document/doh/ohnation/ohncont.htm See also: http://www.ohn.gov.uk/
63. Townsend, P. and Davidson, N. (eds) (1982). *Inequalities in Health*, Penguin Books, London.
64. Traffic Research and Statistics Section, Land Transport Division (1993). *Road Deaths: Official Road Fatality Statistics*, Wellington, New Zealand.
65. http://www.hda-online.org.uk/
66 Cleminson, R. (1995). Health Care History. Anarchists for health: Spanish anarchism and health reform in the 1930s. Part I: Anarchism, neo-malthusianism, eugenics and concepts of health. *Health Care Analysis* 3(1), 61–67.
67 Navarro, V. (1986). *Crisis, Health and Medicine: A Social Critique*, Tavistock Publications, New York.
68. Scott-Samuel, A. (1989). The new public health: Speke neighbourhood health group. In *Changing Ideas in Health Care*, ed. D. Seedhouse and A. Cribb, John Wiley and Sons, Chichester.
69. Parkin, C.W. (1966). Burke and the conservative tradition. In *Political Ideas*, ed. D. Thomson, Penguin Books, Middlesex.
70. Wilson, C. (1978). *The Outsider*, Picador Edition, Pan Books, London.
71. Highsmith, P. (1950). *Strangers On A Train*, Harper and Brothers, New York.
72. Jenkinson, C. (ed.) (1994). *Measuring Health and Medical Outcomes*, UCL Press, London.
73. Eisen, S.V. (1995). BASIS questionnaire. In Andrews, W.G. (1995). Outcome measurement. *Draft discussion paper prepared for APHA meeting*, February 1995.
74. Mental Health Inventory, Rand Corporation.
75. Wright, L. (1994). The long and the short of it: the development of the SF-36 general health survey. In *Measuring Health and Medical Outcomes*, ed. C. Jenkinson, UCL Press, London.
76. Seedhouse, D.F. (1995). The way around health economics' dead end. *Health Care Analysis* 3(3), 205–220.
77. Goulden, P. (1994). Non-treatment orders, including do not resuscitate (DNR). In *Principles of Health Care Ethics*, ed. R. Gillon, John Wiley and Sons, Chichester.
78. Gill, W.M. (1984). Subjective well-being: properties of an instrument for measuring this (in the chronically ill). *Social Science and Medicine* 18(8), 683–691.
79. Chamberlain, K. (1988). On the structure of subjective well-being. *Social Indicators Research* 10, 581–604.
80. Aristotle (1953). *Ethics*, Allen and Unwin, London.
81. Moore, A., Hope, A. and Fulford, K.W.M. (1995). Mild mania and well-being. *Philosophy, Psychiatry and Psychology* 1(3), 165–177.
82. Griffin, J. (1986). *Well-being*, Oxford University Press, Oxford.
83. Large, R.G. and Schug, S.A. (1995). Opioids for chronic pain of non-malignant origin – caring or crippling. *Health Care Analysis* 3(1), 5–11.
84. Seedhouse, D.F. (1991). *Liberating Medicine*, John Wiley and Sons, Chichester.
85. Seedhouse, D.F. (1998). *Ethics: The Heart of Health Care*, second edition, John Wiley and Sons, Chichester.

86. Brown, R.B., McCartney, S. and Bell, L. (1995). Why the NHS should abandon the search for the universal outcome measure. *Health Care Analysis* **3**(3), 191–195.
87. Williams, A. (1992). Cost-effectiveness analysis: is it ethical? *Journal of Medical Ethics* **18**, 7–11.
88. Williams, A. (1988). Ethics and efficiency in the provision of health care. In *Philosophy and Medical Welfare*, ed. J.M. Bell and S. Mendus, Cambridge University Press, Cambridge.
89. Cribb, A. (1993). The borders of health promotion – a response to Nordenfelt. *Health Care Analysis* **1**(2), 131–137.
90. Liss, P.-E. (1990). *Health Care Need. Meaning and Measurement*, Linköping University, Sweden.
91. Seedhouse, D.F. (1994). *Fortress NHS: A Philosophical Review of the National Health Service*, John Wiley and Sons, Chichester.
92. Mill, J.S. (1910). *Utilitarianism, On Liberty, and Considerations on Representative Government*, Dent, London.
93. Whitbeck, C. (1981). A theory of health. In *Concepts of Health and Disease: Interdisciplinary Perspectives*, ed. A.L. Caplan, H.T. Englehardt Jr and J.J. McCartney, Addison-Wesley, Massachusetts.
94. Wilson, M. (ed.) (1983). *Explorations in Health and Salvation: A Selection of Papers by Bob Lambourne*, University of Birmingham.
95. Dubos, R. (1959). *The Mirage of Health*, Harper and Row, New York.
96. Richman, J. (1987). *Medicine and Health*, Longman, London.
97. Sedgwick, P. (1981). Illness – mental and otherwise. In *Concepts of Health and Disease: Interdisciplinary Perspectives*, ed. A.L. Caplan, H.T. Englehardt Jr and J.J. McCartney, Addison-Wesley, Massachusetts.
98. Murray, R.B. (1989). *Nursing Assessment and Health Promotion Strategies Through The Life Span*, fourth edition, Appleton and Long, Norwalk, CT.
99. Fuchs, V. (1981). Concepts of health – an economist's perspective. In *Concepts of Health and Disease: Interdisciplinary Perspectives*, ed. A.L. Caplan, H.T. Englehardt Jr and J.J. McCartney, Addison-Wesley, Massachusetts.
100. Raphael, D.D. (1994). *Moral Philosophy*, second edition, Oxford University Press, Oxford.
101. Moore, B.N. (1994). *Moral Philosophy: A Comprehensive Introduction*, Mayfield Pub. Co., Mountain View, California.
102. Rogers, A., Pilgrim, D., Gust, I.D., Stone, D.H. and Menzel, P.T. (1995). The pros and cons of immunisation. *Health Care Analysis* **3**(2), 99–115.
103. Seedhouse, D.F. and Lovett, L. (1992). *Practical Medical Ethics*, John Wiley and Sons, Chichester.
104. Stilwell, B. (1989). Talking Treatments. *The Health Service Journal*, 14 September, 1130–1131.
105. Matte, N.M. (1980). *Space Policy and Programmes Today and Tomorrow: The Vanishing Duopole*, Carswell Co., Toronto.
106. Stewart, G.T. (1994). Scientific surveillance and the control of AIDS: a call for open debate. *Health Care Analysis* **2**(4), 279–286.
107. Caton, H. (1994). Review article: Alternative models of the AIDS epidemic. *Health Care Analysis* **2**(4), 351–354.
108. Attenborough, D. (1995). *The Private Life of Plants*, BBC Books, London.
109. Moore, T.J. (1989). *Heart Failure: A Critical Inquiry Into American Medicine and the Revolution in Heart Care*, Random House, New York.
110. World Health Organization (1977). *Food Hygiene in Catering Establishments: Legislation and Model Regulations*, Geneva.
111. Chomsky, N. (1992). *Deterring Democracy*, Vintage, London.
112. Slutsky, A.M., Rovin, S., Kaplis, N.A. (c. 1980). Fluoridation: 100 questions and answers. In *The Tooth Robbers: A Pro-Fluoridation Handbook*, ed. S. Barrett and S. Rovin, George F. Stickley Co., Philadelphia.
113. Murray, J.J. and Rugg-Gunn, A.J. (1982). *Fluorides in Caries Prevention*, second edition, Wright P.S.G., Bristol.
114. Glass, R.L. (ed.) (1982). First international conference on the declining prevalence of dental caries. *Journal of Dental Research* **61** (special issue), 1304–1388.
115. Leverett, D.H. (1982). Fluorides and the changing prevalence of dental caries. *Science* **217**, 26–30.

116. Diesendorf, M. (1986). The mystery of declining tooth decay. *Nature* **322**, 125–129.
117. Colquhoun, J. (1988). Decline in primary tooth decay in New Zealand. *Community Health Studies* **12**, 187–191.
118. Gray, A.S. (1987). Fluoridation: time for a new baseline? *Journal of the Canadian Dental Association* **53**, 763–765.
119. Colquhoun, J. (1994). Child dental health differences in New Zealand. *Community Health Studies* **11**, 85–90.
120. Hildebolt, C.F., Elvin-Lewis, M., Molnar, S. et al. (1989). Caries prevalences among geochemical regions of Missouri. *American Journal of Physical Anthropology* **78**, 79–92.
121. Yiamouyiannis, J. (1990). Water fluoridation and tooth decay: results from the 1986–1987 national survey of US schoolchildren. *Fluoride* **23**(2), 55–67.
122. Diesendorf, M. (1995). How science can illuminate ethical debates: a case study on water fluoridation. *Fluoride* **28**(287), 87–104.
123. Goldsworthy, N.E. (1960). Every doctor a dietitian. *Medical Journal of Australia* **1**, 285–286.
124. Silva, M.F. de A., Jenkins, G.N., Burgess, R.C. et al. (1986). Effects of cheese on experimental caries in human subjects. *Caries Research* **20**, 263–269, and references therein.
125. Turner, E. and Vickery, K.O.A. (1966). The wholemeal bread family: a pilot study. *Vitalstoffe-Zivilisationskrankheiten* **11**(3), 99–102.
126. Colquhoun, J. (1985). Influence of social class and fluoridation on child dental health. *Community Dentistry and Oral Epidemiology* **13**, 37–41.
127. Bradnock, G., Marchment, M.D. and Anderson, R.J. (1984). Social background, fluoridation and caries experience in a 5-year-old population in the West Midlands. *British Dental Journal* **156**, 127–131.
128. Carmichael, C.L., Rugg-Gunn, A.J. and Ferrell, R.S. (1989). The relationship between fluoridation, social class and caries experience in 5-year-old children in Newcastle and Northumberland in 1987. *British Dental Journal* **167**, 57–61.
129. Wilson, B. Personal communication.
130. Hunt, S. (1994). Cold hearts and coronaries. *Health Matters* **19**, 16–17.
131. Seedhouse, D.F. (2002). *Total Health Promotion: Mental Health, Rational Fields and the Quest for Autonomy*, John Wiley and Sons, Chichester.
132. Jarvie, I. C. (1970). Explaining Cargo Cults. In *Rationality*, ed. Bryan R. Wilson, Basil Blackwell, Oxford.
133. Jarvie, I. C. and Agassi, J. (1970). The Problem of Rationality in Magic. In *Rationality*, ed. Bryan R. Wilson, Basil Blackwell, Oxford.
134. Kekes, I. (1976). *A Justification of Rationality*, Albany, State University of New York Press.
135. Seedhouse, D.F. (1984). *Rationality*, PhD Thesis, Manchester University (unpublished).
136. Camazine, S. (1992). *Self-organisation in Biological Systems*, Princeton University Press, NJ.
137. Koestler, A. (1979). *Janus: A Summing Up*, Pan Books, London.
138. Lama Norlha (1986). In Kalu Rinpoche, *The Dharma*, Albany, State University of New York Press, p. 155.
139. I thank Joanna Rose, a PhD student at Queensland University of Technology, for her extensive advice and insights into the considerable difficulties faced by DI children. I could not have used this example of health promotion were it not for her academic research and personal experience.

Index

Page numbers in *italics* indicate figures.

Health Promotion, Second Edition: David Seedhouse
© 2004 John Wiley & Sons, Ltd: ISBNs 0 470 84732 8 (HB); 0 470 84733 6 (PB)